Gout

GOUT
The Patrician Malady

Roy Porter and G. S. Rousseau

Yale University Press
New Haven and London

Set in Bembo by Best-set Typesetter Ltd, Hong Kong
Printed in Great Britain

Library of Congress Cataloging-in-Publication Data

Porter, Roy, 1946–
Gout: the patrician malady/ Roy Porter and G.S. Rousseau.
Includes bibliographical references and index.
ISBN 0–300–07386–0 (cloth)
1. Gout – History.   I. Rousseau. G. S. (George Sebastian)   II. Title.
RC629.P67   1998
616.3'999'009 – dc21   98–16881
CIP

A catalogue record for this book is available from the British Library.

2 4 6 8 10 9 7 5 3

Next Gout appears with limping pace,
Pleads how he shifts from place to place,
From head to foot how swift he flies,
And ev'ry joint and sinew plys,
Still working when he seems supprest,
A most tenacious stubborn guest.

John Gay, Fable XLVII, from *The Poems of John Gay*, ed. V. A. Dearing
(Oxford: Clarendon Press, 1974), 364–5

was he Free from the Pain This [the gout] gave him, his Blindness would be
Tolerable.

John Milton, as reported by Jonathan Richardson: Helen Darbishire, ed.,
The Early Lives of Milton (London: Constable, 1932), 203–4

Full soon the sad effect of this [port wine]
His frame began to show,
For that old enemy the gout
Had taken him in toe!

Thomas Hood, 'Lieutenant Lough', in Walter Jerrold, ed., *The Complete
Poetical Works of Thomas Hood* (London: Oxford University Press, 1935), 204

In the happy moment of mirth and conviviality, and the mad career of dissipation,
an epicure, or a voluptuary, little dreams of the gout; which hangs over his head,
like the sword of Damocles, and threatens his destruction. Amid the joys of wine,
and the shouts of the Bacchanals, the still voice of reason is not heard; the sober
dictates of discretion are disregarded; and the friendly warnings of the physician are
either totally forgotten, or treated with ridicule and contempt.

John Ring, *A Treatise on the Gout* (London: Callow, 1811), 3

Contents

Illustrations

Acknowledgments

Gout is notoriously a chronic disease, and it may well have seemed to our friends that, by some malign sympathy, the condition had infected this enterprise; indeed that this volume – the brainchild of GSR back in the 1980s – would become a malady of which the authors themselves would never be relieved. That this has not proved so we owe in large part to their patience and encouragement in the completion of this project.

We also owe a debt of gratitude to the labours of many people over many years: in London notably Caroline Overy, the world's best research assistant, Elizabeth Watts, Sian Field, Sheila Lawler, Sally Bragg, Frieda Houser, Jan Pinkerton, William Schupbach and Brenda Sutton, all at the Wellcome Institute for the History of Medicine; in Los Angeles, Oxford and Aberdeen, Scotland, notably Leila Brownfield, another world-class research assistant, and Michael Dzanko, Clark Lawlor, John Gregor, Keith Bodner and Alison Auld. We also owe debts to numerous scholars and institutions over many continents: Georgia B. Barnhill, Andrew W. Mellon Curator of Graphic Arts, American Antiquarian Association, for sending us illustrations of gouty patients; Margaret DeLacy, Portland, Oregon; Edward E. Harnagel, MD, Pasadena, California; Joad Raymond and Ingrid de Smet of Magdalen College, Oxford; Clive Edward, Research Fellow, Victoria and Albert Museum; Dr John Erlen, Falk Library of Medicine, University of Pittsburgh; Dr Kevin Fraser, Victoria, Australia, who shared his wealth of information on William Stukeley's gout with us; Timothy Huisman of the Boerhaave Museum in Leiden who opened his large collection of prints and drawings; Alan Jutzi and Thomas Lange, Department of Rare Books, and Barbara Donagan, historian of the English Civil War and aficionado of things seventeenth century, all of the Huntington Library, San Marino, California; Professor Antonie Luyendijk-Elshout in Leiden, always eager to share Dutch materials, particularly those associated with Boerhaave and his school; Richard Wolf and his helpful staff, Countway Library of Medicine, Harvard University; the staffs of the Houghton Library at Harvard College and the Bodleian Library in Oxford. We especially relied on the wealth of materials in the Burney-Fraser Collection of Gout and Arthritis, Texas Medical Library and Collection in

Houston, perhaps the largest collection of primary material about gout in the world, and we are grateful to their curators.

We hope we have discharged these debts in the endnotes. And we are also very grateful to the late Leila Brownfield and GSR's colleagues at the Thomas Reid Institute for having read various earlier drafts, offered comments and saved us from the errors that remain our own.

Roy Porter
Wellcome Institute for the
History of Medicine
London

George Rousseau
Thomas Reid Institute
Aberdeen
Scotland

CHAPTER I

Introduction

No apology is needed for writing the history of a malady and its cultural representations. It is now agreed that understanding ailments in historical context requires more than epidemiological and clinical expertise. Discourse about disease goes beyond recognizing the powers of pathogens: it may be freighted with associations like disorder and dirt which embody value judgments and emotive charges.[1]

What diseases are and where their boundaries lie are matters of controversy. Disputes rage as to whether pregnancy, menopause and ageing should be viewed as pathological states. There is still no consensus as to what is to count as *disease*, as distinct from sickness, affliction, weakness or sin: is it a state of mind as well as a process of Nature? – a point underlying Alexander Pope's reference to 'this long *Disease*, my life'.[2] Morbid processes involve certain natural manifestations, but they don't qualify as *diseases* until so denominated by medicine, science and society. Conditions like neurasthenia have come and gone; the same may happen with RSI (repetitive strain injury) and ME (myalgic encephalomyelitis, 'yuppie flu' or chronic fatigue syndrome).[3] Diseases, to employ Rosenberg's helpful expression, become diseases for us only when they are 'framed'.[4]

And even once particular diseases have been framed and named, disputes persist respecting what they *mean* to sufferers, to employers and insurers, to law courts and the community at large, as is obvious from the fact that terms like leper possess solid scientific meanings while simultaneously serving as stigmas ('moral leper'). AIDS has tragically underlined all these truths through the epidemic of infamous victim-blaming clichés like 'gay plague'. One consequence of these verbal imbroglios has been the divergence between arcane professional jargon and the lay languages of medicine.[5]

In recent years, literary scholars, biographers, psychohistorians and other humanists have been drawing attention to illness experience and body awareness as facets of identity and the thread of the narration of one's life.[6] Pathography may be the key to biography:

– I'll tell it, cried Smelfungus, to the world.
You had better tell it, said I, to your physician

I

was Laurence Sterne's comic suggestion – at the expense of the splenetic surgeon and writer, Tobias Smollett, about whom we have much more to say below in Chapter 7 – that a life could be read through diagnosis of its morbific humours.[7] It is needless to labour this point: decoding disease is integral to the understanding of culture, society and biography.[8]

But why a book about *gout*? Is that not (one anticipates the objections) a rather trifling condition? Perhaps comic, a topic tailor-made for the *belles lettres* of a bygone age but not for sober medical history.[9] Nowadays gout provokes the enormous condescension of slimline political correctness. Wasn't it, surely, a disease of the *ancien régime* and the Old World? Didn't the idle and licentious bring it upon their own heads, or rather feet, by outrageous overindulgence, while they shrugged off responsibility by the solemn palaver of dignifying their condition as 'the gout', as if it were some boon companion or noble foe to whom it was a great 'honour' to fall martyr?[10] He and his physician 'were very well satisfied with the proceedings of the Gout', Edward Gibbon explained to his step-mother: 'he had behaved like a fair and honourable Enemy'.[11] Recycling that stock simile, the Revd Sydney Smith quipped that gout was 'the only enemy that I do not wish to have at my feet'.[12] By means of this grim rigmarole, gout's sting was drawn, just as, in Shakespeare's time, one had to jest with death. 'I enjoy all the dignity of lameness,' bantered the gouty Samuel Johnson, making a virtue of necessity. 'I receive ladies and dismiss them sitting. *Painful pre-eminence.*'[13]

Gout thus yields medical anecdotes and biographical insights. Does it offer more? We believe so, as we document in these opening chapters and in more theoretical form in Chapters 11 and 12. For one thing, the glaring neglect of gout draws attention to biases in medical history. Scholars have chiefly studied lethal, epidemic diseases: plague and smallpox, yellow fever and typhoid fever, tuberculosis and AIDS. Such afflictions invite cathartic involvement: we share the horror, we pity the victims.[14] But this concentration on killer epidemics arguably creates an imbalance that needs redressing. For the diseases causing most pain have not been apocalyptic; sickness has typically been less like the Holocaust than an interminable succession of stumbles and muggings – but no less agonizing for that. Historical pathology mainly consists of chronic conditions, attacking the musculoskeletal system, the respiratory system, the nervous system, and of course the brain – not in themselves fatal but incurable, typically debilitating, sometimes crippling and inordinately painful.[15]

Gout falls into the category of non-infectious, non-lethal ailments. Though widely associated with the olden days – with Christmas-card scenes peopled by ruddy-faced Mr Pickwicks drinking toasts[16] – in truth gout is very much still with us; it continues to threaten males in the developed world, and globally it is spreading.

During the last century and a half, epidemic disorders have been receding, resulting in the West being worse afflicted with chronic and degenerative disorders – partly, of course, consequential upon greater longevity. Among the diseases besetting large numbers of people today, articular ailments are highly prominent: arthritis, rheumatism, sciatica, gout and related conditions. Their neglect by historians appears rather myopic.[17]

We also have another goal in this book: to demonstrate why the 'gout diagnosis' triumphed over its competitors. In this respect our project resembles the explanatory agenda of those contemporary histories of science aiming to show why particular theories or paradigms win out over others. Gout had its competitors in dropsy, ague, fever, inflammation, sciatica, vapours, spleen, all the class of rheumatics and many others. Until approximately the mid-eighteenth century it remained such an unstable medical condition that it bled into other diagnoses with such seeming ease that these maladies were to a degree interchangeable.

Yet somehow the gout diagnosis prevailed and established itself. The tensions and resonances implicated in the 'somehow' constitute a major portion of this book. By the nineteenth century gout had installed itself. The upper-crust Regency gentleman who assumed he would in due course become 'gouty' as part of the normal life-cycle made a cultural assumption whose lineage requires unravelling and decoding. In addition to chronicling gout's internal medical histories we attempt to describe the strategies of rhetorical persuasion and figurative and visual representation of those constructing its rise and fall. Gout's cultural representation constitutes one focus of our task, as gout entailed much more than a torment in the toe, painful though those attacks were.

Gout afflicts the joints of the extremities, classically the great toe.[18] They become swollen and inordinately painful (it felt, remarked Sydney Smith, 'like walking on my eyeballs'),[19] and tophi sometimes form, chalky concretions routinely likened to crab's eyes, which, unlike the swellings, are painless. The paroxysm was described by the illustrious seventeenth-century clinician Thomas Sydenham, himself long-suffering. 'The *regular gout* generally seizes in the following manner,' he recorded:

> The patient goes to bed and sleeps quietly till about two in the morning, when he is awakened by a pain which usually seizes the great toe, but sometimes the heel, the calf of the leg or the ankle. The pain resembles that of a dislocated bone . . . and this is immediately succeeded by a chillness, shivering and a slight fever. [The pain] grows gradually more violent every hour, and comes to its height towards evening, adapting itself to the numerous bones of the tarsus and metatarsus, the ligaments whereof it affects; sometimes the gnawing of a dog, and sometimes a weight and constriction of the parts affected, which become so exquisitely painful as not to endure the weight of the clothes nor the shaking of the room from a person's walking briskly therein. [Things worsen] till after twenty-four

hours from the first approach of the fit . . . the patient is suddenly relieved . . . And being now in a breathing sweat he falls asleep, and upon waking finds the pain much abated, and the part affected to be then swollen; whereas before only a remarkable swelling of the veins thereof appeared, as is usual in all gouty fits.[20]

It has been recognized since the nineteenth century that gout is brought on by an abnormally high concentration of uric acid in the blood (hyperuricaemia), which provokes deposition of sodium urate in the joints, either through increased synthesis of uric acid, or through decreased capacity of the kidneys to excrete such acid. Hyperuricaemia may also occur for other, extraneous reasons, for example blood diseases, producing 'secondary gout'.

Not in itself harmful, uric acid is normally absorbed in the bloodstream. But under adverse circumstances it may escape and crystallize, forming monosodium urate crystals in the sinovial fluid and so creating inflammation. It still remains unclear why this occurs predominantly in joints, most commonly in the feet or knee. Various clinical manifestations distinguish gout from other joint diseases. Unlike most arthritic complaints, the great majority of patients are male – ever since the Hippocratic writings it has been observed that gout rarely develops in women before menopause. The first attack typically occurs in middle age. About half the sufferers develop tophi; kidney stones are common. Though the historical incidence is impossible to quantify, contemporary studies suggest that up to one in a hundred males in Europe and North America may be disposed to gout.[21]

There have always been various therapies. Some are essentially prophylactic. Dietetic attempts to prevent or treat the condition have been based on belief in the virtue of moderation and the supposition that gout is caused by rich food and alcohol. Among treatments, colchicum in the form of extracts from the bulb of the meadow saffron (*Crocus autumnale*) was known from Antiquity, though it came into widespread use only around 1,800. It is highly effective in relieving the acute attack.[22]

In the 1910s, cinchophen was introduced. Being not only effective in the acute attacks but, unlike colchicine, also an analgesic, cinchophen virtually replaced colchicine until it became evident in the 1930s that it caused liver damage. Colchicine returned. Two pharmaceutical breakthroughs date from 1951. Probenecid was found to accelerate excretion of uric acid; the frequency of gout attacks diminished and tophi shrank. The other discovery was phenylbutazone, with therapeutic effects similar to cinchophen. It proved toxic, however, particularly hindering blood-cell formation in the elderly. Allopurinal arrived in 1963. That drug lowers uric-acid levels and is effective in renal failure, also decreasing uratic kidney stones. Though acute attacks are thus now more treatable, gout remains incurable; nor can its initial onset be predicted or prevented.[23] Moreover underlying trends are not encouraging, in view of the protein- and fat-rich diets now typical of Western populations. This is borne out by studies revealing highish uric-acid levels and tendencies towards hyperuricaemia.[24] American surveys have found that executives have higher urate concentrations and a greater incidence of hyperuricaemia than blue-collar employees.[25] There seem to be links between hyperuricaemia, hypertension and obesity, findings underscoring the traditional gout profile.

Whatever the First World situation, occurrence of gout is rising world-wide, as a consequence of the Westernization of diet and habits. Though rural Third World peoples have suffered from various arthritic conditions, they have never been gout-prone.[26] There is no evidence till recently of gout in Africa, in South America or in Asia. In 1952 it was said to be unknown in China, Japan and the tropics, and rare among blacks. But non-Western peoples are now experiencing a rising incidence, as a result of 'improved' diets containing higher proportions of fats and proteins. Studies in Tokyo in the 1970s showed uric-acid levels to be the same as in Caucasian populations, and gout in Japanese men has increased. In South Africa the lowest uric-acid values are found in tribal populations, and the highest levels, equal to those of urban whites, in Soweto.[27] Numerous 'diseases of civilization' are currently being exported to the Third World.

So gout cannot be shrugged off as if it were a trivial complaint, an archaic disease, an ailment of the elite, a condition inconsequential because self-inflicted. Gout has been, and remains, a major cause of human suffering, and for that reason it is worthy of attention. Yet it is also, as this book explores, an intriguing example of a malady whose very specification has been marked out with medical, cultural and social meanings. Gout early acquired a personality.

Most spectacularly, gout's ascribed characteristics have been associated with the great and their glamour. The following chapters will probe its mythologies with respect to consumption and luxury, situating it within debates over the relations between wealth and health, civilization and disease.[28] Prophets and politicians have always given medical events moral meanings, changing morbidity has been seized upon as a prime symptom of social progress or pathology.[29]

The framing, naming and blaming of disease involves many other elements, not least gender. It was always observed (or *stipulated*) that gout was a male condition. This may well have been the case; but it was also a conclusion entailed by models of maleness and femaleness and of the gendering of disorders. Thus, if a woman's functions were essentially reproductive, it was natural that disease would principally assail her central organ, her womb: hence hysteria. Men, by contrast, were made for action. Their diseases would more likely hit at their mobility: hence gout.[30]

Another parameter has been rank. In medical discourse, gout has tradition-ally hobnobbed in high society. So pressing has been the ideological need to reinforce hierarchies of social distinction that the upper crust has even been eager to flaunt marks of debility to signal its exclusiveness – a foible inviting satire. Gout thus affords a valuable opportunity to trace the use of illness as insignia.[31] And the links between gout and greatness run deeper, for it has often been maintained that gout goes with genius.[32] Such beliefs tell us about the privileges and penalties of pre-eminence within a Christian moral scheme that took suffering as a mark not just of sin but of superiority, sanctity and spirituality.[33] The story of gout thus throws light on philosophies of disease-meaning and distribution: who falls sick, who gets *which* disease, and why.

A third parameter entails the metaphoric and visual heritages, less 'concrete' than those of class and gender. We show that gout, especially in its 'podagra' incarnations, has borne a particularly complex relation to the development of 'play', the *homo ludens* about which the Dutch historian Johann Huizinga wrote so eloquently in his classic monograph of that title (1944); and we develop this 'cultural history' and cultural profile in Chapters 11 and 12. *Gout: The Patrician Malady* is a book with a 'thesis' about illness and its metaphors.[34] Almost from the start of its discursive representations gout was viewed in ludic – playful – contexts: as if to suggest the internal contradictions between its chronic afflictions and basic insulation from effective calamity. Alone among diseases, gout bore this relation to play. Why so? How did the foot and the limbs become metaphorized and visualized within the tropes of play?

Study of gout is no less interesting for what it reveals about changing ideas of disease.[35] For long, historians took little interest in the history of disease theory, for it appeared easy to posit the progress over time from error to science, from supposedly vague, verbalizing conceptions of sickness (Greek humoralism) to 'specificity'. The new accent on anatomy and physiology fostered by the Renaissance; the mechanical philosophy; Enlightenment tax-onomy and nosology; early nineteenth-century pathological anatomy; the deployment of the microscope in the laboratory; the triumph of bacteriology – all such developments appeared to reveal the true 'scientific' nature of disease and to lead to identifications of specific diseases: it might be called the transition from 'dis-ease' to 'disease', and from 'Disease' to 'diseases'. Armed with Koch's postulates, the twentieth century dawned with the hope of finding the micro-organism that was the cause of each and every individual disease, the vaccine that would prevent it, and the 'magic bullet' to cure it. Books with titles like *Microbe Hunters* and *Virus Hunters* reinforced Whiggish recitations of the advance of medical science.[36]

But, in truth, the definition and understanding of disease remain conten-tious to this day: the rancorous row as to whether HIV is *the* cause of AIDS is only the most spectacular instance nowadays of profound uncertainty.[37] More generally debates as to whether it is possible to be sick without being diseased or to have a disease without being sick still carry major theoretical and practical implications. Doctrines of susceptibility and immunity are highly intricate and, some would say, inherently question-begging. And, in the end, who has the right to pronounce someone ill: the sufferer, the physician or society?

On top of this, the crossing between mind and body in sickness remains a minefield. How far may disorders be thought psychogenic or at least to have a psychosomatic component?[38] Not least, larger questions loom about the organism: what is to count as healthiness and what as sickness? what is 'normal', what 'pathological'? It is no easy matter to judge which biomedical events truly help or harm: is fever a disease, a symptom or the body's (and so Nature's) way of fighting sickness?[39]

As this book will demonstrate, such vexed questions have been endemic to attempts over the centuries to define or design the disease called gout. Was gout to be envisaged as an occasional event ('gutta' means a 'dropping', that is of matter from the body's vitals to the extremities), or was it an underlying fate (being gouty), or was it a disease in the sense of a causal agent? Was it an injury to the body, or a bodyguard, the system's attempt to expel a threat? What were the relations between gout (or goutiness) and the broader health or sickness of the organism and its constitution?

These questions have prompted disparate answers from sufferers or their physicians, from regulars or irregulars. And such responses have hinged upon wider, extra-medical doctrines respecting order and harmony, good and evil, and pervasive beliefs about the economy of Nature, the purposes of Providence and the meaning of life, beliefs articulated in the West within the frameworks of Classical metaphysics and Christian eschatology.[40]

The point of raising such issues is not to challenge the reality of gout or to deny that modern scientific medicine has advanced understanding and provided relief. Old ideas about gout cannot, however, be understood in isolation from wider belief systems; and in certain respects the models and metaphors buoying up those beliefs have continued to shape scientific theories in the twentieth century: much vintage metaphysical port has been poured into new scientific bottles.

Finally, it may be helpful to clarify the relations between gout and other joints diseases that will subsequently be mentioned only in passing.[41] 'Arthritis' is the generic medical term for disorders producing swelling in the joints and pain in the limbs, and 'rheumatism' in lay parlance describes assorted pains associated with the joints and bones. Modern disease classifications distinguish gout from rheumatoid arthritis, osteoarthritis and certain more unusual conditions, such as ankylosing spondylitis, a degenerative syndrome in which the whole spinal column becomes enclosed in a bony casing. Palaeopathological and textual evidence indicates that such diseases of the joints have been present throughout known human history.

More common than gout, rheumatoid arthritis is the major crippling illness among chronic rheumatic disorders. A systemic disease, it affects various joints – hands, feet, hips, knees, wrists, elbows and shoulders – with a lasting inflammatory reaction. Remissions occur, but the illness progresses to produce commonly permanent damage and deformity. Despite intensive study, its cause remains disputed.[42]

The physicians of Antiquity delineated both gout and arthritic conditions. Soranus described a chronic arthritic state affecting people above the age of thirty-five, especially women. Perhaps the earliest known description suggestive of rheumatoid arthritis, however, is in Ayurvedic medicine, discussed in the *Caraka Samhita*, written in the second century AD.[43]

In the thirteenth century, Bartholemaeus Anglicus, describing several types of arthritis, stated that 'one form of the disease is worse for it draws together tissues and makes the fingers shrink and shrivels the toes and sinews of the feet and of the hands'. Only later, however, did the differentiations standard today begin to be drawn. Guillaume de Baillou (1538–1616) and, a couple of generations later, Thomas Sydenham distinguished between gout and rheumatoid arthritis. Baillou used rheumatism not in the original sense (a defluxion of body fluid into one part) but in something nearer its modern meaning: acute joint pains (polyarthritis) independent of gout.[44] Rheumatism, he noted, invades the whole body 'with pain, swellings and a keen sense of heat'. 'The joints are racked with pain,' he continued, describing the attack, 'so that neither foot, hand nor finger can be moved without pain and protest'. Those who suffer from rheumatism, 'unless they take care of themselves, can scarcely hope to escape chronic arthritis'.[45]

Sydenham, who pioneered the nosological idea of a 'natural history of diseases', established that rheumatism and gout were different diseases. He offered a clinical description of acute rheumatism in his *Methodus curandi febres* (1666):

> It begins with shivering and shaking, and presently heat, restlessness and thirst; and other symptoms which accompany Fever. After a day or two, and sometimes sooner, the Patient is troubled with a violent Pain, sometimes in this, sometimes in that Joint; in the Wrist and Shoulders, but most commonly in the Knees; it now and then changes places, and seizes elsewhere, leaving some redness and swelling in the Part it last possessed . . . When this Disease is not accompanied with a Fever it is often taken for the Gout though it differs essentially from that, as plainly appears to anyone that well considers both Diseases.[46]

Sydenham believed rheumatism had affinities to scurvy and other cachectical disorders suggestive of constitutional maladies. An admirer of Sydenham, the great Dutch physician Herman Boerhaave (1668–1738), penned a clear delineation of rheumatism ('a disease ally'd to the Gout and the Scurvy which is very common in England').[47]

From the seventeenth century, evidence accumulated establishing the specificity of gout as a distinctive joint disorder. In 1776 the Swedish pharmacist Carl Scheele discovered an organic acid in urinary concretions which he called lithic acid. From 1848 the London physician Alfred Garrod devised tests for detecting uric acid in blood. Garrod's view that acute gout results from the precipitation of sodium urate in a joint was later confirmed. Over the centuries gout thus became recognized as distinctive from other arthritic conditions, which in turn began to be linked with infections and fevers. In the nineteenth century, both tuberculosis and syphilis were said to cause arthritic conditions, as were scarlet fever, pneumonia, dysentery and brucellosis.

Exemplifying the new French preoccupation with disease localization, rheumatoid arthritis was mapped out early in the nineteenth century as a specific condition, following a clinical description by Augustin Jacob Landré-Beauvais, who dubbed it 'primary asthenic gout', distinguished it from gout proper and significantly deemed it a disease of the poor. Meanwhile William Heberden and Benjamin Brodie described long-term, chronic, debilitating diseases affecting multiple joints, including hyperextension and other deformities of the fingers.[48]

A cacophony of names continued to denominate what we recognize as rheumatoid arthritis: rheumatic gout, chronic rheumatic arthritis, *goutte astenique privative*, *rheumatismus nodosus*, rheumatoid osteoarthritis and others. In 1859, Garrod argued that 'rheumatoid arthritis' should be used to 'imply an inflammatory affection of the joints not unlike rheumatism . . . but differing materially from it'.[49] 'Rheumatoid arthritis' did not become standard usage until the twentieth century: in 1941 the name was recognized by the American Rheumatism Association. Pathognomic signs like tophi and chemical evidence framed gout relatively early; demarcating rheumatoid arthritis (or polyarthritis) was, by contrast, more difficult. For its part, osteoarthritis became recognizable by a process of exclusion and was awarded its name in 1888 by the Bath physician, John Kent Spender.[50] The modern distinction between rheumatoid arthritis and osteoarthritis was established by Archibald Garrod.[51]

Around 1900 it became widely held that a poison-generating focus of infection could produce toxic elements leading to arthritis. This 'focal infection' hypothesis – popular for explaining other conditions, including insanity– led physicians to recommend tonsillectomies, appendectomies and so forth in hopes of halting the development of arthritis.[52] In 1940, however, researchers identified a substance similar to an antibody circulating in the blood of arthritis sufferers and which they named the 'rheumatoid factor'. Its nature remained obscure until it was shown that a group A streptococcus caused rheumatic infections.

In the light of such disease descriptions and definitions that tend to dissolve like clouds it is crucial to avoid prematurely hypostasizing past accounts as though they will map precisely on to our present disease categories. Retrospective diagnosis risks sacrificing historical understanding of past medical mentalities. Such terms as 'gutta' should not automatically be conflated with our disease entity 'gout'. Historically 'gutta' meant the process of flowing or dropping; mention of 'gutta' thus indicated that peccant humour or morbific matter had accumulated in a part or a joint. It described a disease process rather than a disease thing. The same applies to 'rheum' and to 'dropsy'.[53] Similarly, though we may be confident that such terms as 'podagra' and 'gonagra' commonly designated cases of gout as would be diagnosed by modern medicine, their referent was not to 'gout' in the modern sense, but rather to the site of the trouble: podagra meaning a disorder of the foot, gonagra that of the knee.

The following chapters will show the remarkable range of conditions and metaphors referred to by the term 'gout': not least, diseases of the internal organs and the head which have nothing to do with modern hyperuricaemia-based theories. We might, of course, choose to regard this as evidence of the ineptitude of pre-scientific medicine. But it is better seen as epitomizing earlier disease theories, which viewed disorders as fluid.[54] It also provides evidence of a pecking-order or hegemony among disease labels; some have been more 'imperialistic' than others. *Habent sua fata libelli*: the same holds true for diseases. What follows is the history of one such destiny.[55]

HISTORIES

CHAPTER 2

The Classical Inheritance

The disease we call gout has a high pedigree, as the first medical writings giving clinical descriptions of the disorder are supported by still earlier archaeological and palaeopathological evidence. Arthritic conditions have been identified in the skeletal remains of Neanderthal man and in Egyptian burial sites. In 1910 Elliot Smith and Wood Jones described a spectacular case of primary gout with tophi on a mummy found near a temple at Philae in Nubia, Upper Egypt. Further finds followed.[1]

Gout was familiar to the Hippocratic writers of the fifth century BC and was mentioned by Plato. No meaningful estimate is possible, of course, of its prevalence in the ancient world. Roman authors would suggest that in the virtuous days of the early Republic, podagra had been rare, becoming a problem only with the spread of luxury under the Empire. Nero's tutor, Seneca (c. 4 BC–AD 65), for instance, lamented that, long unknown among the fair sex, it had even spread to women: 'their manner of living' had changed, for 'in this age women rival men in every kind of lasciviousness . . . why need we then be surprised at seeing so many of the female sex afflicted with the gout?'[2] Such judgments voice the ritual Silver Age rhetoric against modern decadence; they may even reflect reality.[3]

Though Graeco-Roman physicians identified instances of what we call gout, they did not have one term exclusively matching our 'framing' of the disease. They commonly spoke of arthritic conditions, meaning complaints exhibiting swelling and inflammation of the joints. And within that category they specified afflictions occurring when the trouble fell upon one particular joint. Arthritic ailments were thus anatomically differentiated: in *On the Causes of Acute and Chronic Diseases*, Aretaeus (AD c. 150–c. 200), for instance, referred to podagra as arthritis (swelling or pain) of the foot ('pous' = foot; 'agra' = prey: hence literally foot-trap); chiagra (or cheiragra) as arthritis of the hands; gonagra as the ailment that seized the knees, and so forth.[4] Such joint maladies (arthritis) were understood as the product of 'rheumatism' in the sense of the descent ('rheuma') of body fluid, the consequence being accumulation, congestion and obstruction in the joints. The idea of rheumatic flux hinged upon humoral theory.[5]

Within the humoral model of health and disease set out in the Hippocratic writings and influential till the eighteenth century, the body's state was broadly grasped in terms of natural rhythms of development and change, determined by the major fluids contained within the skin-envelope, their balance determining health and illness. These vitality-sustaining fluids were blood, choler (or yellow bile), phlegm and melancholy (or black bile). Humours served different life-sustaining ends. It made sense to highlight fluids as the clues to the functioning of the body. After all, life itself was something that flowed: fluids and vitality were all of a piece.

The belief that the body comprised a fluid equilibrium thus suggested that sickness could be the consequence of abnormal or excessive flow of ill-digested humours: a 'rheum' or flux. The idea of rheumatism did not apply exclusively to diseases of the joints and could be used for any internal humoral defluxion. Like a traffic jam, a viscous rheum might snarl up around almost any organ.

The Greek notion of rheumatism was to be echoed in the Latin word *gutta*, a drop, the source of the English 'gout' and the French *goutte*. This also drew upon humoral conceptions of disease, implying the falling of humours to a particular body part. With *gutta* as with rheumatism, the pathological pos-sibilities were not confined to joints, there could be a flow (flux) of humours anywhere in the body. Hence it was quite legitimate to specify gouty sciatica, migraine or haemorrhoids, and even gouty epilepsy and paralysis: gout might be implicated wherever humours accumulated.[6]

The major Greek physicians made pronouncements on arthritic conditions and podagra, some of which were to assume canonical authority. Hippocrates (*c.* 460–*c.* 357 BC), or rather the writings by him and his followers now known as the Hippocratic corpus, laid the foundations.[7] The Hippocratic authors differentiated between 'arthritis' and 'podagra' (acute gout). In respect of the former it was stated that 'fever comes on, acute pain affects the joints of the body, and the pains which vary between mild and severe flit from joint to joint; it is of short duration, and often very acute, but not mortal. It attacks the young more frequently than the old': we might regard this as a description of rheumatic fever. Podagra, by contrast, according to *On the Affections of the Parts*, 'is the most violent of all joint affections, it lasts long, and becomes chronic . . . The pain may remain fixed in the great toes . . . it is not fatal.'[8]

The Hippocratic writings regarded podagra as the outcome of excessive accumulation of bodily humour, probably phlegm, which swelled the affected joint. This painful state might result from sexual excess or from a sedentary life with too rich a diet, causing 'indigestion' of the humours. Three Hippocratic aphorisms implicated sexual function. According to Aphorism 28, eunuchs do not take the gout, nor do they become bald.[9] In his later commentary, Galen accepted this as basically true, while maintaining that modern times were so indolent and vicious that even eunuchs occasionally contracted gout.

Aphorism 29 then states that a woman does not take the gout unless her menses had ceased. Galen also glossed this aphorism, saying that now Imperial luxury had superseded republican simplicity, younger women had also become subject to gout. Last, according to Aphorism 30, a young man does not become susceptible to gout until the time of indulging in copulation. These Hippocratic aphorisms thus linked sex with virility, a view underpinning aetiological thinking until the eighteenth century.[10]

The Hippocratic authors characteristically discerned periodicity in the attacks, saying that 'for the most part gouty affections rankle in the spring and in the autumn' (Aphorism 55). Arthritic disorders were reckoned to be diseases of the spring. Later commentators, notably Celsus, explained the apparent worsening of podagra in the autumn as nature's effort to expel to the extremities peccant humours accumulating at the height of summer.

With respect to podagra as so much else, Galen reiterated the key Hippocratic teachings, while revealing preoccupations of his own. In his commentary on the Hippocratic Aphorisms, he alluded to the role of heredity, observing that those inheriting gout suffered more intensely than those acquiring it.[11] He also downplayed general humoral imbalance, suggesting the ailment stemmed from an accumulation of peccant humours in the affected part. Tophi were local concentrations of humours.

Several other Ancient physicians offered observations. Aretaeus (second century AD) gave an account of a condition resembling rheumatoid arthritis. In *On the Causes of Acute and Chronic Diseases*, he also depicted the onset of podagra, ghosting Sydenham's famous later description:

> pain seizes the great toe, then the forepart of the heel on which we rest; next it comes into the arch of the foot, but the ankle-joint swells last of all . . . the disease often progresses to an incurable stage because at the commencement the physician is not consulted, while the disease is feeble and can be brought under control. When it has acquired strength with time all treatment is useless.[12]

Aretaeus maintained that the causes of podagra were internal, although a blow or a pinching shoe was often blamed (the true causes of arthritis, he noted, were known only to the gods). The disease sometimes remitted for long periods – a man subject to podagra had even been known to win an Olympic race during a healthy interval. Above all he drew attention to the tender toe and its ligaments: 'if they become spontaneously painful, as in the gout, no other pain is more severe than this, not iron screws, nor cords, not the wound of a dagger, nor burning fire, for all these may be had recourse to as cures for the still greater pains'.[13] Like his contemporary Galen, Aretaeus suggested the efficient cause of gout might lie not in a humoral plethora but in a specific peccant humour. Nevertheless, he believed in classic manner that disorders arose under the influence of internal factors like temperament, and suggested that podagra often turned into dropsy and sometimes into asthma. Gout was a male disease, and goutiness might be inherited.

Other medical writers discussed podagra without introducing significant new information or thinking. Aulus Cornelius Celsus (*c.* 25 BC–AD 50) – no physician but a country gentleman whose *De re medicina* was a literary labour of love – recognized one basic affection of the joints which he termed arthritis, using a more precise terminology for local sites (podagra, chiagra and so forth). To ward off arthritic conditions, he commended regular exercise and the avoidance of corpulence. Such advice would demand a transformation of lifestyle: in those degenerate times, many recent rulers had suffered from podagra ('whether of their own faults or that of their progenitors I know not'); the Consul Agrippa endured three acute attacks and committed suicide at the onset of his fourth rather than suffer further.[14] Celsus' therapeutic preferences were familiar: blood-letting, diuretics, emetics and hot fomentations. During remission he recommended easy exercise and spare diet, observing that 'some have obtained lifelong security by refraining from wine, mead and venery for a whole year'.[15]

Among the other Classical physicians, Soranus of Ephesus (*fl.* AD 98–138) gave a clear account of tophi: 'These may burst through and jut out. They can be removed surgically, or upon their early appearance may be merely lifted out with a spoon-shaped instrument, though later they will grow again.'[16] His contemporary Rufus of Ephesus mentioned seeing tophi dissolve in course of treatment. He also developed the notion, hinted at in Aretaeus, of visceral or metastatic gout, in which the malady might recoil from the joints, especially in response to hasty cooling, and lay siege to one of the crucial internal organs. 'Such sudden revulsion of the humours from the joints', he judged, 'will provoke pulmonary or cerebral complications, and in the same way failure of the renal and intestinal functions may produce a fatal result, generally preceded by convulsions and coma.'[17]

Paul of Aegina (AD 625–90), the last of the great Greek physicians and a major codifier, recognized there were singular aspects of podagra requiring explanation, not least its periodicity and tendency to remit. In addition to 'a preternatural humour', Paul inferred there must also be some congenital weakness or mechanical inferiority in a joint that would draw and anchor the gouty humour.[18] When the morbid matter was greatly in excess it would ooze through the coverings of the joint and crystallize as tophi. Like other Greek physicians, he believed psychological factors played their part – 'sorrow, care, watchfulness, and other passions of the mind may excite an attack of this disorder'.[19]

The Hippocratics believed diet paramount in the management of gout.[20] While they did not entirely forbid wine, particularly for elderly patients, barleywater drinks were strongly recommended. In stubborn cases, heroic therapies involving purging with white hellebore (*Veratrum album*) were prescribed – to imitate the best natural relief for the malady, which was an attack of dysentery. Where localized pain continued, counter-irritation might be tried by scorching the veins above the affected joint with raw flax (moxibustion).[21]

Celsus, however, voiced doubts, reiterated by almost all subsequent writers, regarding the wisdom of local external applications to affected joints. He counselled great caution with regard to cold compresses, believing these frustrated Nature's efforts to disperse the condition by means of the acute attack, thereby driving it inwards towards the vital organs. His preference lay in moderate bleeding from a vein. This would cause the joints first affected to remain pain free until the next annual recurrence – and often for longer.[22]

Therapeutically Galen advocated a dietetic regime similar to the Hippocratic, while also, as was almost a reflex with him, adding prophylactic bleeding every spring.[23] While approving of strong purgatives alongside extensive bleeding, he held that diet was the key factor influencing health and disease. Though the indications varied according to the individual temperament, he also laid down general rules based upon humoral theory. These prescribed bland, easily digested food: 'Barley bread is a very excellent thing, and a sausage in due season; and a little cabbage half boiled, with a soup of mixed vegetables.' Fruits were to be taken only during the summer and then sparingly. A spring sea voyage could also be very advantageous – presumably because this would entail a Lenten diet and therapeutic sea-sickness.[24]

Following Hippocrates and Galen, a standard therapeutics was thus formulated that long proved influential. It involved depletion of the excessive accumulation of humours that had flowed into the joints. Purging, vomiting, diuresis and phlebotomy were to expel the offending humours. Suspicion was voiced of violent methods of cure, lest these repel the attack, creating the perilous condition of visceral gout.

Some authors, however, had hopes of drastic action. Aretaeus praised hellebore because 'it possessed a quality of no mean description'. If he was thereby stating that hellebore possessed a property specific for gout, it was a perceptive judgment, as hellebore is related to colchicum, so called because it grew near Colchis in Asia Minor.[25]

Indeed, the one therapeutic breakthrough of enduring importance was the recommendation by Alexander of Tralles (sixth century) of a drug he termed hermodactyl, derived from colchicum (*Colchicum autumnale* L., autumn crocus, meadow saffron), as a gout specific.[26] Its medicinal properties were well known. The plant had been discussed at some length in the *De materia medica* of Dioscorides (*fl.* AD 60–77), which prescribed a number of simples for podagra.[27] He recommended decoction of white willow leaves and use of the bark as a warm poultice – this would contain salicin in sufficient amounts to act as an analgesic and antipyretic, bringing some local relief. He also suggested barley, together with quinces or vinegar, for gouty inflammations; cabbage with fenugreek and vinegar 'helps those with gout in their feet and joints', asphodel and colocynth (*Cucumis colocynthis*) were useful.[28] Dioscorides also produced a chapter on the autumn crocus; its sole use, he believed, was as an antidote against mushroom-poisoning. Alexander of Tralles, by contrast, stated that hermadactyl, an extract from the colchicum corn, had purgative properties useful for dealing with a certain kind of arthritis. Colchicum later became controversial, since if taken in large doses it was found to have severe gastro-intestinal side-effects, indeed to be poisonous.[29]

Podagra evidently acquired some notoriety in Antiquity since it made its mark upon folklore and literature. Authors somewhat facetiously identified various mythological figures as sufferers, including King Priam of Troy, Achilles, Bellerophon (who died of it) and Oedipus, King of Thebes. The tradition relating to Oedipus continued into modern times. An anonymous eighteenth-century poetaster captured its essence:

> And where malignant Juices flow,
> Close *knotty Knobs* in Sharpness grow,
> Old OEDIPUS the *Theban* King,
> Felt *swelling Joint* and *Gouty Sting*,
> And tho' the Sage could SPHINX explain,
> The Sage cou'd ne'er unriddle *Pain*.

Pain was inextricably tied to gout in the Classical period. Seneca among others referred to the disease as the rosy daughter of Bacchus (Dionysus) and Venus (or Aphrodite): 'Bacchus pater, Venus mater, et Ira obstetrix Arthritidis.'[30] Podagra, the foot-torturess, was a fury who roused dread even in Jove, attacking her victims when 'the Spring the rising Sap impels':

> Then unperceiv'd she drives her piercing Dart,
> And Wounds the inmost Sense with secret Smart . . .
> Thro' ev'ry Joint the thrilling Anguish pours,
> And gnaws, and burns, and tortures, and devours;
> Till Length of Suff'ring the dire Pow'r appease,
> And the fierce Torments at her bidding cease.[31]

These lines form part of an eighteenth-century translation of a work by the Greek playwright Lucian (*c.* 125–*c.* 190). Author of some seventy-nine prose works and a collection of fifty-three epigrams, Lucian also produced two mock-tragedies on gout. One was entitled *Tragopodagra*.[32] Its cast includes a Gouty Man, a Messenger, a Doctor and a Chorus of Pains, and its (anti-)heroine is the heartless demon goddess Podagra:

> What mortal born on earth but knows of me,
> Resistless Gout, the mistress of men's toils?
> Me no sweet reek of incense can appease
> Nor blood of victims burnt in sacrifice
> Nor shrine whose walls with idols rich are hung.
> Me Paean cannot worst with medicine,
> Though doctor he to all the gods of heaven,
> Not yet his learned son, Asclepius.[33]

In response to this imperious proclamation of her invincible powers, the Chorus of Pains humbly acknowledges Podagra's might and bows down before the tyrannical goddess:

> Prosperous Gout, how great thy power!
> Dread art thou to Jove's swift shaft,
> Fearsome thou to Ocean's waves
> And to Hades king below;
> Bandage-loving Sickbed Queen,
> Speed-impairing Joint-Tormentor,
> Ankle-burning Timid-Stepper,
> Pestle-fearing, Knee-Fire Sleepless,
> Loving chalkstones on the knuckles,
> Knee-deformer, Gout's thy name.[34]

Podagra boasts of her triumphs:

> Great numbers I've o'ercome, as sages know.
> Priam, though Doughty called, had gouty feet.[35]

The hapless Doctor, by contrast, is totally unable to cope and collapses in despair:

> Alas, alas, I'm utterly destroyed!
> I burn in every limb from bane untold . . .
> Have mercy, queen, for neither salve of mine
> Nor other remedy can quell thy course.
> All votes agree you conquer all mankind.[36]

Yet even Podagra shows she can be merciful in her fashion – that is to say, however implacable the goddess, there are remissions in her attacks:

> Ye torments, cease. Relax their suffering
> For now they're sorry that they challenged me.

> Let all men know that I alone of gods
> Do not relent or yield to remedies.[37]

Lucian's other gout play was *Swift-of-Foot*. The title character was distinguished for grace and strength, and a devotee of the hunt and wrestling-school. He would often laugh scornfully when he stared at victims of remorseless Gout, crying that the disorder amounted to nothing at all. Outraged, the jealous goddess assailed him through his feet. When he initially bore up sturdily and denied his plight, Podagra put him on his back, once again appearing as a despotic queen:

> I have a name men dread and loathe to hear;
> They call me Gout, a fearsome scourge to men;
> I bind their feet in sinew-knotting cords,
> When I have swept unseen into their joints.[38]

[★]

In later centuries, Byzantine, Arab and Latin Christian writers were to transmit and gloss Graeco-Roman writings on podagra, without, however, developing major new ideas of their own.[39] The greatest of the Islamic medical writers, Avicenna (980–1037), for instance, reiterated the Greek notion of salutary purgation and argued that to correct from time to time 'the unhealthy state of the temperament which has been produced by the plethora', one should undergo 'a form of evacuation which itself serves to protect one for instance from an attack of gout, or from an epileptic seizure which one knows will occur on a certain date, especially in spring'.[40]

The thirteenth-century Byzantine physician Demetrios Pepagomenos produced a notable manuscript known by the Latin title *Liber de podagra et id genus morbus*, dedicated to his patient, Michael Palaeologus, the Emperor Michael VIII (r. 1261–82). Following the Ancient writers, Demetrios stated that gout was due to a collection of humours in the affected joints which were the product of imperfect digestion. He advocated vomiting, phlebotomy and purging, recommending for acute attacks a pill containing hermodactyl, aloes, cinnamon and scammony, in line with the prescriptions of Alexander of Tralles 700 years earlier.[41]

In Latin Christendom the term 'gutta' became standardly applied to podagra. It was used, for instance, by Ralph Bocking, a Dominican monk and domestic chaplain to St Richard of Wyche, Bishop of Chichester (1197–1258). He recounted that he had been a great sufferer with *gutta quam podagram vel arteticam vocant* (the gout which is called podagra or arthritis), until healed by wearing a pair of the Bishop's boots. Belief grew up that any sufferer slipping his gouty foot within the holy Bishop's boots would be granted a speedy cure. The Bishop's stone effigy still presides over the healing waters at Droitwich, his birthplace.[42] 'Gout' began to make its appearance in the English language. In an account of the Crusade of 1270, one of the leaders is said to have fallen sick in Jerusalem of a 'gote' in his knees and feet. In *Piers Plowman* (1377), Langland writes: 'He . . . gyued me in goutes, I may noughte go at large.'[43]

Gout assumed a certain presence in religious healing. About this time, sufferers with 'gutta' were reported to have been miraculously cured at the tomb of St Thomas à Becket in Canterbury. At least thirteen other saints and holy men possessed similar therapeutic powers, including Andrew the Apostle, St Julian of Alexandria, St Sebastian, St Tranquillanus, the Blessed Autriclinian of Limoges, St Maurice, St Placidus, St Maurus, St Staphinus of Dourgne, St Gallus, Hildegard of Bingen, St Albert of Messina and St Wolfgang.[44]

A fourteenth-century French manuscript describes treatments. It is preceded by the words: 'Pour les goutte Sr Jehan d'Aix'. Jean d'Esch (or Jehan d'Aix) was a magistrate in Metz who died before 1398. Suffering from gout, and having unsuccessfully consulted the local physicians, he addressed a certain Hehan Le Fevre de Metz, who lived at Montpellier, already a great medical centre. The suggested treatment spells out general bans on harmful foods and drink, and gives recommendations of diet and herbal recipes:

1. . . . take care that you do not eat peas or beans or other legumes, or chestnuts; however, you may eat pea-soup or chickpea soup, but not too often.

2. Likewise, guard yourself against eating any food made with dough, that is, dough cooked in foods or beverages; or which has been dried previously and then cooked in vinegar; either with meat or with cheese; or which has been preserved in honey, such as spiced bread.[45]

Medieval English medical writings seem to make rather little reference to gout, though there is mention of kidney and bladder stones.[46] Among medieval physicians and laity alike, joint disorders were clearly well known, but it took the Renaissance to create new thinking about gout. Scientific rebels, like Paracelsus, developed new conjectures about articular inflammation; while concepts of courtesy and human destiny prompted speculations on the relations between civilization and disease.

CHAPTER 3

Prometheus's Vulture:
The Renaissance Fashioning of Gout

... kills us with a lingering death, and like Prometheus's vulture, gnaws
us into fresh torment.

'A Dissertation on the Gout,' *London Magazine* (October 1755),
612, letter from R. Drake to Editor

The invention of printing and the spread of literacy, the growth of towns,
affluence, courts and universities created the conditions sustaining the vast
sixteenth-century proliferation of medical learning and publishing. Elite physicians and surgeons promoted medical humanism, aiming to recover, perfect
and improve the authorities of Antiquity; meanwhile, books began to appear
instructing the laity how to tend their health and treat their ailments.[1]

Among their ABCs of disease and head-to-foot anatomical charts, many
such works included discussions of arthritic conditions and podagra, distilled
and sometimes simplified from the masters of Antiquity and Islam, spelling
out the nature and causes of those afflictions, and informing readers, professional and lay, about prevention and cure. Works even began to appear
devoted exclusively or essentially to gout. The first of these was *Ob das
Podagra Möglich zu Generen oder Nit. Nutzlich zu Wissen Allen dene die damit
Behafft* (On whether it is possible to cure gout. Useful to know for all those
who suffer from it). The work of a German physician, Dominicus Burgawer,
it was printed in Strasburg by Mathias Apiarius in 1534.[2] Little is known about
the author, except that his text shows him to have been an admirer of Rhazes
and Avicenna and familiar with Paracelsus. It may serve as a window upon
Renaissance views.

Asking 'What is Podagra?', Burgawer responded that 'it is a pain in the feet
with or without swelling, which comes from dampness or draught'. The
generic term for the condition was 'ARTHETICA' (sic), which, he said, may
be rendered as 'sickness of the limbs'. In Latin its name was 'GUTTA', which
'means "drop" because it is like the drops running down the roofs to the
ground'.[3] The correct word depended upon the terminus of the flow: 'If the
flux or matter goes into the hands it is called CIRAGIA, into the hip
SCIATICA, into the knees GENUGRA, and into the feet PODAGRA.'[4]

Burgawer then turned to aetiology, for 'prevention is possible if one knows this'. Podagra arose 'from outward or inward sudden changes to extremes of cold or heat' – 'cold' of course meant more within humoral theory than a temperature measurable by a thermometer. This dangerous cold, he explained, 'can be caused by superfluous food, superfluous sleep and constant idleness'. Rhazes had proved that pain did not attack 'those who work, only those who do not have to work'. There were also, he believed, other causes of gout, intelligible in the light of Graeco-Roman teachings on the non-naturals:

> The disease also comes from great sadness, and from excessive venery, especially after meals, for Hippocrates and other philosophers say eunuchs and those who have nothing to do with women do not get it . . .
>
> Similarly harmful is inordinate eating and drinking, mixing one's wines, which stifles natural heat, whereby superfluous fluids are collected in the body, and this happens to the grand gentlemen who have all their heart desires.[5]

The point about gender was especially telling. Burgawer concluded in good Renaissance manner by citing his source: 'All this has been said concisely by Rhazes.'[6]

Burgawer's tract was representative of much contemporary writing. It drew upon the authority of Greek and Arab physicians; it offered a multi-causal account of the disease, grounded in humoral philosophy and the individual constitution; and it stressed temperamental (moral and emotional) as well as strictly physical factors.

Among the fullest discussions of podagra was that presented by the French surgeon Ambroise Paré (1510–90), whose magisterial surgical writings contained a discussion 'Of the Disease of the Joints Commonly Called the Gout'. Paré wrote eloquently, being himself, like Sydenham a century later, a sufferer. 'The paines of the goute', he explained, obviously describing his own case, 'are rightly accounted amongst the most grevous and acute; so that through the vehemency of the agony many are almost mad, and wish themselves dead.'[7] Paré held the natural duration of an acute attack was forty days; it was either inherited or acquired; and, he pointed out in Galenic mould, that what determined its severity was the venomousness of the peccant matter distilled from the humours, as it 'causeth intolerable tormenting paine not by the abundance, because it happens to many who have the gout, no signe of defluxion appearing in the jointes'.[8] Unlike Paracelsus, Paré was diffident about the chemistry of morbific matter: 'It is not of a more knowne, or easily exprest nature than that which causeth the plague, *Lues veneria* or falling sicknesse.'[9]

What triggered attacks? In most cases, Paré suggested, the affected joint must previously have been weakened, either by nature or by an accident. But the predisposing cause lay in over-indulgence and luxury.[10] Discussing diet, he advocated chicken as easily digested – though with the reservation, reflecting Renaissance theories about cosmic correspondences, that 'some of the antients have disallowed of the eating of capons and the like birds, because they are subject to bee troubled by the goute in the feete'. Folklore had it that hawks also, mirroring their aristocratic masters, were subject to this complaint.[11]

Paré recommended a double defence. It was essential to follow a moderate regime – 'such gouty persons as remain intemperate and given to gluttony and venerie (especially the old)', he insisted, 'may hope for no health by the use of medicines'.[12] But he also expressed some faith in medical interventions, chiefly prophylactic: frequent copious bloodletting, vomits, sweating, purging and diuresis, including the use of hermodactyl (colchicum) pills. Gouty subjects should not drink much, lest excess fluid chill the stomach and so check digestion, thereby leaving 'crudities' which would collect in the blood and create fresh poison. Though a surgeon, Paré was circumspect regarding external remedies, except cautery and setons as counter-irritants. One of many practitioners who referred to it as the 'opprobrium medicorum', Paré took the view that, while it might be prevented and treated, gout did not admit radical cure.

With gout as with so much else, the great challenge to humanist orthodoxy came from the Swiss iconoclast Paracelsus (1493–1541).[13] He was the first who radically rejected humoral ideas of gout and renal calculus, regarding the emphasis upon 'catarrh' and 'flux' as mere gammon, lacking anatomical plausibility. If black bile had its seat in the spleen, how could it descend to the legs, causing ulceration?[14] Each was a disease in its own right, though certain diseases, for example syphilis, would, however, develop only on top of others, by 'transplantation'.[15] Syphilis, for Paracelsus, was the pathological expression of the lewdness and luxury rife in those corrupt times, but it was also a 'specific' poison.[16] Thus, there was the risk that gout would change into gouty syphilis.[17]

The image of 'tartar' and 'tartaric disease' occupies a prominent place among Paracelsus' nosological theories. It implied general pathological conceptions. Disease was a concrete entity which could be made visible and tangible, in contrast to disease in the Ancient sense, conceived as a mere humoral upset. It was seen as exogenous – due to indigestible matter introduced with food and drink – rather than endogenous, as with Hippocratic theory. The disease entity could be defined in chemical terms as the product of coagulation, connected with the action of 'salt' on the deleterious substance entering from outside. It was a failure to separate 'pure' from 'impure', nourishment from waste. Furthermore, this process was 'specific', a chemical operation in its own right, departing from the holistic model posited by Classical medicine. Overall disease was a local process.[18]

On the basis of such pathological convictions, Paracelsus advanced in *De*

Morbis Tartareis (1531) a novel explanation of gout, via his concept of the diseases of tartar. Some local factor, such as water supply, probably influenced corporeal chemical depositions of this kind, he suggested, noting that in Switzerland, 'the most healthy land, superior to Germany, Italy and France, nay all Western and Eastern Europe, there is no gout, no colic, no rheumatisms and no stone'.[19] Gouty nodules consisted of calcined synovia or an excremental salt – tartar – coagulated in a joint. The tartar found in wine casks was a result of fermentation. Such material could be compared to certain natural bodily deposits – encrustations on the teeth (still called, of course, 'tartar'), gallstones and kidney stones.

Bodily tartar, Paracelsus believed, was derived from food and released through digestion. In some individuals it failed to be excreted, tending rather to be coagulated by 'spirit of salt' and thereby transformed into stony substances. In the tartarous precipitation of the gout:

> the gluten, which was called synovia by the old wound surgeons, is sticky and gelatinous like eggwhite. Now when salty matter comes into contact with and mixes itself with this, it coagulates at once into a solid . . . The gout of the feet, hands, and knees has its origin in this coagulation.[20]

This theory of 'tartarous disease' – a tendency to retain acrid substances – was one of the earliest attempts at a chemical aetiology for a malady. Paracelsus, however, made no practical advance in therapy. Moreover, the impact of his teachings upon later thinking is somewhat equivocal. Other learned doctors, including Théodore Turquet de Mayerne,[21] the French-trained physician to James I, adopted his views. In his *Treatise of the Gout*, translated by Thomas Sherley and published posthumously in 1676, Turquet de Mayerne considered gout as one of the diseases of tartar, but his views did not prove influential.[22]

This is not to suggest that the Tudor and Stuart era did not bring discussions of gout among English physicians. These, however, chiefly summarized and popularized the commonplaces of learned medicine. Henry VIII's physician, Andrew Boorde (1490–1549), broached the question of podagra in two works, the *Dyetary of Health* (1542), and *The Breviary of Health* (1547).[23] Attempting to reconcile Greek and Latin sources and to find English equivalents for classical concepts, Boorde deplored the slovenly habit of giving the name arthritis to all aches in the joints, 'whether the pain arise from a rheumatic inflammation or a gouty humour': 'all jointe illnesses are not the goute'.[24] He distinguished four types, namely chiagra (of hands, fingers and arms); podagra (of the feet, toes and legs); 'Goute arterycke, which involves jointes elsewhere'; and sciatica.

In matters therapeutic, Boorde endorsed Humanist orthodoxies. Allopathic in his preferences, he aimed at the removal of peccant humours by prophylactic spring and autumn bleedings, as Galen had advocated, supported by a moderate diet. During paroxysms, external remedies should be used. He recommended the wearing of dog-skin hose, perhaps taking a hint from Soranus of Ephesus, who had suggested that gouty feet should be anointed with seal fat and then encased in seal-skin slippers. Boorde also prescribed daily application to the painful joints of baked fermentations of ox-dung wrapped in cabbage leaves. Such external methods could be accompanied by strong scammony purges, followed by generous quantities of treacle to 'weaken the virulency of the gouty malignancy'.[25] He was keen on an infusion of ash bark (*Fraxinus excelsior*), a favourite recipe all over Europe for gout, scurvy and fevers until the introduction of the Peruvian bark (*cinchona*).[26] He favoured assorted diuretics, including sorrel roots, parsley and other herbs stewed in broth.[27] Like many contemporaries, Boorde presented a mixed bag of treatments, evidently responding to the fact that gout itself was protean.

In 1560 there appeared a *Method of Phisicke* by Phillip Barrough, a Fellow of the College of Physicians, *Containing the Causes, Signs and Cures of Inward Diseases in Man's Body from the Head to the Foot*.[28] By 1583 it had run to a seventh edition, dedicated to Lord Burghley, a celebrated martyr to the gout. In his chapter 'Of the Goute in the Feet and the Jointes', Barrough gnawed at the taxonomic problem dogging contemporary physicians: that of distinguishing various joint afflictions, clarifying the terms used for them by Classical authors, and matching up the old authorities against clinical reality. He tended to think of a diversity of words, a unity of disease:

> Podagra and arthritis in Latin be diseases of one kind, and therefore they differ not but in places diseased, for in both of them there is weakness of the joints and unnatural humour floweth to them, and if that the fluxe of the humour do flow to the feet, that is called podagra in Latin, but if the humour flow to the joints, it is called in Greek arthritis, in Latin articularis morbis, the joint sickness.[29]

Precisely what should count as podagra troubled him. Barrough also aired the causes of the disease and mentioned – with what, in the light of the dedication, might be taken as a breathtaking want of tact – that 'this disease is engendered of continued crudities and drunkenness, and of immoderate using of lechery'. Alongside such Hippocratic orthodoxies, he tabulated other precipitants: an attack could come on by 'vehement and swift deambulations and walkings, by suppressions and stopping of accustomed excretions and fluxes and through intermission of familiar exercises. Perturbations of the mind do not only engender this evil, but also do breed hurtful and corrupt humours' – the well-worn mixture of predisposing and exciting causes, physical and emotional triggers.[30]

A popular work was Thomas Cogan's *The Haven of Health* (1584), 'for all those that have a care for their health, amplified upon five words of

Hippocrates, Labour, Meat, Drink, Sleep and Venus'.[31] Alongside attention to the non-naturals, he counselled prudence and moderation: 'Wherefore I say to the gentleman who have the gout, that although the forebearing of wine and women and other things noisome in that disease do not utterly take away the gout, yet it will abate quality and abridge the pain and make it much more tolerable.'[32] Cogan's book traded upon the intimate connections between kitchen and pharmacy, victuals and medicine. Discussing diet, he pointed out that *eating* old and hard cheese was taboo because it bred melancholy – but there was more to cheese than edibility: 'an old hard cheese is good for some things, for Galen showeth that an old cheese cut in pieces and sodden with the broth of a gammon of bacone and made in the manner of a plaster and laid to the joint where the gout is, will break the skin and dissolve those hard knots which the gout causeth'.[33] Without forbidding wine, Cogan urged abstinence at the onset of an attack. The link between gout and excess was clear: he would address 'the Gentlemen that hath the gowt', and them alone, 'for poore men seldome have it, because for the more part it groweth through excesse and ease'.[34]

Much was proposed and used against gout. Drawing upon medieval authors such as Gilbertus Anglicus, who had recommended an ointment made of puppy boiled up with cucumber, rue and juniper, herbals offered remedies,[35] and there was always the wisdom of the Ancients to fall back upon. As Thomas Nash observed in *A Pleasant Comedie, Called Summers Last Will and Testament*:

> And well observe Hippocrates old rule
> The onely medicine for the foote is rest.[36]

The idea that luxurious living would bring nemesis in the form of vengeful maladies was a Humanist commonplace, particularly after the appearance of the new disease of syphilis.[37] 'They foreshorten their lives considerably,' commented Laurent Joubert, adopting the Hippocratic view that gout was the wages of sexual excess,

> just as do lascivious and wanton lechers, who do not live very long but fall quickly subject, prey, and victim to gout, colic, nephritis, apoplexy, paralysis, convulsions, and other disease of indigestion (the cause of phlegm, father of all these diseases).[38]

Pithily in *The Rape of Lucrece* Shakespeare anchored the malady to miserly, masculinist moorings that would hold up through to the era of the Georgians and Victorians:

> The aged man that coffers-up his gold,
> Is plagu'd with cramps, and gouts and painful fits.

This he achieved, as well, by highlighting its pains and perils,[39] implying, through the railings of Falstaff, that it was the old man's version of the pox: 'A man can no more separate age and covetousness than 'a can part young limbs and lechery; but the gout galls the one, and the pox pinches the other.'[40]

In Renaissance times it was a fantasy but also a visible fact that podagra haunted the pre-eminent. The muster of illustrious sufferers was imposing.[41] The Medici in Florence illustrated the links between gout and grandeur upon which many contemporaries remarked. Son of the gouty Giovanni, Cosimo de'Medici (1389–1464) was said to have grown 'old very rapidly as he suffered very severely from the gout, and in his later years became very infirm, which caused him to leave the affairs of the state largely to others'. Cosimo had two sons, one of whom, Piero il Gottoso (1416–69), succeeded him. Piero ('The Gouty') suffered from boyhood onwards with acute attacks; for long spells he was unable to address public business; he became very crippled; and late in life his incapacity was such that he could move only his tongue.[42]

The Holy Roman Emperor Charles V (1500–58) suffered his first gouty paroxysm at the age of twenty-eight. Severe attacks followed in 1536 and 1544–5, when he was immobilized for almost the whole winter. By 1550 he was almost completely physically disabled. Despite increasing incapacity, Charles failed to control the gluttony that fed his disease. Ignoring court physicians, he would follow the latest quack who would promise recovery without the need to curb his appetite. His recurrent bouts of gout influenced the fate of his Empire. Thus in his French wars, plans to lay siege to Metz, the key to Lorraine, had to be postponed in 1552 because he was sick. Physical incapacity was perhaps one reason for his abdication in favour of his son Philip: two years later he died miserably, 'sicke and frustrated of the goute before the High Altar of his chapel in the Escorial'.[43]

What treatments did Charles V try? A temporarily fashionable remedy for gout, as well as for other diseases like syphilis, was a decoction of guaiac wood, or *lignum vitae*, recently introduced from the New World via the Augsburg banking family of Fugger. An alternative was the 'China root', the diuretic extract of the dried rhizome known later as *Smilax china*, brought back from the East by the Portuguese, for which similar virtues were claimed.[44] With both, the patient was put to bed on a low diet in a heated room, and the decoction administered. The Emperor was subjected to each of these 'specifics'; he preferred China root, however, as fewer dietary restrictions were thought necessary. Neither proved effective.[45]

In England, the pre-eminent gout sufferer was William Cecil, Lord Burghley.[46] Assorted letters to him survive in English, Latin, French and Italian, offering infallible cures. A note from a Mr Dyon dated 24 January 1553 recommended a combination of diet and physic. Similar directions came from Lady Harington in a letter dated 4 February 1573; an Italian letter, dated

12 December 1575, concerned a secret gout powder. Four years later Dr Henry Landwer came up with a Latin prescription for medicated slippers, while Dr Hector Nones, or Nunez, a Fellow of the College of Physicians and one of the leaders of London's Spanish Jewish colony, showered him with cures culled from Averroes and others. In 1583 yet another letter from a certain Nicholas Gybberd held out prospects of an infallible cure: an alchemical tincture of gold. The Earl of Shrewsbury also wrote begging His Lordship to 'make trial of my OYLE OF STAGS BLUD, for I am strongly persuaded of the rare and great vertu thereof. I know it to be a most safe thynge, yet some offence there is in the smell thereof'.[47]

In a letter of 1592, Henry Bossevyle, an alchemist living in Calais, offered in return for preferment and a fee of four or five hundred pounds to 'furnish some infallible plaisters to cure the gout':

> Concernynge the applyinge thereof, one water [solution] must bathe the place nere unto the payne, leaving a joynte between the place of payne and the place bathed, if conveniently it maye be. Then must a peece of the sayd lether be cutte convenient to make a plaister, which muste be well moystened in one of the sayde waters, and thereon severall other powerful things spredde, which plaister muste be layde upon the place bathed, there to remayne XII howers; and afterwards there must be freshe bathinge and plaisters.[48]

As cautious with regard to his own health as to the nation's, Burghley sent no answer.

To his son Robert, Earl of Salisbury, Burghley bequeathed not only several of his offices of state but also his affliction, from which Robert died on 24 May 1612 on his return from a 'cure' in Bath ordered by Turquet de Mayerne, the royal physician (not to be confused with Maier, who we mention in Chapter 11). Burghley's eldest son, Thomas (1542–1623), Earl of Exeter, also suffered, leading to his untimely retirement from court and occasional confinement in his house at Wimbledon.[49]

As gout took up residence with ministers and monarchs, it also became identified as the monarch among maladies – often being jocularly referred to, with echoes of Classical lore, as a quasi-deity born of the union of Bacchus and Venus.[50] The explanation as to why gout's abode lay within the palace, or at least the mansion and manor-house, was provided by the popular just-so story of the travels of Monsieur Gout and the Spider.[51] In 'A Tale That is True Enough', Richard Hawes offered readers his *The Poore-Mans Plaster-Box. Furnished with Diverse Excellent Remedies for Sudden Mischances, and Usuall Infirmities, Which Happen to Men, Women, and Children in this Age* (1634), just one of many tellings.[52] The point of Hawes's tale was to explain why the gout 'commonly keepes good company, as Bishops, Cardinals, Dukes, Earles,

Lords, Knights, Judges, Gentlemen, and Merchants'. It was all because of the
wretched entertainment Monsieur Gout had once received at a peasant's cot.
'A great while ago,' Hawes began,

> when Monsieur Gout was not so rich (as now he is), he was forced to
> travel, as other poor men are sometimes. In his travel he met with a spider,
> whose journey lay as Mr. Gout's did. They being both benighted, they
> sought lodging, and came to a poore man's house, which the Gout took up
> for his lodging, for he always being a lazy companion, would go no further;
> but the spider being more nimble, went to a rich man's house, and there
> took up his lodging for the night. The next day they met again, and asked
> each other of their entertainment the past night.
>
> 'Mine', said the Gout, 'was the worst as ever I had, for I had no sooner
> touched the poor man's legs, thinking there to take my rest, but up he gets,
> and to thrashing he goes, so that I had no rest the whole night.'
>
> 'And I', said the spider, 'had no sooner begun to build my house in the
> rich man's chamber, but the maid came with a broom, and tore down all
> my work, and so fiercely did pursue me, that I had so much ado to save
> my life, as ever I had.'
>
> 'Seeing it is so, then,' said the Gout, 'we will change lodging, I will go
> to the rich man's house, and thou shalt go to the poor man's.' They both
> were well and content, and did so, and found such ease and rest in their
> lodging, that they resolved never to remove, for the spider built and was
> not troubled, the Gout he was entertained with a soft cushion, with down
> pillows, with dainty caudles, and delicate broths. In brief, he did like it so
> well, that ever since he takes up his lodging with rich men, where I desire
> that he should take his rest, rather than in my poor house.[53]

With a sting in the tail equally for *Dives* and *Lazarus*, the fable was often
recycled, not least by La Fontaine.[54] Personification of diseases in this
Aesopian manner, endowing them with moral messages, was a common
rhetorical device.[55] Humanists liked to suck sermons out of sickness, and
maladies formed a school of virtue.[56]

Petrarch (1304–74) had pioneered the genre two centuries earlier. In a
letter written around 1338 from his retreat at Vaucluse he had offered his own
rendition of the fable of the spider and the gout, drawing the uplifting
conclusion that while the poor had to stomach certain nuisances – such as
creepy-crawlies – their simple way of life protected them from the terrible
retribution of the gout.[57] In a series of moral letters to a gouty friend,
Colonna, he praised the disease for the opportunities it furnished for moral
edification:[58]

> you will see that like the bridle for the untamed horse a gout was required
> for you. Perhaps it ought to be required for me too so that I might now

learn to stay in one place and settle down. Without doubt, however, it was required for you more than anyone else I know. You would, if you could, have gone beyond the boundaries of the inhabited world; you would have crossed the ocean; you would have gone to the antipodes, and your reason would not have helped you seek a halt though it is powerful in other matters. What more need I say? You were able to stay still only with the help of the gout.[59]

In his *De remediis*, written 1357–60, Petrarch further moralized gout. In that series of dialogues, 'Sorrow' complained of being 'tortured by repulsive gout', made 'unfit' and weakened: 'I cannot stand on my feet.'[60] 'Reason' provided the moral corrective, explaining that it was to be expected that old age brought an 'army of diseases'; but years also brought wisdom: gout encouraged one to be ruled by one's head not one's feet. Not least 'this disease afflicts mostly the rich', providing the perfect inducement to 'declare war not only on the pleasures of Bacchus but of Venus'.[61] In short, 'Reason' counselled that one's shield lay in temperance.[62] The best persuasive to continence, gout was a fate against which the courageous Christian philosopher should fortify himself by strengthening the mind: 'even when you are lying down, your mind can stand up straight'; health of mind and soul paved the way for philosophic meditation, which was of far greater value than the frivolities to which gout mercifully put a stop.[63]

The Petrarchan prescription for extracting philosophy from podagra was pursued by the prince of Humanist scholars, Erasmus. In 1511 his *Encomium Moriae* (Praise of Folly) launched that brilliant genre of Humanist writing, the mock encomium. Tracts in that mould tootled facetious praise for the subject being satirized, the principal 'heroes' of encomia being wicked men, loathsome creatures (lice, for example), various sins and vices, and disease. Among the vices the most popular was drunkenness and, of the maladies, gout – subjects intimately interlinked.[64]

Throughout his life, Erasmus suffered poor health and hypochondriacal tendencies, fretting about ruining his constitution by his dedication to learning, while reading extensively in the medical writings of Antiquity. 'I can see also that my own health is frail,' he wailed as early as 1506, before his first bout of renal colic, 'and has been further weakened to a considerable degree by my laborious studies.'[65] Twenty years later he explained his kidney stones:

I surmise that I know the cause of the illness. For more than twenty years I have been in the habit of standing when I do my writing and hardly ever sit down . . . As it is inevitable that the stomach of one who writes standing is somewhat bent, I surmise that the stomach has begun to remove half-digested food because the gastric juices had been led somewhere else and that is the cause that the stone does not keep enlarging.[66]

In 1522 his friend and fellow Humanist Willibald Pirckheimer, whom we also discuss in Chapter 12 in the context of the visual heritage, after suffering gouty attacks for about a decade published his homage to the *Encomium Moriae: Apologia seu Podagra Laus* (In Praise of Gout).[67] Pirckheimer obliquely alluded to the *Praise of Folly* in the Introduction.[68] In her opening declamation, the maiden Podagra asked: 'For how can there proceed any right judgment when Folly captivates Wisdom, Rashness rules Reason, Impotence of mind cashiers counsel?'[69]

Pirckheimer had earlier written that 'The doctors claim that my excessive studying is the cause of my ailment . . . However, for what does one live when one may not study?'[70] The pair of Humanists thus both experienced wry satisfaction in having acquired the gout, considering it a testament to unstinted scholarly labours. Erasmus voiced their joint feelings to his comrade. 'In agony which usually is unbearable,' he wrote:

> because this tyrant with its cruel retinue moves from the loins through the haunches to the region of the spleen, from there it goes with the intention of breaking through into the bladder, tearing, twisting and throwing everything along the way into disorder; how used to violence are princes who delight more in being feared than in being loved.[71]

Shortly afterwards, in May 1525, Erasmus published an edition of St John Chrysostom's *De Sacerdotio*. Its preface included a brief 'Encomium to the Gout and the Stone',[72] involving an expansion of the letter written to Pirckheimer two months earlier. It expounded a philosophy splicing Stoicism with Christianity, and praising the 'glory' of disease.[73]

Launched by Petrarch and refined by Erasmus and Pirckheimer, the Renaissance gout eulogy continued with Geronimo Cardano's *Podagrae Encomium*. 'What a man gout makes! devout, morally pure, temperate, circumspect, wakeful,' he commented: 'No one is so mindful of God as the man who is in the clutches of the pains of gout. He who suffers gout cannot forget that he is mortal, because it affects him in every part of his being.'[74] The genre reached its elaborate apogee in *Ritterorden des podagrischen Fluss* (Order of the Gouty Humour), an allegorical poem composed by Georg Fleissner in 1594.[75] Further editions in 1596, 1600 and 1611 attest its popularity. Nothing is known about its author, except the information on the title page which indicates he was a captain from Schönberg living in Schlackenwerth, both towns near Carlsbad.

Prefaced by an epigram stating that 'the strong must pay for their frivolity with hardship and must suffer great pain and be martyred for many years', Fleissner's encomium involved elaborate parodies operating upon several assumptions. Podagra was herself noble; those upon whom she bestowed her favours were thereby ennobled; by rendering her devotees sick, Podagra did them a huge favour, by preventing folly and crime and affording leisure for reflection.

Purportedly written by the Order Of Knights of the Gouty Humour, the encomium claimed to tell of the 'delicate maiden and goddess PODAGRA's origin, birth, name, appearance, manner, upbringing, education, position, her playmates and servants, companions, amusement and principal pleasure'. Many aspired to social distinction – but typically they failed![76] 'No one thinks much of such nobility,' the reader is told, hence effort was wasted in pursuit of gold and glory. But not so with gout:

> because the gouty are noble not in pretense but in deed. They do not chase after nobility, nor purchase it for money, but are soon raised to the nobility and gentry by their feet and hands. They then do not presume that there may be a respite from Podagra but realize that she is a noble, delicate maiden, born of the gods, who will not be so forgetful as to have relations with a coarse peasant man.[77]

Who, in any case, would want to be healthy? Good health was hopelessly plebeian, and a sure recipe for disaster: 'Someone who lives in health is not master of his body even though he be of good means, but is unceasingly plagued with others' business. He is almost a serf.'[78]

By contrast, what brought true dignity and distinction was disease and, among diseases, the princess was Podagra. Gout conferred the ultimate aristocratic luxury, ease:

> When friends presently appeal to him for aid, he can counter with the excuse that he really cannot move, because Podagra with a cramp has already challenged him to another fight, or has already attacked him, so that he cannot stand on his feet . . . Now please tell me whether such a person is not without doubt in control of his body – is he not a mighty lord over it? Oh, Podagra, you are justly praised for all time![79]

Podagra did not merely confer ease. She also inspired religious faith and other nobler virtues:

> Podagra also encourages piety at all times: no one is more devout, moderate, or chaste than the gouty because they are always wide awake in bed and are not likely to sleep without prayer. They think much more about the hour of death than healthy people do.[80]

These were not the only pronouncements. Later encomia followed in the footsteps of these familiar twists of didactic irony, typically praising gout on two grounds. It afforded proof of social superiority, while compelling a life of ease preserving the victim from vices and temptation. Cutting the persiflage, the moral message was that gout was a consequence of venery, gluttony and drunkenness, and folks were victims of their own folly. Fools, folly, vice, pleasure: the very stuff of the Menippean tradition of Lucian, as we shall see over and again in the evolution of gout and its representations.

A late instance of this 'Fools' Literature' is *Podagra* by Gottfried Rogg (1669–1742) of Augsburg, Bavaria, a publisher and engraver. An elaborate copperplate engraving, it has some of the features of the modern comic strip.[81] Presenting an apology for the ravages caused by gout, Podagra is praised for her twenty virtues in a text now so uncommonly found that we cite the virtues in their entirety:

1. *The Podagra is a fashionable ailment.* Because he who is burdened by it does not run around all over town with other ambitious persons, but remains elegantly at home.

2. *It takes care of itself all alone.* Since it does not especially care about foreign things, having enough to do by itself.

3. *It is humble.* Because it attaches itself to the patient's feet.

4. *Wakeful.* Because it permits little rest or sleep.

5. *Moderate.* Because the patient is repelled by almost all foods.

6. *Temperate.* Because such a patient often drinks water rather than wine.

7. *Obedient.* In that one in this condition lets himself be greased, have incense burned, and have the feet bandaged.

8. *Taciturn.* One sighs more than one reads, while all conversation becomes annoying.

9. *It is patient.* Because whether such a patient may sit, lie, or stand, it is a constant effort for him.

10. *Prudent.* As long as one avoids or discards all that from which it originates.

11. *Pious.* It teaches the person to pray and to direct his thoughts toward heaven.

12. *Shaming.* When it develops in a patient, he attempts, as much as possible, to conceal his illness and to masquerade under the name of another misfortune.

13. *It helps the person to the greatest virtue.* Because it stimulates him to abide by the commandments of heaven as much as possible, and finally brings him so far that he can derive a steady comfort from their possession.

14. *Chaste.* Since it does not even like to be touched.

15. *It enriches the person in temporal and eternal values.* In that it restrains him from many sins, it deters him from all feasts, toasts, dances, immoderate lovemaking, and so forth, whereby the structure of the human body becomes virtually shattered and decrepit, wherefore the healthy days of life are then frequently shortened by a great many disorders.

16. *It is devout.* Since it creates devout people, teaches them to live piously, and also brings about certain cessation of sin.

17. *It is faithful.* Because it seldom leaves its patient entirely.

18. *It is wise.* Since, in tormenting the person, it teaches him to know himself and to move others to sympathy.

19. *It is loving.* Because it attracts the evil vapors unto itself, consumes the humours, cleanses the body including the head, and thus brings about quite a different disposition in the person, and so proves its faithful services.

20. *It finally is also majestic.* One lies in bed like a king on his throne, one goes to meet no one, one arises for no one, one accompanies no one, and one finally visits no one, even when one has been visited.[82]

Taking all score of such benefits into consideration, only one conclusion was possible: celebration of the blessed malady.[83]

CHAPTER 4

Science and Sydenham

Not all was celebratory in that early self-fashioning: there were *agonizing* sufferers, female as well as male, even if their gout diagnosis may not have been classified as 'gout' later. The prolific Countess of Warwick, Mary Rich (1625–78), for example, left a detailed narrative of her spiritual and corporeal life, tied for most of it to a most pathetically 'gouty husband'. She was born into the star-studded Boyle family, children of the Earl of Cork, and her brother Robert became the world-famous Oxford and London chemist. Mary was 'born-again' by converting to a radical Puritan sect after her marriage at fifteen to the Earl of Warwick, suffered the hazards of chronic illness of every type (spleen, convulsion, hysteria, ague, dropsy) and endured wrenching bereavement throughout her life.

Her own illnesses were bagatelles compared to other dire calamities in her aristocratic household in Essex. First her only daughter died, then her only son, leaving the Warwicks without heirs. She tried to conceive but could not. Their physician, a 'Dr Wright' who also harboured mystical bents, treated both wife and husband but was unable to improve their bodily conditions. Even this barrenness, however, was trivial compared to milord's crippling gout, which lingered for almost twenty years and wore out the Countess to the point of mental derangement. The Warwicks may not have been gouty for generations in the way the Harleys were, but milord's exhausting gout nevertheless turned him irritable, so that he forbade anyone to touch or speak to him.

Mary's pathetic account speaks for the whole seventeenth century. Its audience was her generation itself, the very late Humanism that introduced gout to society and provided it with its calling card. Her main theme was that something had to give if the malady were to progress from its current miseries. This chapter will examine gout against the backdrop of the profound transformations science and medicine were undergoing in the early modern era. How far did understandings of the malady change in the light of alterations in basic perceptions of Nature and natural knowledge? The question requires a brief glance at the so-called Scientific Revolution and its impact on medicine.

The sixteenth and seventeenth centuries have been widely regarded as bringing about a Scientific Revolution, distinguished by the 'new science' of Copernicus, Kepler and Galileo, Bacon and Descartes, Hooke and Boyle, Newton, Huygens and Leibniz, and marked by the founding of scientific institutions like the Royal Society and the Académie Royale des Sciences.[1] The 'age of exploration' also transformed anatomy and what would later be called physiology and biology. Vesalius' *De humani corporis fabrica* (1543) lent impetus to anatomy, which could be represented as the foundation and pinnacle of medical science,[2] and its immense prestige promoted reorientation of the study of the body and its disorders. The holistic view of health and disease was challenged by a new emphasis on bodily mechanisms, which came to fruition in Harvey's studies of the circulation of the blood.[3]

Harvey's revolutionary work was not universally accepted, and he supposedly complained that his medical practice 'fell off mightily' after the publication of *De motu cordis*. Nevertheless, his inspiration spurred and guided further physiological inquiry and a clutch of younger English researchers continued his work on the heart, lungs and respiration.[4] One was Thomas Willis, one of the founder-members of the Royal Society (1662), whose principal work was on brain anatomy. The most brilliant of the English Harveians, however, was Richard Lower, whose *De corde* recognized the heart as a muscular pump.

Physicians met natural philosophers at such venues as the Royal Society and exchanged ideas and techniques. Many believed there was all to gain from making their doctrines more 'scientific'. A new aid was the microscope, whose value for understanding living things was demonstrated by the Dutchman Antoni van Leeuwenhoek.[5] Another lay in the startling contemporary shifts in the physical sciences. The corpuscular and mechanical philosophy promoted by Descartes and others presented the machine as the model for the body, proposing a hydraulic understanding of its vessels and tubes, and denouncing the old humoral theories as empty words.

The mechanical philosophy stimulated new research programmes. In Italy, Marcello Malpighi (1628–94) conducted microscopic studies of the structures of the liver, skin, lungs, spleen, glands and brain. The Pisan Giovanni Borelli and other iatrophysicists (doctors convinced that physics offered the key to the body) studied muscle behaviour, respiration, gland secretions, heart action and neural responses.[6] Giorgio Baglivi represented the culmination of this iatrophysical programme, yet he was aware of the predicament facing pioneers of scientific medicine: their vaunted scientific theories seemed to yield almost nothing that led to effective therapeutics. The relations between research and remedies remained ambivalent.[7]

Another innovative attempt to analyse the body in scientific terms lay in iatrochemistry. Repudiating the humours, certain investigators looked back to the chemical theories of the iconoclast Paracelsus. His Netherlands follower Johannes (Joan) Baptiste van Helmont[8] rejected his notion of a single archeus (or in-dwelling spirit), developing instead the idea that each organ has its own regulating *blas* (spirit). Spiritual chemistry was the key to life and to medicine. Views like these were radical – Gui Patin, leader of the ultra-orthodox medical faculty in Paris, denounced van Helmont as a 'mad Flemish scoundrel'.[9] Franz de le Boë (Franciscus Sylvius), a Harveian who taught at Leiden, disparaged van Helmont's ideas as occult, seeking to replace his gases and ferments with models of bodily process combining chemical analysis with circulation theory.[10] By the late seventeenth century, in other words, Vesalian anatomy and Harveian physiology had created the dream of a scientific understanding of the human body to match the newly prestigious mechanics and mathematics. But did new teachings in anatomy and physiology have any impact on practical medicine?

A particular volume announced in its title *The Medical Revolution of the Seventeenth Century*.[11] But one of the editors insists that, at the bedside, continuity was more characteristic than change. For most practical physicians, humoral models remained paramount, as did the traditional therapeutics of evacuation and dietary regulation.[12] With respect to gout, the latter reading – the stress on continuity – makes most sense.

Continuing a trend developing ever since the invention of printing, the century brought a vast output of medical compendia, mostly pouring old learning into new bottles.[13] Some were aimed at physicians, others at lay readers, like John Archer's *Every Man His Own Doctor* (1671).[14] Our sampling of such standard medical compendia suggests that, despite the 'new science', gout generally continued to be popularly understood in a conventional humoral manner. It was seen as the dropping of a humour upon a joint, accounted for in terms of a dyscrasia (disorder) in the system, possibly provoked by an external cause, such as a fall, jolt or psychological shock. Therapeutics continued to stress prevention (moderation), gentle evacuations, repose and the application of bandages and poultices. Medicines popular since Antiquity were still recommended. William Salmon, for instance, that prolific Stuart medical hack, prescribed Mithridatium for gout – as well as for plague, cancer, 'Sciaticas, Quartans, and other diseases from cold and melancholy humours'.[15]

One of the most ambitious compendia appeared in 1655 under the pseudonym 'Philiatros', purporting to contain 1,720 'Receipts fitted for the cure of all sorts of Infirmities whether Internal or External, Acute or Chronical that are incident to the body of Man'.[16] 'Philiatros' offered gout cures respectively attributed to a Mr Peacock and a Mr John Cornwallis, as well as five or six treatments by unnamed contributors.[17] Of the latter, one, designated the best, contained black soap and the yolks of raw eggs bound to the afflicted part by a plaster of eggwhite and flour.[18] It also offered 'Dr. Stevens' cure for gout', made up of his famous 'water', plus sheep's suet, boar's grease, wax and 'neet's foot oyle'. A prescription contributed by a lay person contained sheep's suet and wax.[19] Among such compendia, gout was quite prominent alongside the stone, dropsy, plague, sciatica and other aches and pains.[20]

Treatments seem to have been fairly empirical, as is borne out by the practice of John Symcotts, a Bedfordshire practitioner, himself a sufferer. In 1653 his brother, a London merchant, wrote to suggest that the physician try the treatment by which he had previously cured himself; this consisted of a paste made from yeast, eggwhite and alum, spread on brown paper and bound round the foot.[21]

Nor is there much sign that the advance guard of seventeenth-century scientists possessed particularly novel views about gout and its treatment. Both Francis Bacon and William Harvey may have been sufferers. 'His infirmitie is given out to be the goute,' it was noted in 1617 of Bacon, 'and the greatest harme or sense he hath of it is in his heele, and sometime he takes pleasure to flout and play with his disease, which he says hath chaunged the old covetous course and is become ambitious, for never beggar had the goute but he.' Whatever his disorder – the heel is unlikely as a site of acute gout – Bacon had his own ideas as to its treatment: a poultice, then a bath or fomentation, and finally a plaster.[22]

William Harvey was also a sufferer, according to John Aubrey, but there is no evidence that his innovative thinking on the heart carried over into his views on gout.[23] He had several patients with joint conditions. Sir John Bramston the younger was treated with purging and sweating, though whether his arthritic condition was gout is debatable; Bramston remained symptom-free for fifteen years, when he again experienced arthritis which 'rann over every joint of my bodie, even my neck'.[24] The same treatment as before was given, but his condition worsened. 'My joints were so benumbed and enfeebled that I could not for a longe time after goe without leadinge, nor could I open or shutt one hand without the help of the other, so that many thought I should be a criple duringe the remainder of my life.'[25] Some friends advised him to go to Bath for treatment, others demurred; so 'I went to Dr Harvey, then newly come from Oxford, and askt his opinion.' Harvey told him to avoid strong drink and to eat sparingly, only once a day. This advice was evidently unwelcome – 'I left him,' Bramston continued,

and went to Sir William Palmer and Mr Coppin, with my brother Robert Addy, unto the Fleece in Cornewell [Cornhill]; who inquiring what Dr Harvey sayd, I told them and Mr Coppin replyed, Dr Harvey hath starved himselfe these twentie years, neither eating nor drinking, but as he hath directed you and yet he hath the gout. To which I returned, if to fast and have gout be all one with eat and have the gout I will doe as I have done. And from that time to this present I have never had any touch of it until this Christmas.[26]

It is clear from this anecdote that Harvey was thought to be a sufferer, but the evidence remains equivocal. He was neither obese nor a wine drinker, nor was there any record of his father or brothers having any arthritic complaint. Neither Harvey nor anyone else described his symptoms. The credulous Aubrey, however, reports Harvey's self-treatment. 'He was much and often troubled with the gowte,' recorded the gossip, 'and his way of cure was thus: he would sitt with his legges bare, if it were frost, on the leads of cockaine-house, putt them into a payle of water till he was almost dead with colde and betake himselfe to his stove, and so 'twas gonne.'[27] It appears that at Harvey's country retreat at Combe in Surrey grottoes were built so that he could retire to a cool place.

Robert Boyle, one of the leading advocates of the mechanical philosophy, was fascinated by the relations between illness and the self. He canvassed the possibility of curing the acute gout attack psychologically, by means of fright, adducing the tale of a villager whose hands and feet had been immobilized with cheesy poultices of the sort mentioned by Cogan and others. 'A sow, finding the door open and attracted by the smell of the poultice, came to devour it, whereupon the man was put into such a fright that his pains decreased that very day . . . and never returned.'[28]

One of Boyle's contemporaries penned the first English treatise on the gout: Dr Benjamin Welles, a Fellow of All Souls who retired, on account of melancholy, to practise near Greenwich. His *Treatise of the Gout, or Joint Evil* (1669) was dedicated to 'My Arthritic patients – who now walk stoutly supported by my Art, as much as by their own leggs.'[29]

Clinical experience was extensively recorded and traded among physicians and the educated public. Every doctor, patient and tittle-tattler had his own tales of causes, crises, cures. One window on to this copious gout lore – endlessly diverse, deeply contradictory – is afforded through the clinical notebooks of John Locke. Not just England's leading empiricist philosopher and friend to the scientific elite, Locke was medically trained and an active amateur physician. It might have been supposed that his jottings and memoranda would have given signals of radical outlooks and teachings on the gout, but that is hardly so. He was certainly well aware of the iatrochemical currents deriving, through a complex lineage, from Paracelsus. He referred to, for example, the fact that Peter Stahl, Oxford's first public lecturer in chemistry, had developed a preparation of spirits of salts (hydrochloric acid) highly regarded in treating gout and the stone.[30] And he was aware of the debate over Stahl's chemical salts discussed in the Royal Society's *Philosophical Transactions*. But Locke had a magpie interest in information from all sorts of sources. Travelling through France in 1678, he observed for instance a particular kind of emetic, apparently useful for gout – 'Mr [. . .] who is now alive in Paris, being crippled by gout, was cured by taking this vomit every old moone for three or four years together, and after that twice a yeare so that he is able to walk and dance etc. as a healthy man.'[31] In July of that year,

Locke observed the prevalence of the disorder in Orleans, and recorded that an informant imputed it to 'their wine which is very strong'.[32]

Six months later, he copied down the details of a cure for a gouty hand, involving a tansy poultice.[33] Spirits of hartshorn, he annotated shortly afterwards, would carry off 'a fit of the gout in 24 hrs', continuing: 'In the gout that falls on stomach, breast or head or any of the viscera give Theriac of Andromachus and it cures for it is noe thing but a weaknesse of the bloud to be strengthened and then the viscera skape.'[34] Therapeutics like that evidently came from the learned tradition. But Locke was not averse to picking up suggestions with an altogether more homely air. 'By eating very litle flesh but abundance of hearbs and drinkeing noething but very well defecated beare,' he recorded in March 1679, 'Mr Welsted is eased of the gout and the stone that formerly tormented him.'[35] Another cure was very much in the same vein:

> Rx. a leg of beef put to it [aqua fortis] in [sufficient quantity], garlic [1 lb], bake it very well drinke of the broth every morning. This cured the gout in a woman of 60 years after being 7 years decrepid and not being able to stir. She takes it now spring and fall 6 or 7 days at a time.[36]

That came from a lay person. So did another, this time for a poultice, containing olive oil and wax, supplied by a Mr Amery.[37]

A small number of Locke's directions drew upon new – indeed, even New World – *materia medica*. Mooting ideas that might have come from his close friend Sydenham, he pondered the applicability of one of the seventeenth-century's wonder drugs:

> Gout is a disease of malnutrition, which gradually but slowly accumulates and finally issues in paroxysms like those of the intermittent fevers; the cure therefore seems to be by Peruvian Bark and other medicines which help the digestion and assimilation of the food.[38]

For the most part, however, Locke copied out everyday tips, for instance a report from Vienna that, whereas wine caused gout, milk-drinking would not only remedy the condition but would cause 'the disappearance of the tophus, so long as it has not yet reached the hardness of chalk'.[39] Yet, pondering the jottings of informants, Locke clearly did not believe wine was automatically harmful, noting how 'Gout and gallstones are rare in Schaffhouse', apparently because of the 'healthy red wine' drunk there.[40] Native herbal remedies also fascinated him, for instance a 'blister' derived from 'speare wort', suggested by an anonymous correspondent.[41] Nettles were another folk cure:

> Mond. 9 Dec. Sam Larkeing of Yukel, a Schiper now 75 years old and very lusty of that age having been troubled with the gout above 20 years . . . did

about 3 years since in the heighth of a fit whip the parts then seized by the gout with nettles till they were all inflamed and blisterd upon which he found ease.[42]

Locke was impressed by the stinging-nettle cure, recording that Mr Larkeing repeated the treatment 'again a day or two after when he found any pain remaining'.[43]

Since England's greatest philosopher–physician seems to have shown little interest in what the new science might have told him about cures, it may not be surprising that the key contributions at this time came not from any path-breaking physiological or chemical discovery, but through bedside observations. Distinctions were being made with greater precision between the different kinds of joint disorders. In the sixteenth century, the great French physician Jean Fernel (1497–1558) and Jerome Cardan (1501–76), the fashionable Pavia physician, had independently pursued the idea – which probably had Hippocratic roots – that rheumatism was associated with fever and was distinct from podagra.[44] Cardan had pointed out the associations of rheumatic fever with children. Relapses of rheumatic arthritis, unlike those of podagra, tended to occur only when fever supervened.[45] This important distinction was emphasized by Guillaume de Baillou (1538–1616), whose *Liber de rheumatismo* was posthumously published in 1642. Baillou developed a new connotation of the word rheumatism, moving away from the literal sense (a flowing of body fluid into one part) to suggest acute joint pains, unconnected with gout; and depicted rheumatism invading the whole body 'with pain, swellings and a keen sense of heat'. Unlike rheumatism, gout was a disease of one single joint. 'Now what articular gout is in any limb, exactly so is rheumatism in the whole body, as regards pain, tension, and the "feeling of burning heat" as I call it. The joints are racked with pain,' continued his description of the attack, 'so that neither foot, hand nor finger can be moved without pain and protest . . . the affected parts are found to be very hot. The pain becomes exacerbated at night . . . the arthritic pains are recurrent, and the patient cannot sleep.'[46]

Baillou's clinical acuity was matched a couple of generations later by Thomas Sydenham (1624–89).[47] Sydenham attended Oxford University but his studies were interrupted by the Civil War, in which he fought on the Parliamentary side. Thereafter he set up in medical practice in Westminster. His subsequent path was rarely smooth. He never acquired a large clientele; and his crippling gout was later complicated by renal calculus, for which he took liberal quantities of small beer. These trials made him a religious, if rather severe, man.

Sydenham rejected hypotheses in examining the perceptible phenomena of disease and, following his hero Hippocrates, maintained that Nature worked cures with a few simple remedies. The remote causes of disease were often beyond the physician's art, and he resisted conjecture. Asked what medical books to read, he allegedly answered: *Don Quixote*.[48] Yet he achieved extraordinary fame after his death, his works going through scores of editions. Successors were impressed by his clinical acuity and the insistence upon precise observation that won him the soubriquet of the 'English Hippocrates'.

At the age of thirty Sydenham experienced his first attack. Seven years later, he developed kidney stones and was subsequently rarely out of pain. Soon his career became almost annually interrupted by lengthy attacks, when he found himself 'unable to indulge in any deep train of thought' for fear of their exacerbation. His *Treatise on the Gout* (1683) was not autobiographical, however, but was written at the request of Dr Thomas Short, Master of Gonville and Caius College, Cambridge. Its graphic account of the acute fit has already been quoted in our Introduction.[49] In a typical fit of the 'regular gout',[50] the joints of the foot, especially the toe, were the 'genuine seat of the morbid matter'.[51] In serious cases resulting from 'wrong management or long continuance', he noted, the natural outlet for the disorder became obstructed, and it would migrate to other regions, turning into 'irregular gout'.[52]

By the time he came to write the *Treatise*, Sydenham had long been a sufferer – a point he twisted into an engaging gibe at his own expense: 'there is no doubt but men will conclude either that the nature of the disease, which is my present subject, is in a manner incomprehensible, or that I, who have been afflicted with it for these thirty-four years past, am a person of very slender abilities'.[53] It was also in the light of personal experience that he insisted that gout did not only seize the 'gross and corpulent'.[54]

So what precisely was it? Sydenham set his interpretation in context of the antithesis between two sorts of diseases, acute and chronic.[55] Acute diseases were infections, essentially due to miasmata arising out of the soil, or what he called epidemic constitutions.[56] Infection had little to do with the individual, who was a victim by accident. Chronic diseases, by contrast, were the disorders of the particular ruined constitution.[57] Gout was one such:

> The *gout* generally attacks those aged persons who have spent most part of their lives in ease, voluptuousness, high living, and too free an use of wine and other spirituous liquors, and at length, by reason of the common inability to motion in old age, entirely left off those exercises which young persons commonly use. And, further, such as are liable to this disease have large heads, and are generally of a plethoric, moist, and lax habit of body, and withal of a strong and vigorous constitution, and possessed of the best *stamina vitæ*.[58]

An individual racked by chronic disease would characteristically be suffering from indigestion, that is, the failure of the humours to be digested.[59] Thus in chronic diseases the '*stamina vitæ* are much debilitated', a phenomenon particularly severe in the case of 'aged persons'.[60]

Having established that gout was a disease of 'indigestion',[61] Sydenham addressed the question of treatment. Ease during the acute attack was possible, and for this opium was his favourite medicament, of which he pioneered a liquid tincture, laudanum, which brought him fame. Between attacks he used Jesuits' bark (quinine) as a prophylactic and to strengthen the blood.[62] But he was sceptical about analgesics[63] and there were no 'cures':

> if it be objected, that there are many specific remedies for the *gout*, I freely own I know none, and fear that those who boast of such medicines are no wiser than I am. And, in effect, it is to be regretted that the excellent art of medicine should be so much disgraced by such trifles, with which the credulous are deceived, either through the ignorance or knavery of authors; remedies of this kind being extravagantly extolled in most diseases by such as make a trade of these trifles.[64]

For chronic disorders Sydenham was sceptical about specifics: in maladies so deep and constitutional, a particular 'cure' was unlikely to work:

> it cannot reasonably be imagined that the cure can be accomplished by means of some slight and momentaneous change made in the blood and juices by any kind of medicine or regimen, but the whole constitution is to be altered, and the body to be in a manner framed anew.[65]

He was above all sceptical about any kind of panacea – 'As for a radical cure – this lies, like Truth, *at the bottom of a well.*'[66] He did, however, at least venture the suggestion, perhaps playfully, that such a 'remedy will be found out hereafter'.[67] Was that just a sop – or a quip? It is hard to gauge the tone of that remark, but the notion of a specific hardly accords with the drift of Sydenham's thinking on chronic disease.

In acute attacks, Sydenham deplored the traditional therapeutics of purges and emetics. Such treatments were undesirable for a particular reason.[68] Gout was the salutary endeavour of nature to drive peccant humours to the extremities. But purges and emetics activated the stomach. Hence their effect would be to draw morbific matter back into the viscera, thereby concentrating the disorder in the innards, rather than beneficially expelling it to the periphery. Purges were therefore unwise:[69]

> *emetics or cathartics* will only invite the *gouty* matter back into the blood, which was thrown off by nature upon the extremities; and hence what ought to be thrown upon the joints hurries perhaps to some of the *viscera*, and so endangers the life of the patient, who was quite safe before.[70]

Violent treatments were so dangerous that 'most of those who are supposed to perish of the gout are rather destroyed by wrong management than by the disease itself'.[71] The preferable therapeutic methods were simple, direct and 'expectant', comprising diet, few drugs and an ample fluid intake (like Hippocrates, Sydenham advocated a barleywater which he referred to as his 'diet-drink').

In gout, the correct therapeutic strategy was to strengthen digestion or, in Galenic terms, 'concoction'.[72] Since gout was generally the product of humours that had accumulated because of gluttony, 'digestive' medicines were recommended:

Whatever remedies therefore, assist nature to perform her functions duly, either (1) by strengthening the stomach so that the aliment may be well digested, or (2) the blood that it may sufficiently assimilate the chill received into the mass, or (3) the solids, so as to enable them the better to change the juices designed for their nutrition and growth into their proper substance, and (4) lastly, whatever preserves the secretory vessels and the emunctories in such a state that the excrementitious parts of the whole system may be carried off in due time and order.[73]

These digestive medicines mainly contained bitters: 'for instance, the roots of *angelica* and *elecampane*, the leaves of *wormwood*, the *lesser centory*, *germander*, *ground-pine* and the like, to which may be added such as are called *antiscorbutics*, as the roots of *horse-radish*, the leaves of *garden scurvy-grass*, *water-cresses* and the like'.[74] Such digestives were to be used not only during the fit itself, but 'chiefly in the intervals of the *gout*'.[75] Above all, doubtful of the effectiveness of medicines, Sydenham urged temperate living, to obviate the build-up of undigested humours. Food and drink intake should be moderated[76] and exercise taken.[77] But no less important was a tranquil life free from excess. As with other chronic diseases, it also helped to seek warmth:

And hence likewise we learn why travelling into *southern* countries is so effectual to conquer those diseases, the cure whereof is fruitlessly attempted in a colder climate. The truth of what has been delivered concerning the general cause of *chronic* diseases will be further confirmed by the remarkable and almost incredible relief obtained by riding on horseback in most *chronic* diseases, but especially in *consumption*.[78]

In the absence of a warm climate, the next best things were 'warm herbs'[79] and a quiet and peaceful mind.[80]

Sydenham's teachings were to prove extraordinarily influential. They offered something for everyone, including for physicians a precise clinical profile. They also provided authority for the inability to cure the condition, indeed for the belief that it was probably incurable. His account strengthened the hand of physicians and sufferers convinced that violent remedies exacerbated the gout. Copeman has maintained that Sydenham's therapeutic caution 'resulted in the use of colchicum being banished throughout Europe for the next hundred and fifty years'.[81]

It can be argued that Sydenham did nothing to further understanding of the chemical and physiological dimensions of the disease,[82] but he helped create a persona for the disorder which squared with ancient medical teachings and appealed to the gouty of late Stuart England. Not least he proffered a social profile with which readers could identify:

> But what is a consolation to me, and may be so to other *gouty* persons of small fortunes and slender abilities, is that kings, princes, generals, admirals, philosophers and several other great men have thus lived and died. In short, it may, in a more especial manner, be affirmed of this disease that it destroys more rich than poor persons, and more wise men than fools, which seems to demonstrate the justice and strict impartiality of Providence.[83]

Sydenham accomplished for gout what no other doctor could. Not until the malady could be seen for what it was in the nineteenth century would this paradigm of culture and illness change. During plague, war and famine, it could appear a blessing in disguise. The gout was to prove an insulation no other condition offered. The early members of the Royal Society intuited what this shield of insulation was but could not fathom why it worked as it did. Sir William Petty's circle of early statisticians saw how it functioned to protect and insulate the numbers of the living from those of the dead. As early as 1662, for example, John Graunt wrote in his observations on the London *Bills of Mortality*, that 'the *Gout* stands much at a stay, that is, it answers the general proportion of Burials; there dies not above one of 1,000 of the *Gout*, although I believe that more die *Gouty*. The reason is, because those that have the *Gout*, are said to be long livers; and therefore, when such dye, they are returned as *Aged*.'[84] When only one in a thousand dies, it was inevitable that the 'glory of the gout' would be socially construed as a blessed plaything to divert the fortunate elderly.

This was the view the eighteenth-century upper crust inherited, with Sydenham crowned as gout's arch-hero. Lady Mary Wortley Montagu, that brilliant champion of inoculation, seems to have uttered the last word about the 'English Hippocrates', though generating her effusive *aperçu* within the context of his work on hysteria. This she casually tossed off in her very first 'letter of consolation' to James Steuart, her new friend made while travelling to Turkey and the Levant – an assessment indicating as much about contemporary feminist views of sex and gender as about Sydenham and medicine. *En fin* it may constitute Sydenham's shrewdest epigraph:

Lady Fanny [James's wife] has but a slight touch of this distemper [hysteria]: read Dr Sydenham; you will find the analyse of that and many other diseases, with a candour I never found in any other author. I confess I never had faith in any other physician, living or dead. Mr Locke places him in the same rank with Sir Isaac Newton, and the Italians call him the English Hippocrates. I own I am charmed with his taking off the reproach which you men so saucily throw on our sex, as if we alone were subject to vapours. He clearly proves that your wise honourable spleen is the same disorder and arises from the same cause; but you vile usurpers do not only engross learning, power, and authority to yourselves, but will be our superiors even in constitution of mind, and fancy you are incapable of the woman's weakness of fear and tenderness. Ignorance![85]

Ignorance indeed! If only she had continued the diatribe to genderize Sydenham and gout in the same vein.

CHAPTER 5

The Eighteenth-Century Medical Debates

'How there can be a doubt what the gout is, amazes me!'

Horace Walpole to William Cole, 30 December 1781
W. S. Lewis, ed. (1937–83) 2, 286.

Sydenham was the hero of eighteenth-century British medicine. Admirers shared his scorn for musty books, dead speculation and rationalism, and endorsed his commitment to experience as medicine's royal road to progress. On matters of gout, his name was ritually intoned, not least by those seeking higher justification for their conviction that gout was incurable. Others for their part seized upon his statement – perhaps incautious, perhaps flippant – that a specific might some day be found, claiming the glory of having made that discovery.

Sydenham's followers were everywhere: in England, Europe, on the shores of the Mediterranean. His almost instant influence in documenting and observing 'the glory of the gout' itself forms a chapter in the history of medicine and its theories. When Dr Pierre Desault, the French author in 1738 of a *Dissertation sur la goutte*, a scarce but comprehensive account hailing Sydenham as its hero, claimed that Sydenham's authority was unassailable he was not exaggerating. One eccentric but nevertheless effective follower was Thomas Dover (1660–1742), who briefly studied with the master. A physician turned privateer, Dover first introduced his 'Diaphoretic Compound Ipecacuanha Powder' (Dover's Powder) as a gout remedy, though this long-lived nostrum, containing opium, ipecac, saltpetre, tartar and liquorice, was naturally sovereign against much else besides. His *The Ancient Physician's Legacy to His Country* (1732) praised Sydenham to the skies.[1]

Sydenham lived in the thick of medical movements to which he was indifferent: iatromathematics and iatrophysics. Fuelled initially by the Cartesians, in England these movements drew renewed inspiration from Boyle, Hooke and Newton. Long before David Hume aspired to be the 'Newton of the moral sciences', many wished to be the Newton of medicine.[2]

The 'new philosophy' changed the parlance and, to some degree, the practice of medicine. Its devotees ridiculed humoral theory as archaic and chimerical. Critics, however, scorned its innovations as but old wine in new bottles. And although this 'new medicine' made an intellectual splash, in practice, faced with crotchety patients, it was easier to rely on soothing old saws familiar to physician, patient and public alike. Indeed, such a course was imperative in the trying world of bedside practice. Needing to earn his living in a lucrative but cut-throat medical market-place, the prudent physician might find occasion to blind his patients with science, but he also had to be able to chat with them, exchanging commonplaces they found plausible and palatable, and all the more so as this was the age when gout was growing more conspicuous among the Quality.[3]

There had been distinguished sufferers in the past, from Florentine princes to Miltonic poets.[4] But in the eighteenth century gout seems to have risen to almost epidemic proportions. This may, of course, partly be an optical illusion, the product of ampler survival of evidence; it might also be a diagnostic artefact, with physicians finding or framing gout in various shapes and forms, to mask their ignorance or milk an eligible diagnosis – rather as with 'hysteria' in the nineteenth century.[5]

The 'gout wave' also suggests that affluence and leisure in the 'first con-sumer society' were exposing more of the population to the protein-rich diets and indulgent habits that provoke the onset of gout.[6] Highly significant was the Methuen Treaty with Portugal (1703), which resulted in the flooding of Britain with port and other fortified wines. As correspondence and cartoons testify, contemporaries had no doubts about the connections between gout and the bottle. 'Mr Hyde, Rr of Wavenden died this Morning,' noted the antiquarian William Cole on 29 September 1767: 'he was a very gross Man & full of Humours, which he had acquired by a very free Life formerly with Mr Selby & his Set, & since by Indolence & free eating & drinking, which filled him with Gout & ill Humours. He had been formerly of Balliol College.'[7]

Moreover the use of lead in casks for such beverages, and the pervasive adulteration of alcohol with lead-based additives, brought on the cholicky symptoms frequently diagnosed as 'visceral' or 'irregular' gout.[8] The role of lead in biliousness was early elucidated by Thomas Cadwalader's *An Essay on the West-India Dry-Gripes* (1745). This New Jersey physician rejected the traditional opinion that the torturing Poitou colic (*colica pictonum*) was due to the acid residues of citrus fruits.[9] Noting the similarity between the dry-gripes and lead colic, he regarded the dry-gripes deriving from rum punch as similar to that arising from the fumes of white lead.

The eminent English physician George Baker substantiated these specula-tions, concluding that lead in cider was the cause of the Devonshire colic. Though he said nothing, however, of gout as a delayed consequence of lead ingestion,[10] the first statement incriminating lead in gout came from one of his staunchest supporters, James Hardy.[11] Rebutting Baker's Devon critics, Hardy maintained that 'gout originates from the action of mineral substances, especially those conveyed into the human system by the medium of adulterated wines'.[12] Hardy was a minor figure and no one paid much attention to his views, but suspicion was clearly growing that alcohol and lead-poisoning were involved in the spread of gout.

Whatever the reasons, gout became a high-profile condition. Physicians began to specialize in the field, treatises proliferated,[13] popular health manuals devoted many column-inches to the disorder,[14] quack remedies were fanfared,[15] and gout became a pet topic of pump-room conversation in Bath and other spas.[16] Certain beliefs acquired almost universal currency.[17] In medical circles, gout had established itself as a clinical condition quite distinctive from other troubles of the joints. Its unique features chimed with social rankings – 'gout is the distemper of a gentleman', insisted Lord Chesterfield, 'whereas the rheumatism is the distemper of a hackney coachman'.[18] Though still sometimes anatomically subdistinguished – as podagra (foot gout), gonagra (knee gout) and chiagra (wrist gout) – such terms grew rarer, as gout (or frequently *the* gout) became the habitual word. Bedside physicians and patients alike customarily spoke of it in terms of a 'dropping' – gout would 'fall upon' a joint; and all agreed that gout could flow, almost at will, around the body. Alongside regular gout – the gout that pinched joints – Georgian medicine made much of irregular gout. Also known by such terms as 'visceral', 'metastatic', 'anomalous' or 'repelled', the irregular kind was gout which, failing to be standardly fixed in the extremities, rebounded to the 'vitals' – head, brain, liver, heart – where it was judged far more menacing. A further type was 'flying gout', where the pain flitted apparently at random around the body. 'Gout flying about me today I think,' recorded Parson Woodforde.[19]

By old-guard and avant-garde physicians alike, gout was read within disease theories premising the unitary nature of health and sickness. All bodily processes should ideally conspire to create health in the individual. The constitution was in good shape if sensible living (respecting diet, exercise, sleep and the other 'lifestyle' features denoted by the 'non-naturals') produced heartiness.[20] Various factors might from time to time bring on sickness. These would include external threats – epidemic fevers, miasmata, weather changes or physical injury[21] – and bodily neglect or self-induced threats to the system, like gross inebriation; while internal imbalances and poisons would express themselves as peccant humours or as surplus bile or catarrh.

The precise sickness outcome would depend upon constitution and attendant circumstances. Fevers might take possession in divers forms – as smallpox, measles and so on, depending upon the individual. A resilient constitution would throw off the disease and restore humoral balance, and its tone would soon reassert itself. In a less robust individual (one with a 'broken' constitution, due to poor inheritance, repeated illnesses or self-destructive habits) such restorative processes might be frustrated, with untoward consequences, for disorders otherwise mild would gather into something far graver, or a passing distemper might have enduring repercussions. It was, for instance, widely maintained that gonorrhoea, if neglected or badly treated, could gravitate into chronic disorders, among them gout.[22]

Underpinning such assumptions lay the idea of a class of 'wasting' conditions, ominous to constitutions and, unless treated, likely to prove lethal: scurvy, scrofula, cancers, marasmus, consumption (tuberculosis) and other such 'cachexiae'.[23] Gideon Harvey designated scurvy the 'disease of London' and consumption the '*morbus anglicus*',[24] and Benjamin Marten pronounced there was 'no Country in the World more Productive of Consumptions than this our Island'.[25] Such wasting ailments were collectively known as the 'consumptions' – though, while including tuberculosis, they were far from confined to it. They were largely attributed to excess,[26] resulting in what Thomas Willis called the 'withering away of the whole body'.[27]

Leading writers like Christopher Bennet, Gideon Harvey and Benjamin Marten were at one with Sydenham in pointing an accusing finger at 'indigestion' of the humours resulting from over-indulgence. In his monumental *Treatise of Consumptions* (1694), Richard Morton ascribed wasting distempers to 'too plentiful and unseasonable gorging of meat and drink . . . not easy to be digested'.[28] This brought on violent purging, diarrhoeas and defluxions,[29] and 'dropsies' might result.[30] Above all, by impeding digestive processes, gastric overload created 'erroneous fermentation', thereby filling 'the blood with Corruption', rendering it 'sharp' and 'incorrigible',[31] and leading to a 'morbid disposition'.[32] In broken constitutions such inflammatory fermentations would provoke ulcers, pulmonary tubercles, schirrosities and cancers; in healthier ones, a salutary attack of gout would hopefully be the outcome.

A comprehensive account of the 'atrophia' (wasting condition) of the constitution was provided by Richard Morton (1637–98). A clergyman ejected from the Church of England following the 1662 Act of Uniformity, Morton tried a second career in medicine, rising to become physician-in-ordinary to William III. *Phthisiologia: Or A Treatise of Consumptions* (1694) was his *magnum opus*.[33] This espoused concepts of atrophia and phthisis derived from Celsus' account of tabes (wasting or consumption).[34] Celsus had distinguished three forms. In the first, the body failed to be properly nourished because nothing was absorbed from the food, and nutrient matter was simply excreted from the body, extreme emaciation being the consequence. Without treatment, atrophia was fatal. The second kind of tabes the Greeks called *cachexia*: so bad was the patient's condition that all foods tended to putrefy. *Cachexia* was predominantly observed in patients already exhausted by a chronic disease. The third form of tabes, called by Celsus *phthisis*, was the most dangerous. It started in the head, proceeding to afflict the lungs, causing fever, bloody phlegms, vomiting of pus and frequent coughs. This was presumably our tuberculosis.

Erected upon these Celsian foundations, Morton's account of bodily decline helps explain notions of goutiness in the context of ideas of 'wasting' that included diseases to us as varied as cancer, jaundice and gout. Using 'consumption' in its literal meaning – a wasting of the body, whatever the cause – Morton acknowledged two basic types: 'original' and 'symptomatical'. An original consumption arose 'purely from a Morbid Disposition of the Blood, or Animal Spirits' – that is, it was not the effect of any preceding disease; the latter, like Celsus' *cachexia*, depended upon some antecedent. Of the bilious diseases – that is, disorders of undigested humours – gout was rated among the preferable manifestations, because, though a malady, it nonetheless attested basic soundness of constitution.

Gout was read as symptomatic of a distempered bodily state. Its outcome would depend upon the encounter between the threat and the constitution, which, like a citadel, would possess a basic soundness but also present targets. 'There is in every Constitution a Propensity or natural Tendency to one Disease more than another,' explained John Cheshire's *A Treatise upon the Rheumatism* (1723):

> and this seems to proceed from the weak Structure of the Fabrick, not equally fortified in every Part from the Inconveniencies, which Man, from the Nature of his Existence, is continually exposed to . . . Thus when any Thing that is offensive to Nature is conveyed into the Blood, it takes Possession, like an artful Enemy, of the weakest Part.[35]

Given this model, it was widely assumed, following Sydenham, that gout was not one of those diseases for which a radical cure should be expected. For one thing, that seemed completely contrary to experience. This gout doctors knew only too well, for, like Sydenham, many who specialized in gout were themselves sufferers: John Cheshire, George Cheyne, William Stukeley, John Hill and others besides.[36] Their evident failure to heal themselves lent their texts a poignant authority. He had applied himself, wrote Cheshire, '*during my Confinement under the last Fit of the Gout, in the Intervals from Pain*'.[37] 'BILIOUS Diseases', opined John Andree, 'are among the most common of the chronic distempers of the inhabitants of England . . . During twelve years, I had too much reason to lament the imperfect state of this part of medical knowledge, having been nearly so long subject to a bilious disorder.'[38]

Experience thus dictated caution about cures, but, as hinted, the idea of incurability in any case had theoretical sanction. For it was believed that gout was not a destructive invasion or a mere breakdown but an integral, protective systematic response: a kind of overflow pipe, Nature's means of evacuating poisons. In a gouty constitution, an attack, though painful, was functional: would not then the idea of seeking to be cured of a beneficial process be downright absurd? Regular physicians gibed at the shallowness of quacks who, too stupid to comprehend the utility of gout, absurdly affected to eliminate it by applications of caustics, hot sand, cold fermentations, ointments, counter-irritants or the knife.[39] It became the creed of regulars that cure was not on the cards. Had not Sydenham deemed that 'a radical cure' lay 'like Truth, *at the bottom of a well*'?[40] Hence, 'in all Chronical Cases', contended Timotheus Bennet, 'neither the Assistance of Medicines, nor Diet, nor Exercise, nor any thing else, can be suppos'd to produce a momentary or sudden Change'. And this was because of the difference between acute and chronic diseases:

> Acute Diseases generally proceed from some sudden Alteration or Attack, and the Effects are quick and violent; Death or Recovery quickly ensues; the strongest and healthiest Constitution is no Guard; the Case is quite different in the GOUT and other chronical Disorder, whether proceeding from the Abuse of the Nonnaturals, or any other Cause, the change brought upon the Constitution is by Steps, slow and gradual.[41]

Hence, it was insisted, often on Sydenham's say-so, that utmost therapeutic discretion was essential. On the very title page of his *A Full and Plain Account of the Gout* (1768), Ferdinando Warner censured 'the Folly, or the Baseness of all Pretenders to the cure of it'.[42] The very idea was ridiculous. 'Art is here too often vainly employ'd to give a new Constitution, and a new Life,' scoffed Timotheus Bennet, dismissing visionary charlatans who promised all and performed naught.[43]

The conventional wisdom on gout, countered one nostrum-monger, was that '*it is better to leave it in Possession of the Body*'.[44] Empirics exposed this denial of curability as self-serving and proof of the regulars' shameful incompetence: parasitic courtly physicians had a vested interest in chronic sickness and in graciously permitting the *beau monde* to continue to indulge. In his *A Treatise on the Gout* (1778), Abraham Buzaglo alleged that none of the regulars had 'yet, been able to discover a radical Cure'.[45] 'After Years of Study', he snarled, '. . . *Flannel, Patience*, and *Sleeping Draughts*, are the only Relief that the Ingenuity of the Faculty has been able to produce.'[46] Physicians fatuously rationalized their failure to cure by spinning the line that gout was all for the best ('*no Disorder whatever will affect them while they labour under the gouty Fit*').[47] What balderdash! 'If the Patient were to allow himself a Moment's Reflection, he would perceive that this Doctrine is big with Destruction to Society . . . Who can refrain from Astonishment, when he sees a Patient so blindly led!'[48] A pretty paradox indeed, wherein the incurability of a disorder was not merely an article of faith for the profession but was represented as a good thing – yet it was a notion, as will be shown in the next chapter, which might also offer solace to sufferers.[49] Those who swore gout was curable were the quacks and some Young Turk physicians who were stirring things up.

The late seventeenth century brought certain attempts to explain gout in the light of the 'new philosophy'.[50] Though without practical consequence at the time, a signal development lay in the first application of the microscope.

Despite his lack of formal scientific training, the Dutchman Antoni van Leeuwenhoek (1632–1723) became a dazzling microscopist.[51] Using a small single-lens instrument, he was one of the first to observe blood capillaries, red blood cells, protozoa, bacteria and spermatozoa. On 11 July 1679, he wrote to Lambert van Velthuysen, regarding the contents of a gouty tophus. 'In your previous letter,' he recounted,

> you asked me to examine the chalk which gouty persons have on their joints or which will break out. Now, although I am familiar with many people suffering severely from gout, the joints of whose fingers are very thick, I never observed a perforation. Consequently I always thought that I could not discover anything worth noting in the chalky matter, imagining that the chalk would consist only of globules.[52]

But then he had a breakthrough that permitted him to make use of his new lenses: he had hit upon the ideal experimental subject, a gouty relative.[53] Leeuwenhoek then delivered an account of his kinsman's illness – the gruesome details go some way to explaining why it was that gout commanded such fascinated attention:

> I asked this gentleman if it had ever happened to him that the chalk came out of his joints; he told me that some time ago the chalk in the heel of his foot, in which there was a large hole, came out in such a quantity that he formed almost a new heel, and that there was also a hole in his arm on his elbow from which the chalk had come during quite six months on end, but not so much by far, nor so thick as from his heel. I asked him to let me have some of the chalk, which he willingly granted me.[54]

Viewing this 'chalky' matter under the lens, the investigator was in for a huge surprise:

> First of all I observed the solid matter which to our eyes resembles chalk, and saw to my great astonishment that I was mistaken in my opinion, for it consisted of nothing but long, transparent little particles, many pointed at both ends and about 4 'axes' of the globules in length. I cannot better describe than by supposing that we saw without naked eye pieces from a horse-tail cut to a length of one sixth of an inch. In a quantity of matter of the thousands of these long figures, mixed with a small quantity of fluid.[55]

Leeuwenhoek had discovered that the matter of the gouty tophus was crystalline in nature. He wrote up his findings, sending them in the form of a letter to the Secretary of the Royal Society, it being published as a paper in the *Philosophical Transactions* in 1685.[56] Over the next couple of centuries, the extraordinary significance of the crystals found in the gouty tophus would eventually become plain. But Leeuwenhoek's microscopic investigations fell into neglect in his own day, and no gout doctor made use of his observations of the gouty crystals. It was through other routes that the new science was to modify the framing of gout.

The most influential of the early Georgian gout doctors was the Scotsman George Cheyne (1671–1743).[57] A follower of the iatromathematician Archibald Pitcairne,[58] Cheyne became, like his mentor, a champion of Newtonian medicine. In 1702, he came to London to establish himself in medical practice, turning in the process into a *bon viveur*. Much of his medical career was passed in Bath, where he attended the Quality while attempting to recruit his own health, ravaged by gluttony, obesity and anxiety.[59] Addressing high-life disorders in an age of pleasure, Cheyne's writings achieved exceptional popularity, speaking directly to sufferers' fears, while blazoning the new scientific theories. Not least, he wittily upbraided the vices of the rich and devised therapeutic regimes with an accent on purified lifestyle. His *An Essay on Health and Long Life* (1724) went through eight editions in ten years, thanks to its plain-speaking recommendations,[60] while *The English Malady; or, A Treatise of Nervous Diseases* (1733) launched the conceit that the English were not just predestined but *privileged* to suffer from 'nervous' ailments.[61] His work on gout achieved equal renown: first published in 1720, *Observations Concerning the Nature and Method of Treating the Gout* enjoyed four editions in its first two years, and eight subsequent editions.[62]

Himself a sufferer, Cheyne's *Observations Concerning . . . Gout* adumbrated a mechanistic theory of the malady that focused on the vascular system. In a gouty person, Cheyne explained in iatrophysical fashion, the arterioles of the extremities were too constricted to permit the blood to pass from the arteries to the veins. Stagnation followed, excess tartrates precipitated out, and tophi developed.[63] Preoccupied with the biliousness of Bath invalids, Cheyne also gave his attention to 'irregular gout' as manifested in headache and abdominal pain. Gout of that sort involved migration of the morbific substance from the vascular to the nervous system:

> The *Nervous* or Flying *Gout* (both which I take to be the same, and to differ from the Windy *Gout*, which is nothing but a *Hypochondriacal* or *Hysterical* Symptom) is owing to the Weakness, Softness, or Relaxation of the *Nerves* of those Persons who labour under it.[64]

What were the underlying causes of those vessel and fibre weaknesses that manifested themselves as gout? The same forces were at work as precipitated the nervous disorders – above all, excess.[65]

Yet while flaying sufferers, Cheyne flattered them too. It was only the elite, he explained in *The English Malady*, whose nervous systems were sufficiently refined to be susceptible to nervous complaints; those in whom surfeit assumed a gouty form were hale and hearty sorts. There was more than a grain of truth in 'the common Observation, that Gouty Persons are People of good Natural Parts, large Feeders, and long-liv'd'.[66] This was because in such beefy specimens 'Strong Health requires liberal Supplies'.[67]

Acquired gout was thus not unpropitious in prognosis, for it was 'produc'd in a Person, otherwise sound, from Ignorance or Negligence of the exact Rules of living'. But it could also be hereditary, a 'Taint (compounded perhaps of Scurvy, Stone and Pox) transmitted to the Patient with the Principles of Life'.[68] That too, however, was no bad diagnosis, since heredi-tary gout ran in good families.

Cheyne outlined various therapeutic strategies. The best plan in irregular gout was to drive the ailment outwards: blistering the ankles might draw ill humours to the feet. Gouty stomach was most perilous; it should be treated with laxatives containing compound spirit of lavender and tincture of hiera picra, snakewood and diambra – 'this may bring on the piles', he confessed, 'but it will discharge the gout of the guts'.[69] As with all violent headaches, he treated gouty head pains by bleeding from an arm vein, or by blistering between the shoulders or cupping the back.

Addressing regimen, Cheyne believed that since the infirmity befell those with thickened blood vessels, exercise and heat would be useful to widen their bore. Purgatives and reduced food intake would relieve the body of 'glewy' substances. Deploring modern luxury, he dictated strict regimen: less meat, and a preference for milk and macrobiotics.

And, attesting his youthful passion for the new science, Cheyne also believed regular gout could be dealt with by metallic medicines:

> THE *Gout*, being also a violent *Inflammation*, first on the *Joints*, and then over the whole Habit, (shifting from Part to Part, till at last it fixes on the *Bowels*, and internal Parts) as much as an *Erysipelas*, or the *Rose*; is never to be greatly lessened, much less *eradicated*, or extirpated, but by *Mercurials* . . .[70]

Mercury purges were sovereign for breaking up gouty concretions – a preference he expressed in the picturesque idiom that won a loyal readership for his books: 'If an *Angel* should propose any other Method, or Medicin, as Nature is now constituted, he ought not to be minded.'[71] With the evan-gelical fervour symptomatic of his intense, if unorthodox, personal piety, Cheyne urged 'total Abstinence from all fermented Liquors, except, perhaps, clear unhopt Small-beer', recommending instead a 'Diet-drink', including 'Guaiac Wood, Juniper berries, Seville Oranges and Honey', used together with gentle laxatives. Even so, he reasserted, '*Quicksilver* and its milder Preparations . . . judiciously manag'd, I truly account the *Elixir Vitae*, in this, and most *chronical* Distempers'.[72]

Overall, Cheyne conveyed mixed messages not easily reconciled – different readers doubtless plucked out what suited them best. Prefiguring William Cadogan,[73] he lent his authority to the reading of gout as a disease of civilization, the bitter fruit of luxury; yet he also stressed, contrary to Cadogan, its hereditary nature, perhaps in deference to his Quality patients. He commended lifestyle changes while also pinning his faith upon violent purgative medicines. Tensions surface in Cheyne between a humoral and holistic concept of gout as Nature's purge – 'disease as remedy' – and a vision of it, derived from the new philosophy, as a mechanical blockage in need of removal: a plumbing problem, so to speak.

Cheyne's contemporary Sir Richard Blackmore (d. 1729) was favoured by William III, developed a considerable London practice, hobnobbed with the great, wrote lofty (if leaden) poetry, and achieved fame with a book on gout, which attracted readers more for its rhetoric than its research. *Discourses on the Gout, a Rheumatism, and the King's Evil* (1726) opened with a dropsical preface assaulting Antiquity and anticomania. In the 'battle of the books', Blackmore fought on the side of the Moderns.[74]

Rather like Cheyne, Blackmore saw the diseases of the day by double vision. They were in some measure symptomatic of overheated imaginations in a hothouse society, and it was the physician's job to bring sufferers and society back to earth. Looking back to the recently abandoned practice of touching for the King's Evil – which, as a supporter of William III, he associated with Popish and benighted Divine Right doctrines – he concluded that its 'cures' were entirely wrought by 'imagination'. This disposed him to be fascinated by the role played in gout by fancy, as both a cause and cure: 'Fright can cause and cure an attack.'[75] Hence gout was a mark of a fevered personality in a disturbed society.

Yet Blackmore also wrote as a champion of the mechanical philosophy: gout arose, he explained, 'from viscous coagulated Salts or cretaceous impurities, caught and entangled in the Ligaments or Glands of the Joints'.[76] While stressing gout's localized symptom profile, he still adhered to the 'physiological' tenet which regarded the distempers of individuals as variants upon general morbid processes.[77] He also likened gout and scrofula, both producing similar symptoms, *viz.* 'Knots and Tumours' – just a few of the 'many odd and surprizing Kernels and Swellings' whose true significance would be plain 'to the experienced Practicer'.[78] Like Sydenham and Morton, Blackmore thus subscribed to the notion that internal disorders were due to undigested humours.

This naturally led him to ponder the status of gout: defect, disease or deliverance? With the *vis medicatrix naturae* in mind,[79] Blackmore was not convinced it deserved 'the Appelation of a Disease', since it seemed a physiological drainage process; yet he was never one for euphemistic flannel, and he repeatedly dramatized its severity, presenting it as a 'Tyrant' that 'lays up his Racks and Tortures'.[80]

Blackmore's text resonates with ambiguity in a further respect, in its characterization of the diseases of high society. Like others, he deemed gout an inheritance of the propertied. Yet he had no mind to indulge in the pantomime of pandering to gouty grandees. 'The Seeds of this Evil are frequently derived from the Parents,' he ventured, going on to describe it as a rampaging tyrant, maiming and crippling.[81] Blackmore also played upon the ludic conceit of gout as a jester, debunking patrician pretence. It fell at, or rather upon, the feet of the great, but in so doing it marked them out for censure. He milked the moral that 'the Great, the Rich, and the most Easy in their Circumstances . . . are . . . reduced to an Equality with the Husbandman, Labourer and industrious Mechanick'.[82] Gout was thus a great leveller, and Blackmore seized every opportunity to reprove elite profligacy: gout 'is not bred in prisons and workhouses, nor engendered in the galley or the mine . . . it is the dissolute and voluptuous indulgence of the sensual appetites' of the wealthy.[83]

The touchstone of that maxim lay in the guts or, to be precise, in the entrenched philosophy of 'digestion'.[84] If gout's pathogenesis lay in failure of digestion, did not this prove the malady was the progeny of 'Immoderate and luxurious Eating'?[85] Debauchery did not merely cause temporary nauseousness but shook the pillars of the constitution:

> When by a long Series of Paroxysms a great Quantity of hard Concretions have from Time to Time been excluded from the Blood and cast off upon the Joints, the cretaceous Matter gradually increasing to a greater Bulk by the Accumulation of new Particles . . . And then we may behold these sad Spectacles, Quarries of chalky Minerals, the Repositories and Hoards where the Tyrant lays up his Racks and Tortures, while it prolongs in a lingering Course the Patient's Sufferings, and manages with frugal Cruelty a dying Life.[86]

The malady grew progressively crippling; but – such was life's comedy – the elderly finally gained pyrrhic relief, thanks to having scarce life enough left to be sick.[87] Such attenuation of pain in the aged was, however, no true remission; and finally even 'the soundest and most athletick Constitution . . . so often stretched on the Rack and crying out in Agonies of Torture' would at last be 'sunk and demolished'.[88] As a devotee of the mechanical philosophy, Blackmore drew attention to the structural damage gout ultimately wreaked upon the body machine: 'It is no Wonder . . . all the fine nervous Cords and animal Threads should become slack and flaccid, and by this Means lose . . . their Spring of Vibration and Power of Self-Restitution.'[89] Indeed the decaying body machine was akin to a disintegrating kingdom, whose government could no longer shoulder its burdens. Finally 'the Spirits themselves, the great Ministers of Digestion', would 'fall at length to Decay and Poverty':

For now every Part of her administration being in Disorder and Confusion, her Government must be unhinged and at length dissolved, since the Blood abounding with Gouty Matter, and its active Principles grown too feeble to separate and expell it, as formerly in their more vigorous State, it makes to the Stomach, the Guts, the Chest, and at length to the Head, the principal Fortresses and Securities of Life, whence it is soon driven out, and quits its Tenement, batter'd and beaten into a Heap of Ruins.[90]

The mechanical philosophy thus led Blackmore to train his imagination on the tangible and local devastation wrought by gout upon the body machine as a theatre of war.

Though upholding traditional morality linking gout and gluttony, there was one key aspect of Hippocratic teachings from which Blackmore dissented – an expression, surely, of his iconoclasm towards Antiquity. He denied that gout was a consequence of *sexual* excess. Exonerating Venus, Blackmore enjoyed parading as an enlightened figure:

I am not unapprised that immoderate Venery is likewise reckon'd another antecedent Cause of this Distemper. But I imagine this has happened through the Inadvertency or Inconsideration of the first Writers on this Subject, and the too obsequious, if not servile Respect paid them by their Successors.[91]

Orthodox, however, in other respects, Blackmore scouted the prospects of radical cure: the mere fact of its commonly being hereditary was almost proof positive that gout was incurable.[92] Yet the physician was not superfluous. His responsibility was not cure but care, and for that he put faith in opiates, 'the patient's chief anchor which enables him to ride out the gouty storm'.[93] In non-hereditary cases, priority must go to prevention. Like Cheyne, Blackmore believed that those most vulnerable were men with 'hail and athletick Constitutions'. They must pursue 'Abstinence . . . in Eating, Temperance in Drinking strong Liquors, and proper Exercise', all of which together were 'great Preservatives against the Invasion of this Evil'.[94] Moderation was the only mitigation.[95]

Possibly crossing swords with Cheyne, who on occasions had advocated alcohol-free living, Blackmore believed wine useful for gouty patients, since 'it aids the concoctive Faculty of the Stomach'.[96] But he hardly pandered to the grandees. Gout might be the escutcheon of the great, but Blackmore portrayed it as a 'cruel-to-be-kind' providential blow, designed to summon the superior to their duties. The physician was a minister of divine justice, rather as, wearing Apollo's mask as poet, he depicted Nature as rewarding virtue, punishing evil and fulfilling the ends of God.[97] Both affliction and admonition, gout was an affirmation of a divine moral order in which the rich would inherit everything, diseases included: it was a spectacle both awesome and repulsive, designed to instil fear and teach stern lessons.[98]

Alcohol represented the most vexing, if ambiguous, of substances in these medical debates. Cheyne and Blackmore permitted wine in modest amounts and of certain types, even distinguishing among colours of wine and nationalities; others decried wine altogether. The ancient British tradition extolling wine and spirits counted for much in these controversies over therapy and possible cure, especially among the upper classes. Class and rank determined preferences for drink, especially within the pervasive mythology then that men drank socially, women medicinally. Contradictions lay everywhere in these positions and prescriptions. Spirits were deemed pernicious, but small amounts of beer permissible. Among the British physicians poking their toes into these controversial waters, one of the most intriguing was William Stukeley. A man of many parts, he was trained as a physician and later ordained, though perhaps best known today as an antiquarian with hobbyhorsical theories about the Ancient Britons, advanced in *Stonehenge, A Temple Restor'd to the British Druids* (1740).[99] In regard to gout too, he fulfilled many different roles.

Stukeley suffered his first attack in 1709.[100] The son of a sufferer, the twenty-two-year-old sensed an ancestral title to the affliction. Initially attacks lasted a week or so, with remissions of up to two years, but they grew more frequent and cruel, especially once (delicious irony) he started dining with his physician, Dr Richard Mead, with whom he 'drank nothing but French wine, so that I was every winter laid up with the gout'.[101] 'After some vellications & preludes the Gout seiz'd upon my right foot in the bones of the Tarsus' – thus opens a graphic description of an attack in 1723, well worth quoting for the apparently indiscriminate therapeutic bombardments:

> I let blood & found it very much inflam'd, & laid a Caustic upon the part, drinking much water & sugar & juice of lemon, fasting, & taking aloes every day. I made a crucial incision & caus'd an issue where the Caustic was laid . . . When I arose in the morning I found a slight touch as a prelude of the Gout in my great Toe of the left foot where it had been most frequently. But at night it went off, Fryday night or rather Saturday following, tho' I went very well to bed. When I gott up I order'd xvi oz. of blood to be taken away & took a good handsome dose of aloes lota as I had done the day before. I likewise order'd a Caustic to be laid upon the part but it prov'd not strong enough.[102]

Stukeley suffered from classic 'articular gout'; but he was convinced it was also a mobile ailment – almost what post-modernists might call a floating signifier – sneaking around the body, attacking weak points more or less at will.[103]

In his thirties, he was assailed at least once a year. While combing the menu of medicines, he put more trust in regimen, moderating his food and alcohol intake and drinking water or milk copiously to aid digestion, particularly during paroxysms. 'I continued to drink water every day,' he noted in April 1724, towards the end of another six-week seizure, 'by small quantitys at a time in morning, noon, after dinner, & night, which kept the gout off.'[104] Observing his urine was concentrated during an attack, it was obviously essential to take ample fluids. And because 'arthritics are slow of making water', it made sense to select foodstuffs with diuretic properties, notably 'turneps, carrots, parsnips, etc.'.[105]

Stukeley heeded the non-naturals – those beneficent angels of clean air, pure water, dependable exercise and sleep – in time-honoured Hippocratic tradition. It was necessary 'to be particularly careful in diet at spring & fall, when the blood & juices take a new turn',[106] but in truth it was winters that worried him, since that was the time of taking cold, blocking the essential 'insensible perspiration' which purged the system of peccant humours. In January 1765, when the Archbishop of Canterbury, the Lord Chancellor, the Duke of Bedford and William Pitt were all laid up with gout as well as himself, he blamed 'severe cold eastern winds, rainy & moist weather succeeding [which] produce the gout epidemically'. By inhibiting perspiration, cold caused ominous build-ups in the gouty toxin which consequently flowed into the joints – or, if repelled, into the belly, breast or brain. To eliminate the gouty matter, he recommended 'oilsocks, diaphoretic medicines, emetics and purges'.[107]

Stukeley thus evolved a regimen upon which he congratulated himself in old age. After all, though a sufferer for over fifty years, he never developed tophi or arthritis, and on his seventy-fifth birthday he could crow, 'I have all my senses perfect & the use of my limbs, in so surprising degree: considering, an hereditary gout began with me at 16 . . . This extraordinary effect is owing to my own management, counter to the notion of all physicians.'[108]

Stukeley must have been referring to the fact that, alongside moderation, his treatment hinged upon use of a specific, Dr Rogers' 'Oleum Arthriticum'. Providence, he mused, had led him to Stamford in Lincolnshire, where one of his parishioners, John Rogers, an apothecary, had for years been crippled by gout. In 1729 Rogers had begun applying oils to the affected joints, which seemed to curtail the attacks.[109] After suffering for much of that year, Stukeley decided, on 11 December 1732, to treat himself with Dr Rogers' oils, 'with success, the first time'. Soon he was writing to Sir Hans Sloane, President of the Royal Society, reporting on this miracle. His letter, 'About the Cure of the Gout, By Oyls externally apply'd', was read before the Royal Society on 1 February 1733, and published that year.[110]

Stukeley's explanation of the efficacy of the gout oils involved some theoretical finessing. After all, nostrums were quackish; Sydenham had warned lest external medicines precipitate repulsed gout; and Stukeley accepted that articular gout had certain benefits – 'relieving the whole by punishing a part'.[111] Hence directly to oppose Nature 'is generally dangerous'. How was Nature to be helped?

Stukeley returned to the iatrophysical writings of Clopton Havers, whose *Osteologia Nova* (1691) had given the first anatomical description of minute bone structure. Havers proposed that the synovial fluid was a mixture of mucilage and an oily matter, its primary function being joint lubrication.[112] Rheumatism and gout were caused by the action of morbific acid humours on the mucilage, producing coagulation and thus preventing lubrication. Building on this concept, Stukeley suggested that the oily substance worked to neutralize the gouty humour. The 'fiery drop' of the gout, he believed, was extinguished in the oil glands causing inflammation, rather as a hot iron bar plunged in oil sets it on fire.[113] If gout were thus a mechanical problem of deficient *internal* lubrication, what better than to treat an attack by *external* application of oils?[114]

Following Stukeley's report to the Royal Society, Rogers issued a statement about the Oleum Arthriticum including instructions for its use; oils (only 7s 6d a bottle) could be bought at his Stamford house or his son's shop in the corner of Chancery Lane. He had not, of course, intended to market the nostrum, but had had his arm twisted by Stukeley, who further publicized it by reprinting his letter to Sloane in a larger work, *Of the Gout* (1734), which proved popular: in 1735, there was a second edition, and it was pirated in Dublin.[115]

Of the Gout opened with pious references to the Bible – '*Let him dip his foot in oil. Thy shoes shall be iron and brass; and as thy days, so shall thy strength be.* Deut. xxxiii.24, 25' – and also to Hippocrates, who 'says well, that the human body is *pervium & perspirabilequid* [sic] somewhat sieve-like'.[116] This pleasantry referred to the body's vulnerability to cold and rain.[117]

An obstinate disease, gout had induced medical fatalism, yet 'many other distempers are but crises; and they admit of medicine'.[118] Physicians could not be exonerated so easily. It was their duty to cure – or rather to aid Nature in making gout 'truly salutary, as doubtless she designs it'.[119] Stukeley would not shirk his responsibility:

> Hence I cannot excuse my self from endeavouring to serve the publick; in notifying after this manner, what I have hitherto observed, in a remedy invented by Dr. *Rogers* of *Stamford* . . . 'Tis a warm oily composition, which he prepared, to anoint the part affected with the gout . . . But since then, it has been try'd, an infinite number of times, as appears by inumerable letters.[120]

Fearing sounding like a quack, Stukeley announced that he took great pleasure in 'being an instrument of benefiting mankind!'[121] He explained gout in terms of the physical and chemical theories fashionable at the time, citing

Musgrave's views on salts.[122] Gout was thus an attempt of Nature to heal, as Walter Harris had earlier observed.[123] Stukeley praised Harris's understanding of the matter,[124] and, following his friend Richard Mead, judged gout a swelling due to poison.[125] With gouty persons, 'our unhappy life is but a continual struggle of nature to drive off that poison from the first vital principle, and fight it as long as it is able':

> I doubt not but the poisonous drop of the gout is similar to that of a venomous bite, as Dr. *Mead* observ'd it upon a microscope glass; a parcel of small salts nimbly floating in a liquor and striking out into crystals of incredible tenuity and sharpness, he calls them *spicula* and darts.[126]

Given these clear 'facts', Stukeley thought that the traditional paraphernalia could be dispensed with – 'all the formidable *apparatus* of bed-cradles, chairs, couches and *automata*, shoes of cloth, cutt or laced, gloves, stockings of various dimensions, sticks and crutches, springs and wheels, and a thousand contrivances of machinery for ease, motion and carriage'.[127] In promoting his radical remedy, Stukeley was not ashamed to adduce testimonials, rather like the quacks.[128] He grew closely involved in marketing the oils; and after Rogers, who died in 1739, bequeathed the recipe to his daughter, Stukeley began to prepare the oils himself. They probably made him rich. In 1743 he acknowledged his gratitude to Rogers by laying a plaque in his garden at Stamford.

Secret remedies, of course, smacked of the charlatan. But Stukeley was far from the only prominent Georgian physician – others included Richard Mead and John Radcliffe – who went in for such practices. Stukeley, in any case, never claimed that the oils would work total and permanent cure, and perhaps for that reason in later life he extended his interest in regimen, arguing in a neo-Hippocratic manner for moderation as a preventive measure. Disapproving of Cheyne's strict vegetarian regimen, considering it would lead to 'a life scarce vital, a languishing, insipid, & unsocial state', his advice was to eat meats, but well cooked and in small amounts, together with vegetables.[129] Like Cheyne, he valued milk as a 'fine, smooth, oleaginous, animal liquor', which 'subdues the acid, corrosive ferments in the stomach'. Apart from small beer, alcohol was to be avoided. Moderate exercise and regular hours were 'absolutely necessary'. While this regimen was hindering the malady, acute attacks were to be treated with the oils.[130]

By 1760, however, Stukeley was accentuating prevention rather than cure, saying that remedy 'must be chiefly left to Natures solution'.[131] He tried to get William Pitt (Lord Chatham) to follow his favoured regimens but the politician followed his own physician, Dr Anthony Addington.[132] Despite these rebuffs, Stukeley was convinced that the nature of gout 'is what I plainly discover'd & publishd to the world above 20 years ago'.[133] Blaming physicians for discouraging curative attempts, Stukeley grew disillusioned with the whole medical palaver: 'bolus's, pills, diet drinks, emetics, purges & the whole pharmacopoea is administerd to little purpose: they touch not the cause, they only depress'.[134] Consideration of the gouty constitution persuaded him that the disease was not radically curable ('a tendency wil ever remain'); it was possible, however, to fortify the constitution by a moderate diet, exercise and temperance.[135]

Overall, Stukeley is an enigma, though one characteristic of his times, and one who in turn inspired another of the greatest paradoxes of the age, the 'will of the wisp' as he was known by his contemporaries, 'Sir' John Hill, that mid-Georgian jack-of-all-trades: actor, poet, playwright, journalist, novelist, apothecary, doctor and man of science.[136]

Like Stukeley, Hill's father Theophilus had graduated in medicine at Cambridge and later taken Holy Orders. He lived in nearby Peterborough and Stukeley often visited him. John, his youngest son, born around 1714, rebelled and left home when young. When Stukeley returned to London in 1748, he became close friends with John Hill, acting as a go-between in 1750 when Hill was banned from the Royal Society. Stukeley published some pieces in Hill's *British Magazine*.

As Hill suffered miserably from gout, Stukeley presumably advised him about regimen. Perhaps as a result, in his book *The Management of the Gout* (1758), Hill stressed exercise, regular sleep and moderation: 'Temperance and a quiet mind are the two great articles.'[137] Often published pseudonymously, Hill's medical works were regarded as puffs for his natural remedies. 'George Crine, MD' was said to be the author of the first five editions of *The Management of the Gout*, in which a chapter was devoted to his pet cure, the burdock root. The book was favourably reviewed and Hill's name finally appeared as the author of the sixth edition (1758).[138]

In *The Management of the Gout* Hill developed the argument that it was 'idle to reason about the gout; since we confess we do not understand it: but it may be useful to others to know how I have softened the agony of the fits; improved the health of intervals; and perhaps prolonged them'.[139] Hill under-lined the cultural reasons for its spread – it was 'an offspring of luxury' – and noted the limited value of medicine.[140] The supposition that medicine would cure was based on a fallacy. Eminent physicians had been 'disgraced', Hill insisted, because their 'absolute' cures had proved worthless – Cheyne, for instance, 'lost credit by believing SULPHUR would cure the gout'. Only a huckster would suggest that a specific was round the corner;[141] the most that could be expected of a 'remedy' was that it would 'blunt the sting'.[142] Regimen, however, would answer the needs of the gouty, for if 'luxury and indulgence be its parents; abstemiousness and exercise will prove a remedy'.[143]

Gout was thus a paradox: as terrifying as 'hereditary madness',[144] yet the endowment of the strongest constitutions – a fact that, ironically, rendered onset all the more likely, for 'as the persons most liable to the gout are the ingenious, active, and rich, their natural course of life contributes also to bring it on: they feed high, and give loose to their passions'.[145] And that in itself involved further irony: the attack (the 'punishment') was also a 'relief', for 'a fit of the gout terminates symptoms which threaten something worse; and the head and stomach are cleared by it, instantly, after long oppressions'.[146] Nevertheless, despite hereditary indisposition, what actually triggered gout among the great was gross gluttony.[147] Hence, even more boldly than Cheyne, Hill advocated return to natural, simple ways of living, commending to the rich the healthier lifestyles perforce led by their inferiors.

In one significant respect Hill sided with the Moderns against the Ancients. Medicine's founding fathers had adjudged sexual activity a cause of gout, and 'reckless youth makes a gouty age' had attained almost proverbial status. Like Blackmore, Hill demurred. The bed of love offered valuable exercise: 'As for a moderate commerce with the other sex, far from enfeebling nature, it preserves her in a right state: it was intended in our construction; and is required by our constitution'. Indeed, sexual bans seemed particularly unjust:

> WHY should any suppose the gouty person denied, in moderation, this supreme delight of the human being? of all men nature prompts him to it most; and here it is no false stimulation: the construction of the body, which makes him liable to the gout, gives him also peculiar strength . . .[148]

★

This sampling of prominent writings from the first two-thirds of the eighteenth century suggests that gout was becoming a more conspicuous problem. The responses advanced shared common ground but reveal differences of emphasis. The last third of the century to some degree turned chaos into confrontation. This was largely (as will be argued in Chapter 7) due to the work of William Cadogan, whose provocative *A Dissertation on the Gout* (1771) concentrated minds. But it is worth briefly noting here that the sharpening of debate also followed from the fact that medical education, the very grammar of medical thinking, fell largely into the hands of Edinburgh University, whose teachers promoted influential doctrines.

The Edinburgh medical school dates from the appointment in 1726 of the Leiden-trained Alexander Monro (Primus) as professor of anatomy. A high proportion of participants in the British gout debate after 1750 shared a common medical education, having been taught there, above all under the illustrious William Cullen.[149]

Cullen was responsible for particular ideas which had deep implications for gout. For one thing, he developed a system of classification.[150] Cullen's nosology took into account the earlier classifiers. His *Synopsis nosologiae methodicae* (1769) proposed a general classification in which diseases were divided into four main groups: fevers, nervous diseases, local diseases and cachexiae ('diseases resulting from a bad habit of the body'). Among the fevers (pyrexiae), he included joint afflictions: rheumatism, arthrodynia, odnotagia (toothache), podagra and arthdopuosis (joint pain). In the last category, alongside all the rheumatic diseases and their subdivisions, he set articular gout.[151]

Cullen subdivided gout into categories destined to become standard. First there was 'regular' and 'irregular' – that being the 'anomalous' gout of Musgrave, Cheyne and others. The 'irregular' category was then subdivided into the 'atonic', which afflicted the stomach and gastro-intestinal tract; the 'retrocedent', in which joint pain suddenly rebounded to some internal organ; and the 'misplaced', in which the gouty lesion was internal from the beginning. Cullen instanced chronic cases in which the joint pains would often alternate with complaints of the stomach or other organs, what he called 'a sort of reciprocal sympathetic action'.[152]

In alluding to sympathetic action Cullen probably had in mind the work of his colleague Robert Whytt. Whytt was particularly interested in the phenomenon of sympathy (body and mind synergism) and the often mysterious pathways between disease sites and pain experience. Hysteria and hypochondria formed the classic cases, but he was also interested in retrocedent ('repelled' or 'flying') gout.[153]

Whytt and Cullen shared the view that some involvement of the nervous system was essential to gout. In their simplified historical sketches, nineteenth-century physicians often presented Cullen as the theorist who decisively broke with humoralism (with its theory of the 'dropping' of some *materies morbi*) and pioneered the nervous theory of gout. Perhaps they were invoking him as a figurehead or a convenient shorthand; but in the next decades the notion of a 'nervous' component in gout became more widely accepted, thanks to Cullen's influence.[154]

Cullen's follower-turned-rival John Brown proposed, by contrast to this nosological drive, a unitary view of disease.[155] Brown's medical system stemmed from his personal experiences with the disorder. Suffering a severe attack of gout in 1771 at the age of thirty-six, he consulted a leading physician, probably Cullen, who diagnosed a gouty plethora. Instructed to abstain from meat and alcohol, Brown tried a strict diet of vegetables and porridge and claimed to have drunk only water for the next twelve months, yet he apparently suffered worsening bouts. Sceptical about his treatment, he conceived the idea that *debility*, not *plethora*, had been the cause, and that the antiphlogistic regimen was the main source of his suffering. Eager to test this unconventional hypothesis, Brown resumed hearty drinking and eating and was rewarded with six gout-free years.

The apparent 'cure' sowed the seeds of scepticism regarding antiphlogistic methods like low diet, purging and bleeding; and when Brown's gouty attacks eventually resumed, he sought assistance in opium. This in turn led him to mistrust the celebrated healing powers of Nature. Instead of Nature, physicians were called on to heal. Within his framework Brown designated gout as asthenic, recommending treatment with large doses of whisky. The influence of these different but related Scottish approaches will be seen below, particularly in Chapters 7 and 8.[156]

CULTURES

CHAPTER 6

Gout and the Georgian Gentleman

Sir, You have the Gout and Stone, with Sixty thousand Pounds Sterling;
I have the Gout and Stone, not worth one Farthing: I shall pray for you,
and desire you would pay the Bearer Twenty Shillings for Value received
from, Sir, Your humble servant,
  Lazarus Hopeful.
    Cripple-Gate, Aug. 29, 1712

Richard Steele, *The Spectator*, no. 472, 1 September 1712

. . . these symptoms are all too slight to make an illness; but they do not
make perfect health, that is sure.

Thomas Gray to Wharton, 21 August 1755
Toynbee and Whibley (eds.), of *Thomas Gray Correspondence'*, vol. 1, (1935), 433.

Eighteenth-century Britain supported a thriving lay medical culture. Relations between patients and practitioners were sometimes cordial, sometimes
contested and always complex: the sick might be far from patient, and doctors
were targets of suspicion and satire. Clients wielded the power of the purse,
presuming to frame diagnoses for themselves and direct their own treatments,
bolstered by scores of 'kitchen physic' books, instructing how all could be
their own doctor.[1] In such circumstances, gout loomed large not just for
sufferers but in the collective mind, discussed over port or at the tea-table
much as plague and pox peppered the conversations of earlier eras. 'Since the
increase of luxury and the good turnpike roads,' grumbled the Hon. John
Byng, extolling bygone rustic seclusion, 'all gentlemen have the gout . . . it
has been found necessary to fly to the bath, and to sea-bathing for relief'[2] –
a migration of the gentry down the new arterial turnpikes mirroring the
gathering of the gouty toxin itself at the corporeal extremities.

Lay views about gout chimed with the judgments of the bag-wigged
faculty. Everyone knew gout was a sign of superiority, with a penchant for
princes, patricians – and even philosophers.[3] Belief in an affinity between gout
and genius remained so entrenched that as late as 1927 Havelock Ellis was still

asserting in *A Study of the British Genius* that the two were more than randomly linked.[4] More broadly, folklore deemed gout a disease of the better sort, a superiority tax, a celebrity complaint 'fit' (so judged the Revd Edmund Pyle) 'for a man of quality'.[5] 'Gout is the distemper of a gentleman,' insisted Lord Chesterfield, 'whereas the rheumatism is the distemper of a hackney coachman.'[6] It was hereditary, running in good families: 'gout loves ancestors and genealogy', bantered the Revd Sydney Smith, 'it needs five or six generations of gentlemen or noblemen to give it its full vigour'.[7]

That it was a disease of the Quality squared with the perception of gout as a quality disease. The 'gout is good' conceit was most exhaustively expressed in a pseudonymous volume purportedly by 'Philander Misaurus' entitled *The Honour of the Gout* (1720).[8] In a facetious humour, its title page flaunted itself as a '*A Rational Discourse* DEMONSTRATING, That the *GOUT* is one of the greatest Blessings which can befal Mortal Man'. Declaring 'all Gentlemen who are weary of it, are their own Enemies', it accused 'those Practitioners who offer the Cure' as being 'the vainest and most mischievous Cheats in Nature'. Rather than looking to physicians for deliverance, the wise sufferer would count his blessings, and raise up a thanksgiving hymn upon the first visitation:

> Welcome, thou friendly Earnest of Four-score!
> Thou that alone hast got the Sov'reign Pow'r
> T'attend the Rich, unenvy'd by the Poor!
> Thou that dost *Æsculapius* deride,
> And o'er his *Gallipots* in triumph stride![9]

The jesting author exonerated gout from all aspersions that unmindful tormented readers might vent:

> Why, Sir! I am inform'd that your Worship, not having a right Sense of Things, nor the Fear of God before your Eyes, should, to the Disgrace of your own Virtue, give your Tongue the Liberty, in an open *Coffee-house*, to speak ill of the *Gout*. Of the *Gout*, Sir! which, if you look on as a Disease, you ought to welcome as the most useful and necessary Thing that could have happen'd to you. But if you consider as becomes you, then, with me, you must reverence it as a Power Divine.[10]

There was a specious notion among the thoughtless that gout was a diabolical evil.[11] The opinion, however, was vulgar and shallow, to be brushed aside in favour of the fiendish alternative that 'if the Devil ever created any Thing, it was the *Doctor*'.[12] If the physician was thus the sick man's foe, gout, by contrast, was his 'best friend'.[13] Was it not therefore preposterous for any man of sense 'to speak ill of the *Gout*',[14] which had been 'sent in mercy down from Heaven, to lengthen wasting Life'?[15] Not ignominy but honour was due:

'BLESSED *Gout*; most desirable *Gout*; Sovereign Antidote of murdering Maladies; powerful Corrector of Intemperance; deign to visit me with thy purging Fires.'[16] Indeed, despite puritan prejudices, it might be fitting to promote gout as a candidate for beatification.[17]

What was it that made gout such a handsome if unlikely benefactor? For one thing, it gave '*Pain without Danger*', because its sting offered salutary warnings that the body was in a parlous state.[18] Furthermore, as folk wisdom proclaimed, gout kept other diseases from the door. Its inoculative quality formed a further reason why it was folly to contemplate cure; for then, other diseases – *truly* dangerous ones – would rush to fill the gap:

> AND now, Sir, let me tell you a Story; the famous *Willis* shall be my Voucher, who dissected the Body of the Reverend, Learned, and Pious Dr. *Hammond*, kill'd purely by his Friend; who unhappily taught him a Medicine to cure the *Gout*; upon the success of that Medicine, the Doctor's old Nephretick Pains return'd, and in a fortnight dispatch'd him.[19]

A similar anecdote later retailed by Robert Southey shows that such ideas were far from idiosyncratic. Gilbert Sheldon, Archbishop of Canterbury under Charles II, reportedly offered '£1,000 to any person who would "help him to the gout", looking upon it as the only remedy for the distemper in his head, which he feared might in time prove an apoplexy; as in fine it did and killed him'.[20] *Want* of gout could thus prove fatal.

The hereditary sufferer, confided *The Honour of the Gout*, should be regarded as a 'fit Object for the Envy of thinking Men'.[21] It was thus a blunder to consider gout a disease; it was, on the contrary, a cultural crest, a veritable heirloom. The genuine threat to health was the 'cunning, conniving practitioner' who, 'purely to force a Trade, impos'd upon the People, That the *Gout* was a Disease'. And once that perverse conviction was implanted, the self-serving physician would plague his patients 'with real Tortures: All which he was pleas'd to christen by the general Name of the *Therapeutick Method*'.[22]

> FIRST, *Phlebotomy*, then *Catharticks, Emeticks, Hypnoticks*, the – and all . . . And when all is done, I'll give them my Body to practise on . . . if plain Cathartick Gruel, and the Cataplasm of a fresh Cow-Turd, do not work greater Wonders than any Thing they can pretend to.[23]

By forming cabals, sustained by 'hard Names, exotick Cant, and baneful Poyson',[24] physicians had long been able to uphold all this palaver. But happily this was an enlightened age, and things was changing, 'now that it is so plainly discover'd that the *Gout* needs no Remedy; not being in Truth, and proper speaking, a Disease, but a sovereign Antidote'.[25]

The Honour of the Gout reiterated the conventional wisdom that one of gout's great merits lay in furnishing protection against other ailments.[26] It was a specific against lunacy. Hence it was absurd for mad-doctors to treat the insane with '*Purging, Bleeding, Cupping, Fluxing, Vomiting, Clystering, Juleps, Apozems, Powders, Confections, Epithems* and *Cataplasms*'.[27] Nor was this all, for '*Gout preserves its Patients from the great Danger of Fevers.*'[28] Overall, insisted the author, borrowing the terminology of the occult, gout should be welcomed as auspicious: 'The *Gout*, if it be lawful to call it a Disease, is a good and useful Disease, a *White* Devil: The Fever, a bad and hurtful Disease, a *Black* Devil; the Devil of a Disease, or a Disease that is the Devil.'[29] Not least, it was the sterling virtue of gout – though the shallow might not fathom this – that '*It is not to be cur'd*': 'For why, Sir, would you *Cure* (as you call it) the *Gout*, which gives you Pain without Danger?'[30] So how preposterous to suppose that any man of parts 'should wish to be rid of the *Gout*'.[31] But the liberty of this desirable disease was daily menaced (continued the author, lending his lampoon a political slant) by a class of men notoriously without a shred of reverence for English liberties – those vandals, the doctors:

> therefore I would wish all unhealthy People, who have bought their Misery of the *Professors*, and all honest Gentlemen, who are preserv'd by the Salutary *Gout* in the Land of the Living, to prefer a *Bill in Parliament* against this destructive order of Men, that by a strong *Cathartick* Act they may be purg'd out of his Majesty's Dominions.[32]

If the liberties of ancient English families were to be upheld, their gouty inheritance had to be preserved. In short, gout was a 'Noble' condition, safeguarding the highborn from all manner of hazards, above all the physicians.[33]

We need not believe sufferers soaked up the persiflage of *The Honour of the Gout*, except in the gallows-humour spirit sometimes essential to make the frailty of the flesh bearable. But there is much evidence that gout was not treated as any old faceless affliction striking out of the blue; rather sufferers treated it as a familiar preserve, potentially amenable to management.

Mirroring the opinions of physicians, educated sufferers seem to have perceived gout as part and parcel of an extremely labile physiology, change-able as the weather. The body's interior was understood as a scene of ceaseless alteration, in which health was always liable to slip into sickness, which in turn, thanks in part to the restorative powers of Nature, should rectify itself into recovery.[34] Many antecedent events might lead to gout, which itself could trigger other complaints. Like a general marshalling depleted troops or a gambler hedging his bets, the sufferer had a finite range of health options at his disposal, each with its pros and cons: 'By drinking too freely of cooling Liquers in order to dilute my Blod and put off the Gout (which it did effectually),' William Abel revealed to Lord Fermanagh, 'I flung myselfe into a diabetes, much the more dangerous distemper of the two, and I am here at

Bristol for a cure.'[35] Care was needed that the remedy should not prove worse than the disease: no one would willingly have parried an impending attack of gout had the anticipated consequence been 'diabetes', which meant in contemporary parlance a threatening kidney disorder marked by excessive urine discharge.

Gout was viewed in a mixed light. Popular lore taught that it was indeed a kind of punishment, just deserts for topers and gluttons – though the distributive justice of affliction did not always seem very precisely administered. 'A Fit of the Gout!' exploded Lord Herbert to a friend: 'how in the name of God, could the Gout seize hold of your little thin person!'[36] But if gout could be a corrective, it might also be viewed positively – in other words, harking back to Philander Misaurus' parlance, a 'white' disease rather than a 'black' one.

Above all, gout was framed within a natural teleology of healing. It was an 'effort of nature' to cope with indisposition by imparting a specific resolution.[37] Gout was thus a cloud (the system was awry) with a silver lining (it was responding positively). Indeed it might paradoxically be a heartening proof of basic health, a safety-valve assuring future wellness.[38] Gouty omens were thus propitious. 'We have been for some days in much inquietude for the Count de Vergennes,' wrote Thomas Jefferson in 1787. 'He is very seriously ill. Nature seems struggling to decide his disease into a gout. A swelled foot, at present, gives us a hope of this issue.'[39] In contrast to other determinations of morbidity – for instance, diabetes or dropsy – *regular* gout was a reassuring sign, for attacks lasted only a few weeks and did not prove mortal.

Gout was viewed as one of Nature's solutions to depravities of the humours. If not entirely expelled, peccant humours or morbific matter were exiled to far-flung parts. Hence it should be left to do its work. 'He that is subject to it', observed Prebendary Pyle, 'had better bear the fits as nature throws them out, than strive to put her out of her way, which if you do *furca licet, usq. recurret.*'[40] This reading of gout as a prophylactic was deeply entrenched. 'I could heartyly wish instead of a Merry Christmas that you might have a smart fit of ye gout,' Sydenham had advised one of his patients, 'which would quickly dissipate your other fears, and those symptoms which, if I mistake not, doe naturally desire a discharge.'[41] He obviously expected that his unseasonal greetings would make sense to his patient. And shared confidence about gout's sanitive properties reverberated down the century. 'I have so good an opinion of the gout', commented the long-suffering Horace Walpole, 'that when I am told of an infallible cure I laugh the proposal to scorn and declare that I do not desire to be cured ... I believe the gout a remedy and not a disease, and being so no wonder there is no medicine for it.'[42] Gout could be seen as a desideratum, a life insurance not a death sentence. The poet William Cowper congratulated a friend on developing the disorder, 'because it seems to promise us that we shall keep you long'.[43] In short, being gout-ridden was preferable to the chimera of being rid of gout. For, reflected David Hume, 'it is itself a Physician' – though that philosophical sceptic slyly added, 'and of course, sometimes cures and some-time kills'.[44] 'All the World', he affirmed, 'allows that Privilege to the Gout, that it is not to be cur'd.'[45]

The relations between gout and the physicians were expressed through various conceits. As in *The Honour of the Gout*, it could be seen as preferable to the doctors' medicine – or as itself a physician. In Benjamin Franklin's playfully didactic *Dialogue*, 'Gout' reminds 'Franklin' that 'it should not be forgotten that I am your physician . . . your real friend'.[46] Its presence was considered a mascot. 'Mr Piozzi has had no regular fit of the Gout this whole year,' his wife complained in 1806, 'and he begins to feel alarmed at it.'[47]

So long as it was properly managed, gout was a bodyguard, inoculating against worse – a view that drew upon the proverbial wisdom that diseases were mutually jealous and exclusive. While gout was in possession of the body, no truly *deadly* enemy could strike. 'To the Gout my mind is recon-ciled,' Samuel Johnson informed Mrs Thrale, being convinced, partly on his physician's advice, 'that the gout will secure me from every thing paralytick'.[48] 'It prevents other illnesses and prolongs life,' enthused Horace Walpole, 'could I cure the gout, should not I have a fever, a palsy, or an apoplexy?'[49] 'I have a touch of Gout Spring and Fall,' Jeremy Bentham was apprised by a friend, 'which I look upon as highly salutary.'[50]

In these circumstances, the approved response was philosophical phlegm. Best opinion forbade reckless shots at curing. For Matthew Bramble, Smollett's irritable yet benevolent squire in *Humphry Clinker*, as we shall see in the next chapter, it provided the basis for an entire way of life. As gout was thought congenital and recurrent, once an attack began, the judicious sufferer was meant to accept that meddling with Nature was the height of folly. One of the eighteenth-century's most articulate sufferers, Horace Walpole, was firmly of this persuasion.

Walpole experienced his first attack in 1755 at the age of thirty-eight. 'Never was poor invulnerable immortality so soon brought to shame!' he confessed on 16 November. 'Alack! I have had the gout!'[51] From the earliest episodes it appears as though Walpole, a timorous man, had decided to treat gout with proper respect. 'Thank you for all your concern about my gout,' he complimented the same correspondent a couple of months later, 'but I shall not mind you; it shall appear in my stomach before I attempt to keep it out of it by a fortification of wine.'[52]

Gout was to become a regular guest at Strawberry Hill, his gothic mansion outside London. Its visitations were a cruel irony, since Walpole was in fact temperate and thin (by consequence he was in no position even to contem-plate saving himself from further attacks by embracing a sparer lifestyle). It returned in August 1760, and he soon became inured, accepting his fate as gout-ridden and warming to his immobilized invalid state. 'In short, my Lord,' he greeted the Earl of Strafford, 'I have got the gout – yes, the gout in earnest. I was seized on Monday morning, suffered dismally all night, am now wrapped in flannels like the picture of a Morocco ambassador, and am carried to bed by two servants. You see virtue and leanness are no preservatives.'[53] Walpole mused upon the irony of his condition, simultaneously supine and stately; there was paradox too in the fact that, in physique, he was not at all like the conventional sufferer gripped by the 'alderman distemper':

> Come, laugh at once! I am laid up with the gout, am an absolute cripple, am carried up to bed by two men, and could walk to China as soon as cross the room . . . since Tuesday I have not been able to stir, and am wrapped in flannels and swathed like Sir Paul Pliant on his wedding-night . . . Nobody would believe me six years ago when I said I had the gout. They would do leanness and temperance honours to which they have not the least claim.[54]

It struck Walpole, a passionate antiquarian, as paradoxical indeed that he could not in fact lay hereditary claims to gout, since it did not run in the family:

> If either my father or mother had had it, I should not dislike it so much; I am herald enough to approve it if descended genealogically – but it is an absolute upstart in me; and what is more provoking, I had trusted to my great abstinence for keeping me from it.[55]

By 1762, he was confessing to Horace Mann that he feared he had even got 'flying gout'. Though this was dangerous and might have been expected to prompt drastic counter-measures, he was still a model of circumspection:

> I treat it with water and the coldest things I can find, except hartshorn; fifty drops of the latter and three pears are my constant supper, and my best nights are when I adhere to this method. I thought for three weeks I had cured myself, but for these last ten days I have been rather worse than before.[56]

Rarely did Walpole mention seeking the services of a physician. He had evidently decided that a life of temperance would ensure that the foot sieges he would inescapably suffer would never be given the chance to descend into anything worse. 'It is true,' he explained in 1775 to George Montagu, 'I have had a terrible attack of the gout in my stomach, head, and both feet, but have truly never been in danger, any more than one must be in such a situation. My head and stomach are perfectly well; my feet far from it.'[57]

Walpole's philosophy was crystal clear as he engaged in his 'dance' with gout (it proved a 'shocking partner').[58] The perils of gout in the stomach or the head could be obviated by making sure that one fixed it in the foot. With such thoughts in mind, he was pleased to report in the same year to the Countess of Suffolk that 'the gout has been a little in my stomach, much more in my head, but luckily never out of my right foot'.[59] Gout was a kind of health insurance, and, in the manner of a policy premium, its charge, or discharge, had to be renewed every so often: 'The gout, they tell me, is to ensure me a length of years and health, but as I fear I must now and then renew the patent at the original expense, I am not much flattered by so dear an annuity.'[60]

Yet it would be a mistake to simplify his responses. He could use the jokey image of a dancing partner or regard it as a 'harlequin';[61] he could think of it as a preservative; yet he could also represent it in more gloomy terms, as a tyrant, no confederate but an enemy. 'I will impose any severity upon myself, rather than humour the gout and sink into that indulgence with which most people treat it,' he blustered to Horace Mann:

> Bodily liberty is as dear to me as mental, and I would as soon flatter any other tyrant as the gout, my Whiggism extending as much to my health as to my principles, and being as willing to part with life, when I cannot preserve it, as your uncle Algernon when his freedom was at stake.[62]

He certainly suffered. 'I have been extremely ill indeed with the gout all over, in head, stomach, both feet, both wrists, and both shoulders,' he groaned in 1765 to his antiquarian friend, the Revd William Cole. 'I kept my bed a fortnight in the most sultry part of this summer, and for nine weeks could not say I was recovered.'[63] Yet he also felt reasonably confident he knew what was likely to bring it on – notably 'cold' – and how to manage its 'caresses'.[64]

Walpole in fact grew proud of his expertise ('I can talk gout by the hour'). This partly stemmed from the fact that, as he confided to Thomas Gray, gout had become a favourite topic of society conversation, and a kind of sufferers' freemasonry had grown up. In Paris:

> There is not a man or woman here that is not a perfect old nurse, and who does not talk gruel and anatomy with equal fluency and ignorance. One instance shall serve: Madame de Bouzols, Marshal Berwick's daughter, assured me there was nothing so good for the gout, as to preserve the parings of my nails in a bottle close stopped. When I try any illustrious nostrum, I shall give the preference to this.[65]

Judging gout one of the two things he most dreaded – the other was Parliament[66] – he set to devising methods for making himself snug. He developed thick, flannel sleeve-like 'bootikins' within which, mummy-like, he sheathed himself.[67] He used this flannel swaddling both as a prophylactic –

it shielded against the cold that he surmised precipitated attacks – and to aid recovery. The bootikins embodied a logical strategy, since there was nothing to be gained by trying to evade gout altogether – 'if you resist it, it is such a Proteus, that it will slip into the shape of a palsy' – but 'you may take out its sting by the bootikins'.[68]

Walpole was pleased as punch with his invention, singing their praises to his friends. 'Happily the torture did not last above two hours,' he crowed to Henry Conway during one attack in 1774:

> the bootikins demonstrably prevent or extract the sting of it, and I see no reason not to expect to get out in a fortnight more. Surely, if I am laid up but one month in two years, instead of five or six, I have reason to think the bootikins sent from heaven.[69]

They were, however, no panacea; their role was at best auxiliary. 'I had kept off the gout for two months by the bootikins,' he confided to Horace Mann, 'but the mighty has prevailed, vanquished me and my armour, and bound me hand and foot above a fortnight.'[70] Nonetheless the mittens at least mitigated. That they would not *prevent* attacks did not unduly concern him because he believed that gout was a condition that 'prevents everything else' – hence 'would not one have something' that hindered other conditions? Why prevent a preventative?[71] 'The bootikins do not cure the gout,' he conceded, 'but if they defer it, lessen it, shorten it', who would not wear them?[72] Putting on a brave face – 'My gouts, as they never attack my head or stomach, are not alarming'[73] – Walpole remained remarkably enthusiastic about the good done by his whimsical invention:

> It is amazing what the bootikins have done for me by diminishing the mass of gout. I have had no fit for near two years, and the three last were very inconsiderable. As I have worn the bootikins constantly every night ever since my great fit, it is demonstration how serviceable they are to me at least.[74]

Above all, the device had cosseted his gout safely in the extremities, allowing him to boast that though 'I have been so often afflicted with severe fits for these twenty years, I never had it but one half-hour in my head, and never once in my stomach'.[75]

Ageing worsened the disorder,[76] inducing him to apply his quirky gothic aesthetics to his own frame. He was 'mouldering', he confided to the Countess of Upper Ossory in 1779 – he was by then sixty-two – 'like a joist of an old mansion'.[77] Such architectural visions of picturesque corporeal ruins alternated with another conceit, the idea that his body had weathered into a landscape feature. The eruptions of tophi called to mind volcanoes and caverns. 'I cannot write more now,' he apologized to the Revd William

Mason, 'for one of my fingers, which has long been a quarry of chalkstones, and has been and is terribly inflamed with this last fit, has burst, and is so sore that I can scarce hold the pen.'[78] For several years chalky tophi exacerbated fears. 'This has not been a regular fit of the gout,' he confided to Lady Browne in 1785, 'but a worse case: one of my fingers opened with a deposit of chalk, and brought on gout.'[79] Such chalkstónes precipitated a quite spectacular topographical event, to which Walpole was narcissist enough to do justice:

> A finger of each hand has been pouring out a hail of chalk-stones and liquid chalk; and the first finger, which I hoped exhausted, last week opened again and threw out a cascade of the latter, exactly with the effort of a pipe that bursts in the street: the gout followed, and has swelled both hand and arm; and this codicil will cost me at least three weeks.[80]

Nevertheless, just as Blackmore had predicted, eventually gout grew less troublesome. 'Never was so tractable a gout as mine,'[81] he boasted to Miss Berry; a subsequent attack was but a 'pigmy fit';[82] and as an old man he was indeed, like Stukeley, strikingly proud of having managed his precarious health so well:

> my clock is on the stroke of seventy-four – and after so many years of gout, have not I cause to be content and thank God that I can creep about my own small garden? . . . I do not believe there is in the whole map of medicine a fountain so salutary as my own temperance and regimen, and cold system . . . In short, I would not be cured of *my* gout, if I could.[83]

Ironically, one of the banes of his later years was rheumatism, which he dreaded far more, 'as it is not so sure of quitting its hold'.[84] It was with almost erotic amusement that he could imagine gout and rheumatism vying for possession of his ancient body: 'the gout is come to assert his priority of right to me, and when he has expelled the usurper, I trust he will retire quietly too'.[85] Overall 'quietness' was thus the keynote with Walpole's affliction: let sleeping gouts lie. It was a tranquil disorder dictating a regime of serenity that perfectly matched the Addisonian ideal of polished urbanity and restraint.[86]

Quite different strategies were pursued by Walpole's contemporary Samuel Johnson – as might be expected, since their personalities were chalk and cheese. Johnson suffered all his life from a battery of ailments, picking up in the process much medical learning and a bluff confidence in his capacity to medicate himself. A bearlike man disposed to vehemence, he could not resist self-treating.

Johnson's general view of gout was conventional enough, as may be seen from the definitions in his *Dictionary* (1755), in which gout was glossed as 'the arthritis; a periodical disease attended with great pain'.[87] His orthodoxy also shows in his response to William Cadogan's *Dissertation on the Gout.* 'At supper, Lady McLeod mentioned Dr Cadogan's book on the gout,' Boswell reported on 14 September 1773:

> Mr Johnson said, 'Tis a good book in general, but a foolish one in particulars. 'Tis good in general, as recommending temperance and cheerfulness . . . 'Tis foolish, as it says, the gout is not hereditary, and one fit of the gout when gone is like a fever when gone.[88]

In conventional manner, Johnson thus deemed it 'folly' to deny gout's hereditary nature or to fancy it curable.

His personal encounters with the disorder somewhat belie this stance. The first hard evidence regarding Johnson's sufferings dates from 1775, when he was almost sixty-five, late for gout to appear. 'This sorry foot!' he grumbled on 29 August to Mrs Thrale,

> and this sorry Doctor Laurence who says it is the Gout! But then he thinks every thing the gout, and so I will try not to believe him. Into the sea, I suppose, you will send it, and into the sea I design it shall go. – Can you remember, dear Madam, that I have a lame foot? I am sure I cannot forget it, if you had one so painful you would *so* remember it. Pain is good for the memory.[89]

It is notable that, at that juncture, Johnson showed not the slightest sign of being glad to join the club of the gouty – taking the opportunity rather to voice his usual distrust towards the physicians' pretensions and his preference for precipitate therapeutic action.

A further attack followed in early 1776, and on 6 July that year Johnson sent news of it north to James Boswell.[90] More attacks followed in 1779, 1781 and 1783. After the last he told William Bowles that 'the Gout has treated me with more severity than any former time, it however never climbed higher than my ankles'.[91]

Johnson handled his attacks with customary gruff humour. In June 1776, for instance, he wrote to Henry Thrale that 'I creep about and hang by both hands . . . I enjoy all the dignity of lameness. I receive ladies and dismiss them sitting. *Painful pre-eminence.*'[92] Occasionally he voiced the platitude that gout would drive out other ailments. 'To the Gout my mind is reconciled by another letter from Mr Mudge' (a physician friend from Plymouth), he confided to Mrs Thrale on 6 October 1783, 'in which he . . . tells me that the gout will secure me from every thing paralytick, if this be true I am ready to say to the arthritick pains – Deh! venite ogni di, durate un anno.'[93] He was, or he made himself out to be, obviously rather taken by Mudge's perfectly orthodox opinion. 'By representing the Gout as an antagonist to the palsy,

You have said enough to make it welcome,' he thanked him three days later.[94] And on occasions he hoped that gout was a desirable discharge which should leave him in better fettle, rather as he was later to believe that his stroke improved his general health.[95] In general, however, he was sceptical of gout lore. 'I have had no great opinions of the benefits which it is supposed to convey,' he snarled to Dr Taylor in 1779. And that led him to various efforts – quite the reverse of Walpole's *quieta non movere* policy – to evict it, once it invaded. 'I made haste to be easy,' he informed Taylor, 'and drove it away after two days.'[96] Johnson's physician friend Thomas Lawrence believed gout would have a beneficial effect on his breathing, and so he resisted his pleas for his preferred procedure – phlebotomy. Like Mrs Thrale and Lawrence, the clergyman Dr Taylor disapproved of such headstrong action, provoking Johnson to counter-punch:

> My Gout never came again. You blame me, but I think very well of myself. Dr Laurence does not seem much to like the trick, but he does not deny that it was very dexterously performed. That the Gout is a remedy I never perceived, for when I had it most in my foot I had the spasms in my breast. At best the Gout is only a dog that drives the wolf away and eats the Sheep himself, for if the Gout has time for growth, it will certainly destroy, and destroy by long and lingering torture. If it comes again I purpose to show it no better hospitality.[97]

It is no surprise, then, that friends believed that Johnson was acting rashly in gratifying his 'haste to be easy'. Mrs Thrale later concluded that his medical troubles all went back to 'repressed gout', repelled into his heart. 'My Fear is lest he should grow paralytick,' she wrote on 17 December 1781, 'he will drive the Gout away so when it comes, and it must go *somewhere*.'[98] Some ten years after his death, she wrote, 'I am persuaded Dr Johnson died of repelled Gout – You may remember the trick he played at Sunninghill putting his feet in cold water. He never was well after.'[99]

The divergent strategies of Walpole and Johnson highlight the doctrines and dilemmas of Georgian gout. Prudence dictated sitting and suffering; only blockheads lost patience and ventured desperate remedies. George IV – dubbed by Shelley 'Swellfoot the Tyrant' – was of that ilk. 'We left the King very ill,' recounted that prize gossip, Dorothea Lieven, in 1822: 'he is tortured by gout and employs the most violent remedies to get rid of it. He looks ghastly.'[100] The King mutinied against the royal physicians, Sir Henry Halford and Sir William Knighton: 'Gentlemen, I have borne your half measures long enough to please you; now I shall please myself, and take colchicum.'[101] Gout folklore had always regarded such quacking as the road to ruin. 'On Thursday last Ralph Ld Grey Baron of Warke died of an Apoplexy,' recorded the Oxford antiquarian Thomas Hearne. 'Tis said he took something for ye Gout wch struck it into ye Head and Stomack, wch immediately caus'd his sudden end: whereby the Honour is Extinct.'[102] The dangers of forcing gout to become (so to speak) introspective had even been jingled out by Jonathan Swift:

> As if the gout should seize the head,
> Doctors pronounce the patient dead,
> But if they can, by all their arts;
> Eject it to the extreamest parts,
> They give the sick man joy, and praise
> The gout that will prolong his days.[103]

★

The stereotype of the gouty male was thus riddled with ambiguities. The heroic course was to have a showdown with the podagric foe, but discretion led the prudent, like Horace Walpole, to accept the sufferer's lot rather than venture upon Johnsonian draw-can-sir extremes. Instincts and counsels were thus at odds: to be active or patient? to treat gout as disease or deliverance, friend or foe? The perfect literary device for negotiating such alternatives was of course the dialogue, permitting simultaneous expression of contradictory views; not surprisingly gout produced a notable instance of that form, one penned by Benjamin Franklin. The paunchy American was a self-confessed *bon viveur* (God clearly intended us to be tipplers, he told the Abbé Morellet, because He had made the joints of the arm just the right length to carry a glass to the mouth). He recognized that he paid the penalty in crippling gout attacks that would immobilize him for up to a fortnight at a time.[104]

While resident in Passy on diplomatic business at Versailles, Franklin composed his divided-self 'Dialogue Between Franklin and the Gout'. Appropriately, the curtain rose to a tumult of torments:

FRANKLIN. Eh! Oh! Eh! What have I done to merit these cruel sufferings?
GOUT. Many things; you have ate and drank too freely, and too much indulged those legs of yours in their indolence.
FRANKLIN. Who is it that accused me?
GOUT. It is I, even I, the Gout.
FRANKLIN. What! my enemy in person?
GOUT. No, not your enemy.
FRANKLIN. I repeat it; my enemy; for you would not only torment my body to death, but ruin my good name; you reproach me as a glutton and a tippler; now all the world, that knows me, will allow that I am neither the one nor the other.[105]

Cruel only to be kind, the strict mistress instructed Franklin to follow sense not his stomach, shape up and slim down. The accused attempted to exculpate himself:

> FRANKLIN. I take – Eh! Oh! – as much exercise – Eh! – as I can, Madam Gout. You know my sedentary state, and on that account, it would seem, Madam Gout, as if you might spare me a little, seeing it is not altogether my own fault.[106]

If business demanded that 'Franklin' must lead a sedentary life, 'Gout' rejoined, 'your recreations, at least, should be active. You ought to walk or ride; or, if the weather prevents that, play at billiards.'[107] 'Franklin' failed to exercise when the opportunities were offered:

> GOUT. What is your practice after dinner? Walking in the beautiful gardens of those friends, with whom you have dined, would be the choice of men of sense; yours is to be fixed down to chess, where you are found engaged for two or three hours! ... What can be expected from such a course of living, but a body replete with stagnant humours, ready to fall a prey to all kinds of dangerous maladies, if I, the Gout, did not occasionally bring you relief by agitating those humours, and so purifying or dissipating them?[108]

The sluggard having thus been arraigned and found guilty, 'Gout' inflicted deserved 'corrections'. 'Franklin' protested – to no avail ('No, Sir, no, – I will not abate a particle of what is so much for your good').[109] 'Franklin' riposted that he did indeed take exercise –

> GOUT. Flatter yourself then no longer, that half an hour's airing in your carriage deserves the name of exercise. Providence has appointed few to roll in carriages, while he has given to all a pair of legs, which are machines infinitely more commodious and serviceable. Be grateful, then, and make a proper use of yours.[110]

Further exchanges led to 'Franklin' demanding, 'How can you so cruelly sport with my torments?'[111] – provoking the inevitable response:

> GOUT. Sport! I am very serious. I have here a list of offences against your own health distinctly written, and can justify every stroke inflicted on you.[112]

In other words, the much vaunted relation between genius and gout was supported by 'Gout', but twirled on its head, or rather its feet: philosophers *were* indeed liable to become gouty, precisely because they were so stupid! 'Ah! how tiresome you are!'[113] the exasperated 'Franklin' complained, to which 'Gout' predictably responded with wounded professional dignity:

GOUT. Well, then, to my office; it should not be forgotten that I am your physician. There.

FRANKLIN. Ohhh! what a devil of a physician!

GOUT. How ungrateful you are to say so! Is it not I who, in the character of your physician, have saved you from the palsy, dropsy, and apoplexy? one or other of which would have done for you long ago, but for me . . . my object is your good, and you are sensible now that I am your *real friend*.[114]

Like the Devil, 'Gout' evidently had the best tunes, and 'Franklin' was aware that he had brought bitter medicines upon himself. In words more candid than those of the *Dialogue*, Franklin elsewhere confirmed his addiction to high living. 'On Monday the 15th I dined and drank rather too freely at M. Darcy's,' he noted, 'Tuesday morning I felt a little pain in my right great toe.'[115]

All the views just examined were backed by the humoral theories of the time and the matching model of the fluid body economy. But the doctrine of gout – especially the image of it as a necessary evil – also had a further prop, in fundamental social, moral and political beliefs. To understand the inflexions of gout in the English-speaking world[116] we must take into account high politics and legal theory. The body was traditionally viewed as an analogue of the state, figuring centrally in narratives of political anatomy, especially insofar as it deployed concepts of flow and freedom, obstructions and checks, and the fluid balance of conflicting vital forces. In eighteenth-century English political argument, notions of political pathology, as classically formulated by Polybius and Machiavelli, were deeply entrenched, while talk of inheritance and entail loomed large, culminating in Burke's notion of the prescriptive constitution.

Ever since Plato, the body natural and the body politic had been superimposed as micro- and macro-cosm.[117] It used to be scholarly orthodoxy that such correspondences dissolved with the new philosophies of the Scientific Revolution, Cartesian rationalism and Lockean empiricism, but closer acquaintance with eighteenth-century idioms has demonstrated that such a 'breaking of the circle' hardly took place: metaphoric juxtaposition of body and nation remained integral to the rhetoric of power.[118] Late in the seventeenth century, Matthew Hale maintained that 'the texture of Humane affairs is not unlike the Texture of a diseased body labouring under Maladies'.[119] Shortly afterwards, the 'commonwealth' political writer Walter Moyle deemed Parliament the 'true physician' of the state, whose business was to 'foresee the seeds of state-distempers'.[120] Such idioms were still alive and well nearly a century later when the radical David Williams, reviewing the American troubles, argued that 'the constitution of a state is in many things analogous to that of the human body'.[121]

In a thought-world interleaving the body politic and the body human, gout was fleshed out through political language and concepts, and this was, at bottom, because it was conceptualized as a *constitutional* disease. As stressed by historians of political theory, political controversy in Britain after the Glorious Revolution and in the newborn American Republic was largely conducted in terms of constitutionality, its origins, nature and hazards. The fabric of constitutionalist ideology was intricate, interweaving traditions of 'civic humanist' thinking deriving from Machiavelli; the common law notion of the Anglo-Saxon 'ancient constitution', later modified into Edmund Burke's vision of a political order continuously evolving and thereby acquiring legitimacy ('our constitution', he asserted, 'is a prescriptive constitution'); the tenets of seventeenth-century classical 'republicans', notably James Harrington, fearful of the subversion of liberty by corruption (that is, by political pathology); and foreign commentators like Montesquieu.[122]

As a political creed, constitutionalism gave voice to a stark realism, at once gloomy and auspicious. Constitutionally regulated states, it was claimed, were clearly preferable to dictatorship, despotism and anarchy: the rule of law preserved liberty, property, rank and degree. Yet the unvarnished truth was that even a constitutional polity was necessarily honeycombed with evils and liable to decay. Politicians were ambitious and rapacious; gold corrupted, as did luxury, nepotism, patronage, party and, above all, power itself. Through its checks and balances and the separation of powers – the *locus classicus* of such doctrines was to be the *Federalist Papers* – the political constitution would hopefully counter the fissiparous forces of faction and prevent dissolution into despotism or demagogy (that 'euthanasia' of the state, according to David Hume). Representative government was a political organism from which some degree of depravity was inseparable (all polities were more or less debased); nevertheless, argued its apologists, a sound constitution would preclude corruption spreading like a cancer, and causing its quietus.[123]

Let no one be deceived, commentators insisted: politics was a dirty business. The British scheme of government was at best a lesser evil; and – herein lay its hard-headed appeal – it would therefore be quixotic idealism or arrant nostrum-mongering to vest trust in schemes of radical regeneration. Politics, as understood by Georgian governing circles, should be the art of the possible not the pursuit of perfection; it was utopian and futile to seek to supplant unclean politics with the millennium of virtue; political evil could not be eradicated, merely palliated. Luxury was lambasted,[124] but David Hume and others berated its would-be exterminators by arguing that the progress of commerce and refinement secured civil tranquillity and political order.[125] Here Hume was echoing views more jauntily advanced in the *Fable of the Bees* (1714) by that arch-cynic Bernard Mandeville – it was surely no accident that he was both a physician and a political pundit. Private vices, Mandeville had insisted, were public benefits, and 'Avarice then and Prodigality are equally necessary to the Society.' Certain malaises within the body politic were entirely compatible with a healthy overall prognosis:

> Thus every Part was full of Vice,
> Yet the whole Mass a Paradice.[126]

And such realist views were underpinned by the widely held theodicy (it has been called 'cosmic toryism'), spelt out most popularly in Alexander Pope's *Essay on Man* (1732–4).[127] Proclaiming 'whatever is, is right', such metaphysical Optimism rationalized the ineradicability of (lesser) evils by demonstrating how particular and apparent defects were compatible with the greater good.

In short, the pith of post-1688 politics lay in the balanced constitution, which was praised for its complicated system of checks and balances establishing an equilibrium between the executive and the legislature.[128] Whereas pure forms of government would collapse of their own excess, lacking internal counter-balance, it was believed that 'only a mixed or balanced constitution, combining the qualities of all three forms, could hope to escape the doom of degeneration'.[129] Under such circumstances, Hume emphasized, subjects had a duty to 'conform themselves to the established constitution'.[130] Blueprints for radical change excited grave suspicion. 'Some innovations', Hume continued, 'must necessarily have place in every human institution . . . but violent innovations no individual is entitled to make.'[131] And this train of thought was given its rhetorical flourish by Edmund Burke, who made much of 'the great mysterious incorporation of the human race'.[132] In the light of such doctrines, political radicalism could readily be ridiculed by its Burkean opponents as the nostrums of arrant quackery.

The constitutionalist doctrines just discussed provide a wider framework for grasping gout. The idioms of politics and those of bodily physiology and pathology were of a piece. Theories of gout were reinforced by the fetishism of the constitution – surely it was no accident that gout was endemic at St Stephen's? The human body was represented as governed by a constitution of its own. Its operation was not without trouble – the motions and commotions of different humours often produced disturbance; imbalances arose, now a plethora, there a weakness. There were occasional obstructions when the animal spirits – those 'Great Ministers of Digestion', in Blackmore's telling phrase – proved incompetent, resulting, so ran his prognosis, 'in Disorder and Confusion', whereupon the body's 'Government must be unhinged and at length dissolved'.[133] Not least, over-consumption in the emergent consumer society caused critical motions in the animal economy.[134] Hence the human body could never be altogether disorder-free: in fact, it was rather beefy, John Bullish, to be pincered by pain.

It made sense to assume that ailments, just like Sir Robert Walpole's House of Commons, had to be managed, through prudent regimen.[135] Gout was doubtless an illness, albeit a by-product of desirable manly, magnate living. But as an evil it was partial, capable of being successfully handled, precisely because it was a *constitutional* disease, integral to physiological order, passed down through the blood from generation to generation, predictable and periodic in its outbreaks – akin, one might say, to the chronic septennial electoral violence which allowed a certain letting off of steam while perpetuating the system. In other words, gout was a disorder of hale and hearty constitutions. In *Some Observations on the . . . Gout* (1779), William Grant thus insisted that gout be regarded as a hereditary disease 'of the whole constitution'.[136]

Constitutionalism, in most ways conservative, was given a very different reading by political radicals, who dismissed such renderings as panglossian blather, and argued that the constitution was sick and in urgent need of fundamental therapy. Thus the Whig historian, Catharine Macaulay, insisted that the architects of the Revolution settlement of 1688 had accepted half-measures, but that this timidity had endangered the nation's health.[137]

Somewhat later, James Mackintosh, an early supporter of the French Revolution, was determined to prove that reform would usher in greater liberty: 'Who will be hardy enough to assert, that a better Constitution is not attainable than any which has hitherto appeared?'[138] Constitutional reform could be transferred by implication to the natural body, an upshot that occurred in the wake of the writings of William Cadogan, as will be explored in Chapter 7.

Another sufferer who, like Horace Walpole, was a Member of Parliament was Edward Gibbon; it is not surprising that the personification – indeed politicization – of gout came readily to him.[139] Gibbon was furthermore deeply sensitive to the imperfections of his own body; so short and fat that he became known as 'Mr Chubby-Chubb'. His later years were marred by the growth of a hydrocele (swollen testicle) as large as a melon which he did his best to ignore. By picturing himself as a thinker and writer, he was able with a certain nonchalance to disregard, or make the best of, his corporeal self.

After a sickly childhood, Gibbon chose to portray himself (with, one imagines, at least a touch of self-mockery) as possessing a rather hardy constitution – or at least a manly disregard for the pains of the flesh. 'It might now be apprehended that I should continue for life an illiterate cripple,' he mused in his *Memoirs*, looking back to childhood illness:

> but as I approached my sixteenth year, Nature displayed in my favour her mysterious energies; my constitution was fortified and fixed: and my disorders, instead of growing with my growth and strengthening with my strength, most wonderfully vanished. I have never possessed or abused the insolence of health: but since that time few persons have been more exempt from real or imaginary ills: and till I am admonished by the Gout,

the reader shall no more be troubled with the history of any bodily complaints.[140]

The rationalization behind this sentiment seems to be that, unlike other ailments, gout was an acceptable, virile, almost genteel condition.

Gibbon was first stricken in 1772 at the age of thirty-five, describing it to his step-mother as a 'dignified disorder'.[141] In succeeding years the trouble grew more frequent. 'The Gout has attacked my left foot,' he informed his friend Lord Sheffield in December 1774, as he was completing the first volumes of the *Decline and Fall*, 'and that imperious Mistress if I presumed without her permission to dispose of myself [sic]. However, she seems inclined to pardon and to leave me.'[142] If to his buddy he toyed with sexual banter, the ex-captain of the Hampshire militia dispatched to his step-mother the more seemly military metaphor. 'The Gout has now asserted his rights in an unquestionable manner,' he told her, 'but on this occasion he has exercised them in a very gentle manner, and I can say with truth that I find myself rather benefited than injured by his transient visit.'[143]

The sceptical historian continued his more risqué tone to male confidants. 'I arrived last night,' he informed Sheffield early in the following year, 'laid up with the gout in both my feet I suffer like one of the first Martyrs, and possibly have provoked my punishment as much.'[144] While engaging in this mild impiety, he soldiered on to his step-mother with martial metaphors, reassuring her that 'the enemy appears to be raising the siege, and that he makes a regular and gradual retreat'.[145] Perhaps out of relief at the diminution of pain, he tried it on his comrade as well:

the Gout has behaved in a very honourable manner; after a compleat conquest, and after making me feel his power for some days the generous Enemy has disdained to abuse his victory or to torment any longer an unresisting victim. He has already ceased to torture the lower extremities of your humble servant; the swelling is so amazingly diminished that they are no longer above twice their ordinary size.[146]

In Gibbon's metaphoric arsenal, gout might be an honourable enemy, but it could be an inexorable foe. 'So uncertain are all human affairs', he explained to his step-mother a couple of months later, 'that I found myself arrested by a mighty unrelenting Tyrant called the Gout.'[147] A further epistle to her, a week later, was less than complimentary,[148] but, as if to compensate for his earlier want of esteem, on the occasion of his next attack Gibbon was almost fulsome in his tribute:

if the name of agreeable can ever be applied to the ugly monster, my Gout has deserved it on this occasion. It lasted in the whole no more than ten days, attacked only one foot, was [not] attended with any feaver, loss of appetite, or lowness of spirits, and has left me in perfect health both of mind and body.[149]

If that assault was almost 'agreeable', that was presumably because Gibbon could envisage it within the theory construing gout as a relief agency: 'This fit of the Gout, though severe, has been short and regular, and I think beneficial.'[150] Shortly afterwards, he implied that a gout fit had set him on to the road to health:

the body Gibbon is in a perfect state of health and spirits as it is most truly at the present moment, and since the entire retreat of my Gout. The state of public affairs is Anarchy without example and without end and if the King does not decide before Monday the consequences in the House of Commons will be fatal indeed.[151]

The juxtaposition of the salubrity of the 'body Gibbon' and the misery of the body politic – a typically polished Gibbonian antithesis – shows that the political implications of gout were in the author's mind.

Gibbon could at least pass gout off, if not as a positive boon, then as one of the many bearable evils of mortal life:

When I was called upon last February for my annual tax to the Gout, I only paid for my left foot which in general is the most heavily assessed: the officer came round last week to collect the small remainder that was due for the right foot. I have now satisfied his demand, he is retired in good humour, and I feel myself easy both in mind and body.[152]

One of the ostensible reasons for migrating in 1783 to Lausanne was to recruit his health – the Swiss mountain air would supposedly be beneficial – and, once there, high above the lake, he presented himself as reaping the rewards.[153] Gout had, admittedly, pounced soon after his arrival in Lausanne, but its onset had been the result of an unlucky accident – 'carelessly stepping down a flight of stairs, I sprained my ancle and my ungenerous enemy instantly took advantage of my weakness'.[154] As was his wont, the historian put on a brave face, demonstrating that, even if all was not for the best, at least every cloud had a silver lining, and that he had been acting prudently:

I have enjoyed a winter of the most perfect health that I have perhaps ever known, without any mixture of the little flying incommodities which in my best days have sometimes disturbed the tranquillity of my English life. [Tissot] assures me that . . . the dry, pure air of Switzerland [is] most favourable to a Gouty constitution: that experience justifies the Theory, and that there are fewer martyrs of that disorder in this than in any other country in Europe.[155]

It may have been true, and this was the same famous Tissot, of course, who also expounded on the notion of gouty figures as solitary literary types, of which Gibbon was a prime candidate. A letter later in the same year gave his step-mother an equally flattering prospect of his improved health, attributing it to his compliance with the regime advocated by William Cadogan:

> the air though sharp is pure, it may be dangerous for weak lungs; but is excellently suited to a gouty constitution, and during the whole twelfthmonth I have never once been attacked by my old Enemy. Of Dr. Cadogan's three rules, I can observe two, a temperate diet and a easy mind.[156]

(The absent third was exercise: Gibbon was notoriously lazy.)

In the same vein he could crow to his old parliamentary crony Lord Eliot that in the 'healthy' climate of Switzerland 'during the whole year of my residence I have not once been visited by my old enemy the Gout'.[157] Yet he spoke too soon. He liked to boast to his step-mother – presumably to convince himself – that 'my health has perfectly sustained the rigour of the season, good spirits, good appetite, good sleep are my habitual state and though verging towards fifty I still feel myself a young Man'. Though he had been 'in hopes that my old Enemy the gout' had given over the attack, 'the Villain, with his ally the winter convinced me of my error, and about the latter end of March I found myself a prisoner in my library and my great chair'. No matter, Gibbon continued, showing the philosopher triumphant over the patient: 'my gout . . . respectfully confines itself to the lower extremities of the Machine'.[158] Sanguine as ever, if also lonely, Gibbon flaunted to his step-mother the frugality of his living and the success of his strategy through 'confining myself to a mess of boiled milk' for supper: 'This regimen appears to have succeeded; I have passed the winter without hearing of the enemy, and last month after a short and slight visit or rather menace, he politely retired and has left me free to enjoy the beauties of an incomparable spring.'[159]

Was he primarily concerned to cheer the old lady? Or was he wilfully deceiving himself? Things certainly worsened the next year, forcing him to grumble to Lord Sheffield, 'This fit is remarkably painful: the enemy is possessed of the left foot and knee, and how far he may carry the war, God only knows.'[160] A subsequent epistle confirmed its severity, with Gibbon's 'finer feelings . . . suspended by the grosser evil of bodily pain': 'On the ninth of February I was seized by such a fit of the Gout as I had never known, though I must be thankful that its dire effects have been confined to the feet and knees without ascending to the more noble parts.'[161] And the tale of woe worsened still further.[162] Almost like one taking his cue from the philosophizings of Philander Misaurus, Gibbon demonstrated how affliction was the mother of fortitude: 'My patience has been universally admired.'[163]

Towards 1790, his health was deteriorating fast, although what finally killed him was not gout but a septicaemic wound following surgery for his swelling hydrocele. The ambiguity of his mode of life, or rather the discrepancy between reality and self-image, is captured by passages in letters written towards the end. 'My MADEIRA is almost exhausted,' he informed Lord Sheffield, 'and I must receive before the end of the autumn, a stout cargo of wholesome exquisite wine.'[164] Meanwhile this man, so desperate for drink, was reassuring his step-mother: 'My health is remarkably good: I have now enjoyed a long interval from the gout; and I endeavour to use with modera- tion Dr Cadogan's best remedies.'[165]

Gibbon's gout bespeaks the self-image of an eighteenth-century gentleman, but also of a very distinctive individual. Deeply embarrassed about his body, gout was the only one of his maladies he could parade. It could be turned into a joke or a performance; since it spared his 'nobler parts' it was not unaccept- ably demeaning; and it called up hidden reserves of character. So long as he could banter about gout, the historian did not need to address himself to more serious complaints.

This chapter has shown that eighteenth-century sufferers and writers situated gout within stories of sickness that were normally secular. And we shall see in the next that a great comic novelist like Tobias Smollett – himself a doctor and sufferer – could tranform the figure of the gouty hero into the protagonist of his last and probably most original narrative, *The Adventures of Humphry Clinker* (1771). Parallel to such understandings there was also a much more traditional cultural approach, deploying a religious frame. The most elaborate attempt to inscribe gout within the Christian master narrative was produced by Cotton Mather, the principal preacher in early eighteenth-century Massa- chusetts.[166] Chief among his medical writings was *The Angel of Bethesda*, completed in 1724, the first systematic American medical treatise. Seeing gout as a disease of the dissolute, Mather found it easy to sermonize upon, which he did at great length and in spectacularly baroque prose. His text is fasci- nating, not least for its utterly Protestant union of divine chastisement and human remedy. But it is difficult to imagine a clergyman of eminence in eighteenth-century England – as distinct from New England – writing in that guise. It was within a human and moral economy, rather than the divine, that gout was perceived among Old World educated and articulate classes. Its meanings remained powerful but they vibrated essentially within the natural rather than the providential order.

CHAPTER 7

Smollett, Cadogan and Controversy

As the eighteenth century wore on all manner of men, great and small, rich and less rich, calibrated their lives according to their aches and pains. Voltaire's enemies, for example, made much of his various maladies, satirizing his gout as Dubois did; and there is a biographical school of the persuasion, perhaps with justification, that the segments of his life can be measured according to his wellness.

In England the same held true. Robert Dodsley, the popular London publisher and bookseller, endured chronic gout all through the 1750s, during his maturity, for weeks at a time (he says never less than four), while continuing to keep a most vigorous routine and cluttered diary. His constant correspondents – the poets William Shenstone, Edward Young, William Warburton, Richard Dyer and many others in the ranks of the Republic of Letters – were less gouty but nevertheless understood his predicament. Indeed, gout was a sign system for something else. In early November 1755 Dodsley had been confined for five weeks, all the while complaining that others are 'lovers of Ease' whose true names should be 'indolence'.[1] A month later he wrote to Shenstone, 'Your Letter found me confin'd with the gout, & to this I hope you will attribute my idle-headedness in scribbling so much stuff.'[2] To John Hylton, another constant correspondent who understood gout's interior signs, Dodsley pathetically railed 'The Gout is the *opprobrium Medicinae*, and past the Art of Me, or My Brethren, to eradicate; but I hope you are at Liberty to walk about, & enjoy Life again.'[3]

Later, in 1757, Dodsley's gout grew worse – or so he said – yet he managed to keep up the same active pace. He complained to Shenstone that he was daily growing worse and wrote to him describing how 'I have sate in a chair near three months & cannot yet set either foot to the ground,'[4] this totalling no less than seven years of gout, all in the language of the tyranny and chains of the disease. 'In this wretched situation, for Charity's sake have some pity upon me; send from your Pharmacopeia of Wit some cordial drops to cheer my spirits.'[5] His correspondents included women, to whom he confided his 'Philosophy upon Crutches': he wrote, 'I am now practicing Philosophy upon Crutches: & you cannot conceive what a complacency & respect I grow to have for my self, on the contemplation of my own virtues of Patience and Resignation.'[6] Living the good life in the flannel dressing-gown nailed him down to his chair, and though unable to walk he worked away as if a predestined Calvinist, giving up drink and pleasure and having 'quitted the bottle for the pail, and become a toper in Milk'.[7]

Milk-drinking Dodsley yoked gout and wit as any gentlemen of the period did, the one the guarantor, or insurer, of the other – so much so that if 'the gout may dread to approach you, wit will'.[8] Robert Lowth, the great biblical exegete of the period, was a fellow sufferer during those years. Dodsley calmed him with assurances that gout was entirely beneficent. 'I hope it [gout] will prove all for your Good, & that it has left you in good spirits, with a stock of health that may last you a great while, before it shall think proper to discipline you again.'[9] Three years later, in 1763, Dodsley was still 'in the gout', having been unaided by the waters of Bath, and descanting to his young cousin Elizabeth Cartwright that gout is something 'to submit to', because it 'serves a very good purpose in weaning us from the World'.[10] Quaffing immortality, Dodsley sang its virtues, claiming how much the big G had done for him and counting his blessings that gout had been his true god in whose temple he worshipped. To the end gout bound these men together, who understood its code as well as the intense homosocial cults of friendship of the age.

William Cowper's correspondence also demonstrates thorough familiarity with this code language among gentlemen. But this was a different understanding from Cheyne's (earlier) and, as we will see, Conrad's (later). For these men, gout was the great enabler, and illness implied creativity above all. Cheyne's creativity was filled with terror: he had swelled up with the gout, then drastically reduced his weight, to the tune of hundreds of pounds. At his peak, he swelled to over 400 pounds, only to reduce to little more than one hundred. Still, his gout was the virtual maker of his creative imagination. For Dodsley and Cowper and many others, gout was the gentleman's code: proof of pedigree, class and rank, insurer of accomplishment and a hard work ethic. But for Tobias Smollett (1721–71), the novelist – physician, gout was something else again: terror compounded by fear and trembling; the constant worry that the disease in his lungs and the ceaseless asthma and consumption were gout in another form.

Smollett's concern over his lungs became an obsession, as did the larger state of his health. While still a middle-aged man, his obsession prompted him to quit his country in search of a warmer climate, where his sickened lungs could recover and his care be abated. But he never lost his sense that his whole life was tied into 'the natural history of gout' and into what we are calling the psychological 'fear and trembling' over his lungs, as is evidenced, we think, in his last and perhaps greatest novel, *The Adventures of Humphry Clinker* (1771).

This work is also the last novel in any language to select the gouty old man as its hero. This is an extraordinary fact, given the rise of the novel and the novel's date, and poses for literary and medical historians a more complex artefact to explain than has been acknowledged. Every socio-economic feature of this typology is finely drawn in Smollett's brilliant caricature proving the joke in the podagra conceit: that they who have been well born pay for it. There can be no doubt whatever about the hero's specific medical malady: it frames the novel at either end. In Matthew Bramble's opening letter – Smollett's epistolary novel is composed in an innovative technique of five sets of correspondences the most prolific of which contains the letters from Bramble to his fictional 'Dr Lewis'[11] – Bramble recounts how 'A ridiculous incident that happened yesterday to my niece Liddy, has disordered me in such a manner, that I expect to be laid up with another fit of the gout – perhaps I may explain myself in the next.'[12] By the very end of the book Bramble's gout is cured by the journey 'northward' to health that enables him to integrate himself through this imagined Caledonian idyll. As Matt writes in his concluding letter to Dr Lewis:

> My sister and her husband, Baynard and I, will take leave of them at Gloucester, and make the best of our way to Brambleton-hall, where I desire you will prepare a good chine and turkey for our Christmas dinner. – You must also employ your medical skill in defending me from the attacks of the gout . . .[13]

The copula of gout and its cock-and-bull story is finished only when Bramble lays down his pen in the concluding words of the book, not fortuitously penned from patient to doctor: 'I intend to renounce all sedentary amusements, particularly that of writing long letters; a resolution, which, had I taken it sooner, might have saved you the trouble which you had lately taken in reading the tedious epistles of . . .'[14] So closes your obedient servant's sinewy epistolary tale, his charming series of loosely connected vignettes about the picaresque road to health.[15] The biographical Smollett was himself gouty, had learned that *to be gouty* was *to be literary* – a scribbler. He was also a qualified medical doctor, trained in the Edinburgh medical school at the beginning of its Enlightenment flowering, and when he moved to London it was among 'the doctors' first that Smollett-the-Scot established his *English* reputation as a medical practitioner.[16]

Smollett also wrote quickly, profusely, almost never having time to revise anything, and wrote around the clock for economic and professional reasons.[17] Little wonder then that both historical author (Smollett) and fictional hero (Bramble) were exhilarated at the prospect of finishing, respectively, their novel and epistolary correspondence. Both were ailing, both chronicly gouty, both acutely aware that the completion of their books – *Humphry Clinker* and Bramble's long letters to Dr Lewis – would herald at least the possibility of a new chapter in their lives.[18] But virtually none of this literary criticism and interpretation even mentions Bramble's emblematic gout, the one specific malady whose images and stereotypes lend such valence to Smollett's book.[19] Smollett's delineation of Bramble as gouty is airtight. Male, elderly; twisted, swollen; benevolent, misanthropic; irritable, sensible, sensitive; melancholic, cynical; ludic, abrasive; chronically suffering, a compulsive scribbler; driven by cares, as we shall see again later, that turn out to be bagatelles initiated by mundane chaos and confusion; a squire of the manor whose gout insulates him from dire illness and encourages him to cultivate the sedentary life without exercise. Bramble's ludic ebullience within an ingrained melancholia remains one of his most striking paradoxes.

Not surprisingly Smollett's contemporaries never mentioned Bramble's illnesses. For example, William Mudford (1782–1848) – a popular literary journalist in the generation after Smollett's – wrote lengthy 'Critical Observations on *Humphry Clinker*' which he published in the Regency; so too Walter Scott: neither mentions Bramble's gout as an integral aspect of his ridiculously comic personality.[20] The result was that eventually Matt's gout evaporated – it disappeared – as a matter of any concern until it was retrieved in our time.[21] The critics of our century have noted that his 'fits' and 'flying attacks' could arise at any time; it seems to have been present but dormant from the start of his life. 'I have for some time been of the opinion, (no offence, dear Doctor),' Bramble writes to his confidant Dr Lewis, 'that the sum of all your medical discoveries amounts to this, that the more you study the less you know.'[22] The discussions in his novel are explicit: 'Now we talk of the *dropsy*, here is a strange, fantastic oddity . . .'[23] Matt is also a spectacular 'gout observer'. In Bath 'we consisted of thirteen individuals; seven lamed by the gout, rheumatism, or palsy; three maimed by accident; and the rest either deaf or blind'.[24] 'So far from being dropsical,' he writes to Dr Lewis, 'I am as lank in the belly as a grey-hound; and, by measuring my ankle with a pack-thread, I find the swelling subsides every day – From such doctors, good Lord deliver us!'[25]

Every 'attack' is analysed, pondered for its effects, and genderized: 'What the devil had I to do, to come a plague hunting with a leash of females in my train?'[26] Now, in old age, he suffers for the sins of profligacy, but he 'suffers' as poignantly as any mock-epic patient, and 'consumes' medication with a scepticism wholly his own:

> It must be owned, indeed, I took some of tincture of ginseng, prepared according to your prescription, and found it exceedingly grateful to the stomach; but the pain and sickness continued to return, after short intervals, till the anxiety of my mind was entirely removed, and then I found myself perfectly at ease.[27]

'As for the water,' he tells Dr Lewis, 'which is said to have effected so many surprising cures, I have drank it once, and the first draught has cured me of all desire to repeat the medicine. – Some people say it smells of rotten eggs, and others compare it to the scourings of a foul gun.'[28] At Harrogate he endures another gouty assault and recounts to his dear doctor:

> I was moved to bed and wrapped in blankets. – There I lay a full hour panting with intolerable heat; but not the least moisture appearing on my skin, I was carried to my own chamber, and passed the night without closing an eye, in such a flutter of spirits as rendered me the most miserable wretch in being.[29]

If these descriptions abound with the legendary features of nervous and ebullient Smollettian prose, they also dramatize gout's inherent inconsistencies: the onset of attack as the guarantor of insulation; exposure and vulnerability within social rank; the yoking of illness to its narrative encodements, clearly evident in the continuation of this bustling letter. Finally, the old man who is to become thematically so crucial in the visual heritage (as we demonstrate in Chapter 12) speaks out:

> . . . I propose to brace up my fibres by sea-bathing, which, I know, is one of your favourite specifics. There is, however, one disease [that is, other than gout], for which you [doctors] have found as yet no specific, and that is old age, of which this tedious unconnected epistle is an infallible symptom: – *what*, therefore, *cannot be cured, must be endured.*[30]

Disease, geriatric realism, fragmented neo-Lucianic writing: the sequitur is predictable. The narrative is as broken, or fragmented, as it is disease-specific and obsessed with old age: these were the gouty man's obsessions too. Perhaps that is why both patient and doctor refer to themselves in this extraordinary correspondence as 'humorists'. 'But', Bramble writes in his nonsensical letter to Dr Lewis of 4 July, 'to return from one humorist to another . . .' The fraternity of 'humorists' is not gratuitous. Gout, whatever it really represented in the minds of the Brambles of Georgian civilization, entailed an ongoing 'spectacle' of interruptions from the realms of the already ridiculous. Adventure in the gouty world partook of this counterpoint between 'fit' and its deviations into 'interruption'. This is why action is so crucial to Smollett's inherently comic book. 'You must know,' Bramble wrote later to Dr Lewis, 'I have received benefit, both from the chalybeate and the sea, and would have used them longer, had not a most ridiculous adventure, by making me the town-talk, obliged me to leave the place; for I can't bear the thoughts of affording a spectacle to the multitude . . .'[31]

As the travellers proceed north towards the homeland – Scotland – Matthew's health improves but not before he realizes his true 'condition': a comic state of affairs indeed. Bramble had persuaded himself that his 'chronic' gout was irremediable; now he learns otherwise as his pieties are overturned, not least the paradox about health: 'my health [is] so much improved, that I am disposed to bid defiance to gout and rheumatism. – I begin to think I have put myself on the superannuated list too soon.'[32]

Remedy for the Georgian gentleman lay in action, ambition, aggression – those values that had been instilled from boyhood. The very definition of a 'gentleman' thrived on these capacities, gout its insulatory proof. Life's wheels were held in motion by deeds rather than words, and motion required vigorous activity and spatial displacement – even jarring geographical dislocation for its attainment. Hence Matthew's conclusion as the travelling caravan crosses the Scottish border into Arcady and Health: '– I am persuaded that all valetudinarians are too sedentary, too regular, and too cautious – We should sometimes increase the motion of the machine . . .'[33] The end of the healing journey is thus predictable: all but Bramble and his ward Jery Melford marry. They too, in turn, are restored to complete health despite continuing celibacy: the protagonist from his perpetual gout, the ward – Jery – through his transformation from the state of innocence to experience.

The fact that Smollett could sustain this gout in his protagonist for the duration of many hundreds of pages is testimony to more than his narrative skill. He was, of course, a consummate writer of comic prose, as the critics have noted for two centuries. But he also wrote in an age when the interpretation of illness had a more vigorous resonance than it does in our epoch. Illness then was the ordinary, not the anomalous, condition of life, gout its most visible insignia in the upper class. The idea of a gentry without gout was then as unthinkable as monarchies without kings and queens, or bodies without dualistic kingdoms. This difference has been one of the major themes of our book: to show – culturally, politically, narratively, visually – how this insignia arose, was culturally inscribed and eventually fell. But proof also requires the demonstration of the ways in which illness was then represented in the popular imagination. As Lawrence Rothfield has astutely commented of the early modern imagination: 'illness, far from appearing as a sudden stroke of fate, constitutes an abiding state of being'.[34]

Elsewhere George Rousseau has argued that Smollett's breakdown in the early 1750s represented near total collapse;[35] that it entailed more than gout no matter how broad the classification. This has been a controversial position, attacked by certain of the Smollettian biographers, but whether spot on or not it makes evident how fragile Smollett's health was even before his thirtieth birthday. 'I am still an Invalid', he wrote in exasperation to John Wilkes from Chelsea on 19 October 1759.[36] His condition was indubitably gouty, as his letters make perfectly clear: 'I have had no attack of the Asthma these two months, but I am extremely emaciated, and am afflicted with a tickling Catarrh, and cough all night without ceasing . . . But neither my Indolence nor my occupation will permit me to persevere in these Endeavours.'[37] No wonder he advocated 'exercise, cold bathing, and plunging into the ocean'.[38]

Smollett's word is consistently 'asthma' and he uses it to indicate all those umbrella conditions under which the gout was classified in his century. 'Your last found me in the Country,' he wrote from Chelsea in a letter dated 19 August 1762 to his real-life medical confidant, John Moore,

> to which I had repaired for the Benefit of a purer Air; but whether it was too keen for my Lungs, or the change of Bed produced a fresh Cold, I was driven home by the Asthma; and soon after I went to Dover with a View to bathe in the Sea, and to use the Exercise of riding on Horseback, and sailing in a Vessel alternately.[39]

The connections of illness and work, sickness and its literary representations, play as large a role for the historical Tobias as the literary Bramble. We suggest then that there is another set of correspondences to be considered: two sets of four-way letters, from Matt to his doctor, his doctor to Matt; and then from Tobias to his doctors, and his doctors to Tobias. This is no bouillon algebra but the very stuff of case history in which the self is represented by narrating in time its conditions of alternating health and illness. Tobias, like Bramble, thinks nothing of dedicating the greatest part of his letters – those that survive – to his health. He wrote minutely from Bath to the great anatomist of the time, William Hunter: 'My Health was so indifferent during the whole Journey that I was obliged to get out of Bed every night and sit two hours untill the Difficulty of Breathing abated . . .'[40]

But by the 1760s his constitution could no longer hold up, his only recourse to flee England in the same search for health as Bramble. Or did Bramble precede Tobias? Was Bramble the inner life of Tobias himself, Tobias merely the fictional persona of that far more real figure? Once gone from London Tobias–Bramble dedicated himself to those remedies touted in *Humphry Clinker*: anti-luxury, the life of pastoral simplicity, spartan diet, cold-water bathing. 'This is the twentieth day of my bathing in the sea,' he wrote in another letter to William Hunter from Boulogne-sur-mer dated 11 August 1764.[41] Later, '. . . still the Tuber continues. I grow thinner and thinner; but I am not without hope of recruiting in the spring.'[42]

During these years Smollett performed one of the most intricate self-diagnoses of the century to a French professor of medicine in Montpellier, Antoine Fizes.[43] We shall not discuss it here except to note that its representations of gouty temperament are of a piece with Tobias's own letters and *Humphry Clinker*. Chronicity and interruption form the main rhythm of these patterns: an endless cycle of illness and health within the counterpoint of verbal productivity. The pattern is constant. 'With respect to my own Health,' Smollett wrote to John Moore, 'I cannot complain. I have not lately lost any Ground; but, on the contrary, have gained some flesh since coming to Bath, where I have been these five weeks.'[44]

Corpulence and matter were essential in these concerns, as they always were to the gouty. 'My Disorder is no other than weak Lungs and a Constitution prone to Catarrhs, with an extraordinary irritability of the nervous System,' he continued in this lengthy analysis to Moore. But constancy lay only in the fact of his condition, not in its disappearance – this constancy was precisely its comedic factor and accounts for the ludic results it produced: 'I do not, however, flatter myself that I shall continue to mend, for I have always found myself better for about a month after any change of air, and then I relapse into my former state of Invalidity.' It was the lack of geographical change and the sheer labour of writing that kept him 'in the gout' for this – as Pope would have said – 'long *Disease*, my life'. Hence, his conclusion to Hunter in the same letter: 'Nothing agrees with me so well as hard Exercise, which, however, the Indolence of my Disposition continually counteracts. If I was a Galley slave and kept to hard Labour for two or three years, I believe I should recover my Health intirely.' Perhaps, but a 'Galley slave' was no landowning gentleman of Georgian England.

There were moments when Smollett thought he had miscalculated these taxonomies; when he was not 'in' a fit of the gout at all. 'To tell you the Truth,' Tobias wrote to Hunter, 'I look upon my being alive as a sort of Resuscitation; for last year I thought myself in the last stage of a Consumption.'[45] But the shades between a consumption, dropsy and gout; between rheumatics and asthmatics – as we have seen above – were subtle, even to a medically trained writer like Smollett. What counted for more was the condition's chronicity and the fact – thank God! – that Tobias repeatedly could represent it narratively in letters.

We have been suggesting that the culture of illness is a homology of the whole: that is, that whether in a Smollett or Cadogan or any representative, illness is configured according to predictable cultural patterns rather than exclusively narrative or rhetorical ones. The narrator of *Humphry Clinker* could have written this passage to Dr Lewis; it happens to have been written to another doctor, John Moore:

> I have for some weeks resolved to write you an account of my Health, about which I know your friendly sollicitude . . . You must remember the miserable way which I was at parting from you in August last. At my return to Bath, I caught Cold, in consequence of which my Rheumatic Pains retired, and the Disorder in my Breast recurred, namely an Orthopnoa, with an ugly Cough and spitting, exclusive of a slow fever from which I had never been free. But these Symptoms gave me little Disturbance in Comparison with the ulcer on my fore arm, which continued to spread untill it occupied the whole space from about three inches above the wrist to the Ball of the Thumb so that I was intirely deprived of the use of my right hand, and the Inflammation and Pain daily increased[46] . . . the Rheumatism again invaded me from the neck to the Heel. In a word, I despaired of ever seeing the End of Winter, and every night when I went to bed, fervently wished that I might be dead before morning . . . In a word, my cure is looked upon as something supernatural; and I must own that I now

find myself better in Health and spirits than I have been at any time these seven years . . . Between Friends, I am now convinced that my Brain was in some measure affected; for I had a kind of *Coma vigil* upon me from April to November without Intermission . . .[47]

★

This detailed analysis might itself seem excessive were it not for the extraordinary coincidence that within weeks of publication of *Humphry Clinker* in January 1771 the controversy of the century broke out over the medical status of gout. The gout diagnosis had remained a bone of contention, but it was not until the 1770s that fierce polemical debate erupted. Smollett's novel was in proofs by Christmas 1770; by March Dr William Cadogan's bombshell was launched.[48] There can be no question of precedence or influence: Smollett had been living in the Mediterranean since the mid-1760s. He began to write *Humphry Clinker* long before 1771 and had been writing the book for years, conjuring it mentally for decades. It summed up his life-plight in more ways than one. Likewise, any possible influence of Cadogan on Smollett is out of the question: cultural homology, the unitary nature of culture, not influence, is our point. Whether the new gout crisis of 1771 was comic or tragic depended, naturally, on the beholder's point of view during 1771; and whether the severity of crisis was abetted in any way by Smollett's immensely popular novel then being read we will probably never know, as there is no evidence one way or the other. Yet there is something extending beyond contingency in the homology of *both* fiction and medical crisis erupting within a few months of each other; and there can be no doubt whatever of the reading public's interest in the psychological, as well as medical, implications of the controversial gout theory being debated, whether construed in the terms of fictional heroism (as in Matthew Bramble) or medical controversy (Cadogan's Everyman).

Cadogan's *Dissertation on the Gout* drew upon some highly emotive views to assail established orthodoxies. For a man of such moment, surprisingly little is known of 'the Dissertator' – in this sense, Cadogan and Smollett are opposite. Born in 1711 of a South Wales family, he attended Oriel College, Oxford, graduating BA in 1731. Studying medicine, he visited the Continent and received his MD degree at Leiden in 1737, perhaps being taught by Albinus, Boerhaave's successor. After army service, he settled in Bristol and published *An Essay upon Nursing, and the Management of Children* (1748); shortly after being elected a Fellow of the Royal Society in 1752, he removed to London, where in 1754 he was appointed physician to the Foundling Hospital, lately established in pastoral Bloomsbury.[49] In the following June, he was granted his Oxford MD; in 1758 the College of Physicians elected him to membership, and six years later he delivered its Harveian oration.

Cadogan glided up the professional staircase, acquiring a house in fashionable George Street, Cavendish Square, and mingling in society. 'Dr Cadogan and his agreeable daughter have spent a day and a night here,' reported the blue-stocking Hannah More in 1777, writing from David Garrick's villa at Hampton; 'the Doctor gave me some lectures on Anatomy and assures me that I am now as well acquainted with secretion, concoction, digestion and assimilation as many a wise-looking man in a great big wig.'[50]

Cadogan's first significant work, *An Essay upon Nursing, and the Management of Children* (1748), proved hugely popular, nine editions appearing over the next twenty years. Building on Locke and other Enlightenment thinkers, he urged that delivery should take place in well-ventilated rooms; he forbade swaddling; above all, mothers should avoid wet-nurses. The tract thus deplored the threats to infant health created by ignorance and extravagance and urged a return to Nature.[51]

Cadogan's most celebrated if controversial work was to come: *A Dissertation on the Gout* (1771) became the talk of the town and sold ten editions in just two years.[52] Its message was simplicity itself: the causes of gout were idleness, intemperance and vexation. Contrary to conventional wisdom, the disease was thus neither hereditary nor incurable; it could be averted, remedied or at least relieved by adoption of a temperate regimen.

Cadogan's opinions created a furore. Precisely why is not immediately apparent since, though his views were quite radical, similar opinions had long been in the air, and physiological puritanism enjoyed a prestigious Hippocratic pedigree. Ever since Luigi Cornaro in Renaissance Venice, health enthusiasts had maintained that well-being hinged upon attention to regimen and the pursuit of frugality.[53] So long as man had tilled the soil and avoided pampering himself 'there were few or no Diseases', Richard Drake asserted in 1758; 'but when Luxury, Intemperance, and Indolence, came in Fashion, Diseases sprang up and multiplied'.[54]

As already discussed, in *An Essay on the True Nature and Due Method of Treating the Gout* (1722) and elsewhere George Cheyne maintained in the same vein that it was 'the *Rich*, the *Lazy*, the Voluptuous, who suffer most by the gout', revealing 'what astonishing Miseries *Wealth* and *Vice* bring upon Human Kind!'[55] That Cadogan echoed these refrains was pointed out by none less than the Great Cham of literature, Samuel Johnson, who considered his *Dissertation* was only 'Dr Cheyne's book told in a new way'.[56] Robert Campbell had similarly argued that in their primeval state humans were hearty and 'their Diseases were few',[57] but:

> as Vice and Immorality gained Ground, as Luxury and Laziness prevailed, and Men became Slaves to their own Appetites, new Affections grew up in their depraved Natures, new Diseases, and till then unheard of Distempers, both chronick and acute, assaulted their vitiated Blood.[58]

Gout occurred as 'Nature grew weak, and sunk under the Load of various Evils, with which Vice, Lust, and Intemperance had loaded her'.[59] Thus civilization begat disease, a theme echoed in John Wesley's popular *Primitive Physick* (1747).[60] In short, the temperance case was widely circulating and must have been utterly familiar to Cadogan, even had personal dealings not put two exponents of such views in his path.[61] One was 'Sir' John Hill, who, as noted in Chapter 5, viewed gout primarily as the wages of over-indulgence.[62] It is likely that Cadogan had direct links with that versatile medical botanist, since Hill's loyal friend William Stukeley was rector of St George's Bloomsbury, the parish church for the Foundling Hospital where Cadogan and Stukeley's associate Charles Morton were physicians.[63] As will be discussed below, on publication of Cadogan's *Treatise*, Hill was stung into response.

Another friend of temperance presumably known to Cadogan and upon whose writings he surely drew was William Buchan.[64] A health-care manual intended for popular consumption, Buchan's *Domestic Medicine* (1769) proved one of the evergreen medical bestsellers. Ordinary people, its author insisted, were capable of looking after their own health, precisely because infirmities were mainly self-inflicted. Let the sick observe modest lifestyles and they would mend.[65] Before Cadogan, Buchan blamed gout on over-eating, laziness and mental agitation:

> There is no disease which shews the imperfection of medicine, or sets the advantages of temperance and exercise in a stronger light than this. Few who pay a proper regard to these are troubled with the gout. This points out the true force from whence that malady originally sprung, *viz. excess* and *idleness*. It likewise shews us that the only safe and efficacious method of cure, or rather of prevention, must depend, not upon medicine, but on *temperance* and *activity*.[66]

Buchan also implicated psychological factors, notably 'intense study' and 'grief or uneasiness of mind'.[67] He tendered a clinical account derived from Sydenham[68] before proceeding to therapies. Orthodox in his view that 'there are no medicines, yet known, that will cure the gout', he confined his observations 'chiefly to regimen'.[69] It was 'dangerous to stop a fit of the gout by medicine', Buchan insisted, and so attempts should be made to recuperate the constitution 'by diet and exercise, as to lessen or totally prevent its return'. But by what means?

> In the first place *universal temperance*. In the next place, *sufficient exercise*. By this we do not mean sauntering about in an indolent manner, but labour, sweat, and toil . . . All strong liquors, especially generous wines and sour punch, are to be avoided.[70]

Buchan's sobering counsels appeared just two years before Cadogan's. It is hard to believe the latter had not read them, particularly in view of the fact that Buchan held an appointment at the Foundling Hospital's regional school at Ackworth in Yorkshire.

Echoing the philosophy of his baby-care book, Cadogan's *Dissertation* was a moralizing Enlightenment attack on luxury: following Nature's ways would produce not just bonny babies but gout-free adults too. Indeed, he intimated that intemperate habits were to blame for all chronic diseases whatsoever, promising in passing a comprehensive study, 'intended to take in the whole circle of Chronic Diseases', which it is tempting to suggest he proved too indolent to deliver.[71]

It was Cadogan's charge that the Quality lived dissipated lives while entertaining exaggerated expectations that medicines would rescue them from the bitter fruits of their vices. They must be schooled out of such stupidity.[72] Attitudes towards the body had become twisted by a feckless fatalism. The sick blithely renounced responsibility for their health, expecting medicines to do the trick, a strategy encouraged by mercenary physicians and their apothecary sidekicks, since it suited them that clients should regard diseases as predestined – curable, if at all, solely by professional ministrations. Disparaging the nostrums of practitioners who had puffed up their art into a solemn mystery, Cadogan offered pearls of wisdom: 'To enjoy good health is better than to command the world, says a celebrated practical philosopher.'[73]

It grieved him that folks – 'not the ignorant vulgar only, but the sensible, the judicious, men of parts' – should be so heedless of health and pursue the thousand and ten thousand idle arts and tricks of medication and quackery'.[74] In truth, men were fathers of their own fortunes, and they equally sired their own woes.[75] The *beau monde* contracted gout almost without a second thought, cheerfully embracing the libertine philosophy of 'a short life and a merry' and duping themselves into believing that the malady was foreordained by heredity and constitution.[76] Countering with his own diametrically opposite philosophy, he dispelled the legends:

> The gout is so common a disease, that there is scarcely a man in the world, whether he has had it nor not, but thinks he knows perfectly what it is. So does a cook-maid think she knows what fire is as well as Sir Isaac Newton. It may therefore seem needless at present to trouble ourselves about a definition, to say what it is: but I will venture to say what I am persuaded it is not, though contrary to the general opinion. It is not hereditary, it is not periodical, and it is not incurable.[77]

The paradigm-shift framing his entire theory – his personal Newtonian revolution – was that gout (and, by extension, all other chronic diseases) was not inherited. Had it been, 'it would be necessarily transmitted from father to son, and no man whose father had it could possibly be free from it: but this is not the case'.[78] Cadogan thus sought to demonstrate that the common model (hereditary, constitutional, periodical, incurable) flew in the face of facts – indeed, was at bottom a smokescreen: 'And as bankrupts, undone by idleness and extravagance, for ever plead losses and misfortunes; so do we inheritance, to exculpate ourselves.'[79]

Gout, Cadogan insisted, was curable – not by arcane medicines but by painstaking adherence to a proper regime based upon the simple recognition that the ailment was 'no more than each day's indigestion accumulated to a certain pitch'.[80] If gout was thus Nature's effort to disperse the dregs of intemperance, surely there was a better road to health.[81]

Believing gout stemmed from self-inflicted troubles, Cadogan itemized the factors particularly responsible. The first was 'indolence' – to counter which he offered elegant readers a somewhat diluted dose of Buchan's stiff medicine:

> It seems to have been the design of Providence that all men should labour, every one for himself . . . The rich and great have so far forgot this first principle of nature, that they renounce all bodily labour as unworthy their condition, and are either too lazy or too inattentive to substitute exercise instead of it.[82]

Without adequate exertion, the body stagnated, the humours putrefied and the insensible perspiration so crucial for keeping the body sweet ceased. There was no fathoming the quirks of fashionable folks who would 'chuse rather to take a vomit or a purge than a walk'.[83]

Alongside indolence, the second cause of gout was intemperance. Bingeing led to a secondary form of debauch, the craving for stimulants to brace the system:

> we want the whip and spur of luxury to excite our jaded appetites. There is no enduring the perpetual moping languor of indolence; we fly to the stimulating sensualities of the table and the bottle, friend provokes friend to exceed, and accumulate one evil upon another; a joyous momentary relief is obtained, to be paid for severely soon after; the next morning our horrors increase, and in this course there is no remedy but repetition. Thus whoever is indolent is intemperate also.[84]

Following a train of argument already spelt out by Cheyne and soon to be refined by Thomas Beddoes, Thomas Trotter and others, Cadogan condemned the epicure's enslavement to his stomach:

> He has recourse to dainties, sauces, pickles, provocatives of all sorts. These soon lose their power; and though he washes down each mouthful with a glass of wine, he can relish nothing. What is to be done? Send for a physician. Doctor, I have lost my stomach; pray give me, says he, with great innocence and ignorance, something to give me an appetite; as if want of appetite was a disease to be cured by art.[85]

Cadogan was thus firing broadsides against luxurious lifestyles in general, but he also sniped at individual targets, including mustard, vinegar and pickles; bread (too acid); and above all wine.[86]

He then divulged his third cause, albeit one less menacing in gouty than in other chronic conditions: 'every great degree of vexation, whether in the shape of anger, envy, resentment, discontent or sorrow, has most destructive and deleterious effects upon the vitals of the body, whether sudden and violent, or slow and lasting'.[87] Moral causes produced physical effects, anxiety destroyed the stomach.

What remedies did he have to offer? Prevention was better than cure. Given that 'whoever will reflect with some degree of intelligence and sanity' could 'trace his complaints and diseases up to one or other of these three causes', it was clear that recourse to quack medicines must be hopeless.[88] Medicines might palliate, but too often at the cost of permanent constitutional damage. In view of this, Cadogan inquired: 'What then is to be done?',[89] before revealing that solutions were fortunately to hand:

> I have already shewn that the causes of these evils are Indolence, Intemperance, and Vexation: and if there be any truth or weight in what I have said, the remedies are obvious: Activity, Temperance, and Peace of Mind. It will be said the remedies are obvious, but impracticable. Would you bid the feeble cripple, who cannot stand, take up his bed and walk? the man who has lost all appetite, abstain? and the sleepless wretch racked with pain enjoy peace of mind? No certainly; I am not absurd. These must be assisted by medicine.[90]

These almost utopian prospects (simple means, sensational results) created quite a stir. Cadogan was promising deliverance for sufferers – but hadn't boosters and quacks long done that? He was proposing a new regime based upon diet, exercise and tranquillity – but surely nobody could have any quarrel with such time-honoured truths: time out of mind, simple living and plain fare had been the regimen-mongers' stock-in-trade. The article of faith that truly put the cat among the pigeons was Cadogan's denial that gout was destiny: 'It is not hereditary, it is not periodical, and it is not incurable.'[91] Far from being a constitutional disorder, gout was thus an upstart, an intruder lacking title deeds. 'It is by their own fault that they are ill,' Cadogan accused the gouty point-blank.[92]

It may seem perverse that objections rang up to heaven against the *prima facie* good news that deliverance was to hand. Did the gouty, used to Cheyne's playful badinage, resent Cadogan's no-nonsense victim-blaming? Moreover his views surely smacked of radicalism, with their insinuation that the malady was not to be humoured but rather eliminated through a bold moral purge. No inescapable 'disease of progress', gout was the price of profligacy – and not gout alone, but a Pandora's box of other misnamed constitutional conditions. 'I say this to invalids in general,' Cadogan boldly pressed, 'for thus may be cured not only the gout, but very bad rheumatisms, ischiaticas, rickets, stone, jaundice, dropsy, asthma, cachexies, and complications of many kind; not excepting even cancers, if they are not too far gone.'[93] But there was to be no redemption without reform.

The *Dissertation on the Gout* stirred up a hornet's nest. It was one thing to propose the blessings of moderation, another to assert that temperance would stave off a specific disease, and more presumptuous still to fly in the face of podagric pedigree, and deny gout was hereditary.

Cadogan did not want for critics. In questioning the hereditary principle and the mores of magnates, he touched a nerve. As with modern anti-smoking campaigns, the wisdom of the advice might be hard to rebut, but extenuating circumstances could be pleaded, defiance asserted and black humour extracted from desperate dicing with disease. 'My belly is as big as Ever,' exclaimed the gouty David Garrick,

> I cannot quit Peck and Booze. – What's Life without sack and sugar! My lips were made to be lick'd, and if the Devil appears to me in the Shape of Turbot and Claret, my crutches are forgot, and I laugh and Eat . . . A Dr. Cadogan has written a pamphlet lately upon ye Gout, it is much admired and has certainly It's merit – I was frightened with it for a Week; but as Sin will outpull repentance when there are passions and palates, I have postponed the Dr.'s Regimen.[94]

Others were doubtless frightened for a week, and they too perhaps displaced their fears through nervy railery at Cadogan's expense. 'Burn the books of Hippocrates, Galen, Celsus, Sydenham, Musgrave, Boerhaave, Hoffman, and all other rubbish of Greek, Latin, Arabic and modern physicians,' bantered John Shebbeare, author of a *Candid Enquiry*:

> And then, let every regular, semi-regular and irregular practitioner, whether he be mounted in a chariot, on a stage or walk on foot; whether he advertise his medicines or himself, be hanged. Yes, my good readers, hang Wintringham, hang Heberden, hang Addington; but for *honest Will. Cadogan*, real *Will. Cadogan*, Liberal *Will. Cadogan*, rational *Will. Cadogan*, and therefore the more *rational*, being as he is, new *Will. Cadogan*, hang not him; save honest Will. And hang all the rest.[95]

Shebbeare's rodomontade accused Cadogan of astonishing conceit in expecting to destroy with a fusillade of blanks a medical citadel that had stood for centuries.[96]

The Cadogan brouhaha is captured in miniature by a droll anonymous poem entitled *The Doctor Dissected: or Willy Cadogan in the Kitchen. Addressed* to all *Invalids, and Readers of a late Dissertation on the Gout, etc. etc, etc. By a Lady,* carrying the equivocal byline: 'The best of all Doctors is sweet Willy O'. This carving up of Cadogan contemplated the revolution in kitchen politics his writings would wreak:

> The Town are half mad (you have heard without doubt)
> For a book that is called *Dissertation on Gout,*
> That king of diseases, no longer endure,
> Adhere to its rule − fee a radical cure![97]

The poet (apparently a Mrs Ireland) made the observation that, in protest against Cadogan's counsels of temperance, all the high-livers in town had mutinied:

> The author, to Styx, in a sulphurous flame,
> They'd waft, and extirpate the breed and the name:
> But, least he poor wight, shou'd oblivion lie snug in,
> Without further preface − 'tis *Willy Cadogan.*[98]

Stressing Cadogan's heretical views, the rhymes drew attention to the subversive pseudo-political implications of his medical admonitions:

> 'And tho' his opinion is, *contradicente.*'
> To those of the faculty, nineteen in twenty:
> 'He still will maintain, that from father to son,
> 'Like estate that's entail'd, it by no means doth run . . .'[99]

   She made play of the fact that Cadogan looked to a levelling down of lifestyle − a transformation that would not only spell the end of gourmet living for the *bon viveur* but also require a collective forswearing by the Great of their dignity and superiority: farewell to civilization, back to native wildness:

> This first state of nature you now must pursue,
> For medical aid, it is plain, will not do;
> Use manual labor, walk many a mile,
> Or pester'd you'll be, − with gout, cholic, and bile.
> For nature alone by brisk exercise thrives,
> A new lease it will give the most desperate lives.[100]

If, as the rather Mandevillian poetess noted, the implication of accepting Cadogan's creed was the overthrow of good society, similarly revolutionary consequences were in store for medicine too: Cadogan was brandishing a new broom, sweeping away traditional Galenic physicians and quacks alike, and so wrecking careers:

> Beware of pretenders to physical myst'ry,
> Nor let 'em phlebotomize, sweat, or e'en blister ye,
> Avoid, like a pestilence, ignorant Quacks,
> From those in gild chariots, – to plain simple hacks.
> Disciples of Galen, all shut up your shops,
> No need, have we now, of your balsams or drops;
> Dear volatiles, cordials, and bracers, adieu!
> Ye all must give place, to a system quite new.[101]

In short, here was a medical vandal, bringing down the pillars of the temple of Aesculapius.[102]

Above all, the poet found it shocking that Cadogan's revolutionary doctrines presumed to challenge ancestral gracious living and the civilized arts of cuisine and cellar:

> All lovers of goose, duck, or pig, he'll engage,
> That eat it with onion, salt, pepper, and sage,
> Will find ill effects from't, and therefore no doubt,
> Their prudence shou'd tell them – best eat it without.[103]

Cadogan was thus a killjoy in pursuit of idiosyncratic puritanism.[104] No friend of the table, in truth he wanted the tables turned – not (as with the Wilkite artisan radicals vocal in the 1760s)[105] in the name of Justice or Liberty but in the cause of health:

> Physicians, I beg, of all rank, and degrees,
> You'll learn the new method of getting your fees:
> Politeness discard, and adopt in its stead,
> The manner now practis'd of being well bred:
> Tell your patients their folly deprives them of health,
> And prefer honest bluntness to fame and to wealth . . .[106]

Amid the commotion, one who with customary perspicacity grasped what was distinctive about Cadogan was Samuel Johnson: he had denied that gout was hereditary.[107] Johnson hit the nail on the head. Despite being a fashionable, wealthy London physician, Cadogan was committing a social *faux pas*, almost as bad as questioning a gentleman's parentage, by tampering with the hereditary system in disease and impugning gout's honour. No wonder rebuttals came thick and fast.

One volley was fired by John Hill, who took the view that, insofar as Cadogan was correct, he was a plagiarist and, insofar as he was original, he was mistaken. To spike Cadogan's guns, in 1771 he reissued his 1758 book, *The Management of the Gout*, under the revised title, *The Management of the Gout in Diet, Exercise and Temper*, thus incorporating reference to Cadogan's trinity to create the impression of having pre-empted him.[108] While these elements had indeed been present in previous editions, Hill now gave them, especially temper, higher prominence. Thus the 1758 statement 'Altho' rich food and little exercise naturally will in time bring on the gout; they have not this effect universally' became, in the 1771 edition, 'Although rich food, little exercise, and sorrow, may often in time bring on the gout originally; they have not this effect universally.'[109] The ploy amounted to a practised art, part and parcel of Hill's masterful techniques of self-puffery. He was evidently seeking to convince readers that it had been he all along who had emphasized vexation as well as indolence and intemperance.

Voicing familiar arguments, Hill also stressed that gout victims tended to be people of the '*best constitutions*', gout being an inheritance:

> Will any conduct, any application of the powers of the mind, or any regimen of life and diet, keep the man always sober, in whose family there is *hereditary madness*? Has any one seen *hereditary Leprosies* kept from appearing to the latest generations? Men therefore smiled with equal reason at the venerable and honest ancient, who thought the Gout was not hereditary; and thought it could be cured.[110]

Some were more disposed to gout than others, and from that the educated and elegant classes should learn a lesson, for 'LABOUR preserves the poor from the gout by the assistance which it gives the circulation . . . What the peasant finds from labour, and the nobleman seeks from exercise, is to prevent thick fluids stagnating and lodging on particular parts.'[111] In the light of this state of constitutional affairs, Hill pointed to three possible avenues to health: labour (for the poor); exercise (for the earnest among the wealthy); and his favourite Burdock tea, for everybody, but above all for the *beau monde* disinclined to exercise. Burdock root was not a 'cure', Hill conceded, for gout 'never can be cured'; all the same, 'assisting nature in any degree this way, must and will, and does alleviate that which nothing can cure'.[112]

As well as demonstrating that he had anticipated Cadogan, Hill relished exposing his errors. Cadogan had, for instance, contended that meat was more digestible rare than well cooked because it was thus closer to the natural state. For Hill, following Stukeley, such reversion to Nature was silliness, a sure sign that Cadogan did not know where to draw the line.[113]

While concurring with Cadogan on temperance, Hill believed he had committed one cardinal error: he had denied the condition was hereditary. He responded by including an additional defence of his longstanding belief that gout was, on the contrary, bequeathed:

> We bring the seeds of it often into the world with us, together with the materials of that strength; and though intemperance encreases it always, and

often brings it on before its time; no regularity of life can obviate its appearance, where there is that parental taint, at some time or other.[114]

Most of the other rejoinders – like John Berkenhout's *Dr. Cadogan's Dissertation on the Gout Examined and Refuted* (1772), William Carter's *A Free and Candid Examination of Dr. Cadogan's Dissertation on the Gout* (1772) and William Falconer's *Observations on Dr. Cadogan's Dissertation on the Gout* (1772) – also focused on the succession question.[115] All upheld the disease's hereditary title; all rebutted Cadogan's claim that gout was essentially caused by lifestyle – and so could by the same means be eliminated. The anonymous *Reflections on the GOUT With Observations on Some Parts of DR. CADOGAN'S Pamphlet*, for instance, hit the mark:

> The next bold and different opinion of Dr. Cadogan, is, that the gout is not hereditary. One would expect from a man thus differing from all others, something new of the nature or history of the disease, that would to sound reasoning and just philosophy, seem to support such an opinion, but Dr. Cadogan puts forth his original doctrine of his own, naked and defenceless . . . The gout must be looked upon as a hereditary disease.[116]

The pamphleteer thus believed that the anti-hereditary tirade was empirically flawed.[117] He also attacked Cadogan for singling out 'vexation' – a most implausible view given that gout 'is mostly found with those, on whom the heavy hand of fortune has not heap'd affliction'.[118]

Marmaduke Berdoe's *An Essay on the Nature and Causes of the Gout* (1772) similarly countered Cadogan by declaring there was 'an hereditary disposition to the disorder we are treating'. Hence traditional therapeutic caution was wise: 'How absurd all attempts to cure a confirmed gout.' Berdoe restated the ensconced belief that 'cure' was worse than the disease. 'Who indeed would wish for a cure, when the consequence might produce either a dropsy or consumption?'[119] Gout was simply one of those afflictions, symptomatic of superiority, which 'sprightly and sensible persons' had to learn to bear.[120] Like other traditionalists, he pointed out the advantage in the disadvantage: 'The gout may, and does often supply the place of the hemorrhoids . . . it screens the patient from other dangerous diseases.'[121] As Nature's escape duct, gout should be welcomed, and supplemented by other depletive methods.[122]

Physiologically functional, gout was thus a blessing, and 'far from dreading the appearance of the gout, we ought on the contrary to consider it as a salutary effort of nature'.[123] Overall, according to Berdoe, it was thus an eligible affliction, 'For if this disorder is once properly characterized, the patient is out of danger.'[124] Better piles than gout, but better gout than the 'various inconveniences [which] depend then upon the surcharge of the abdominal viscera, one of the most frequent disorders incident to the human constitution'.[125] Gout was thus, he insisted, an inherent condition, 'produced, therefore by any circumstance which changes the functions in the organs of the body'.[126] Once gout had taken root, 'the cure cannot be attempted but with danger'.[127]

Further reinforcements for orthodoxy came from William Carter. His *A Free and Candid Examination of Dr. Cadogan's Dissertation on the Gout, and Chronic Diseases* (1772) warned readers against slavishly following 'the Dissertator' – not least, he waggishly urged, on those vexatious and momentous questions of salt, vinegar and mustard: evidently Cadogan's crusade against condiments was collapsing into a dinner-party joke.[128] Like other critics, Carter took umbrage at Cadogan's setting himself up as the man to expose his profession while delivering the tablets of health to the people. Once the ballyhoo had died down, there was nothing so very 'oracular' about 'the Doctor's speech', with all its sententious pronouncements to the effect that *'health is not to be established by medicine'*.[129] The worthwhile bits were all old hat and its novel teachings were fallacious. Above all, Carter countered, gout must be understood as *'sometimes hereditary'* and *'periodical'*.[130]

Furthermore, Cadogan's programme was severely limited in applicability: only to the as yet untouched might it prove serviceable, for what he 'has hitherto published to the world, seems rather *calculated to prevent, than to cure the fit'*.[131] What point preaching spartan temperance to *bon viveurs* in bathchairs? For 'persons afflicted with the gout are generally joyous; love their bottle and their friends, and to take them off intirely from *wine*, must be a penance, few, or none, will submit to'.[132]

What's more, it was queer that Cadogan had been so puritanical about venison while silent about vice: 'Can a man be intemperate in victuals, and drink only? May he not riot, and revel in company with Venus, as well as with Bacchus, and Ceres?'[133] He had no doubt that 'excess in VENERY contributes not a little to frequent returns of the gout'.[134]

In recalling gout's venereal roots, Carter was departing from the new Enlightenment exonerations of erotic permissiveness proclaimed by Blackmore and Hill, and reinstating Hippocratic orthodoxy. Even so, he eschewed Cadogan's Welsh censoriousness: pleasures and pains were interwoven in life's rich tapestry, and strict Cadoganian physical puritanism was in error, for *'the abuse* of things, *not the use* of them, is to be condemned'.[135] Carter liked to parade as a realist: Cadogan's creed might suit utopia, but in this sublunary existence it was vain to expect *l'homme moyen sensuel* to trade vice for virtue overnight. Rather than offering counsels of perfection it was more sensible to furnish palliatives.[136] The physician should not mount the pulpit, his place was at the bedside.[137] Cadogan's sanctimonious sermons were mocked by Carter: he had become fixated on footling dietary foibles. Foodstuffs harmlessly eaten for centuries (indeed, those hallowed in the Christian sacraments) had now, all of a sudden, in his holier-than-thou scaremongering, been revealed to be amazingly injurious:

The Author of the Dissertation has been so lucky as to discover, that BREAD and WINE *are pernicious*, and destructive of health; another gentleman has lately found out, that NATURE has made *water too impure* . . . and great pity it is, that nobody has hitherto arisen to speak in favour of ACORNS.[138]

Take your pick, Carter implied: you could, if you please, go back to Nature and pursue, with Jean-Jacques Rousseau and Cadogan, the thorny life of the healthy savage; or, he implied, you could follow plain common sense. Though Cadogan's heart was doubtless in the right place, he concluded on a note of cheery condescension, his feet weren't on the ground: 'what is said of Homer, that *the good man sometimes nods* is applicable to the Author of the Dissertation'.[139]

As is by now obvious, the first commandment in anti-Cadogan circles was the hereditary nature of gout. The anonymous *Reflections on the Gout* maintained along these lines that 'the gout must be looked upon a hereditary disease',[140] as did Sir James Jay's *Reflections and Observations on the Gout* (1772), which declared that 'in a genuine Gout, it is evident, there is a disposition in the constitution,' on account of which 'radical cure is not to be expected' – radicalism evidently spelt quackery.[141] Jay furthermore accused Cadogan of indulging in extravagant speculation and *a priori* system-building – errors symptomatic of intellectual adolescence – and surveyed the long-running curability debate. Indirect evidence that, *pace* Cadogan, gout truly was incurable lay in the array of quack nostrums on offer – he could thereby hint that Cadogan was a distant cousin to the mountebanks.[142] His denial of natural pathogenesis and predilection for nurture were erroneous. Not all blame could be laid on lifestyle; gout was more than an acquired disease, for 'in a genuine Gout, it is evident, there is a disposition in the constitution . . . to produce and accumulate gouty matter'. Proof lay in the fact that 'if there was not such a disposition in the body, a person, after he had got rid of one fit, would not fall into another'.[143] The gouty predisposition was thus real. Yet this might find expression quite distinctly in different individuals. In line with humoralism, Jay emphasized gout's protean personality, which meant that a zodiac of symptoms could all stem from it.[144] Jay thus fully subscribed to the 'healing power of the gout' creed. Yet, despite its lability, he condemned as fatalistic the prejudice that, because gout was constitutional, all treatments whatsoever were automatically trivial or counterproductive. Far from it.[145]

Jay would hobble along with Cadogan so far as to censure *The Honour of the Gout* and insist that, though 'a radical cure is not to be expected', something could and should be done; but he parted company on the importance of the physician's intervention, arguing that 'it seems not unreasonable to think, that Gouts . . . may be greatly palliated, if not intirely cured, by the judicious application of medicine, and a suitable way of life'.[146]

Similar sentiments were digested in Richard Kentish's *Advice to Gouty Persons* (1789). Countering Cadogan he advised arthritics – he was one himself – to cling fast to their 'tenure' upon their 'enviable possession'; gout was a 'patrimony', the 'hereditary right' which had been denied by the levelling Cadogan and his followers.[147]

As these overtly political allusions make clear, the gout war was being waged in a climate of mounting alarm respecting threats to the British constitution. In the 1760s, George III and his favourite sometime Prime Minister Lord Bute seemed to Whigs like Edmund Burke to be sabotaging the constitution; Bute in turn provoked Wilkite radicalism, with its accusations that the constitution had been undermined by the King and his secret cabinets – though others deemed the true threat to the constitution lay in street-fighting mobs. The American Revolution followed, and 'constitution in danger' anxieties then culminated in the shockwaves following the French Revolution. In the 1790s, new-broom Whigs called not for the defence of the existing constitution – it had already, they claimed, been fatally compromised and was little more than a mouldering ruin – but its resurrection in the name of political reformation and authentic liberty. 'Who will be hardy enough to assert', demanded Sir James Mackintosh, 'that a better Constitution is not attainable than any which has hitherto appeared?' Ministries and their supporters leapt to constitutional rescue. In such electrically charged ideological climates it became a badge of loyalism to vindicate the 'honour of the gout' as supportive of the status quo, and rally to the defence of its ancient constitution no less than the British.[148] It was not hard for conservatives to descry in Cadogan's almost Rousseauvian call for an end to high living and a grand purge of luxurious lifestyles an assault upon everything English, a threat to the established constitution, and a questioning of the old order.

Cadogan also had his supporters, or at least physicians making reinforcing contributions to the controversy upon gout and other diseases of civilization. One intervention worth examining in some detail came from the Aberdeen practitioner William Grant, whose Scottish sensibilities clearly paralleled those of Cheyne and Buchan while also apparently giving vent to certain distinctive tenets deriving from the Scottish Enlightenment.

Though fundamentally differing from Cadogan on certain doctrines, Grant's *Some Observations on the Origins, Progress, and Method of Treating the Atrabilious Temperament and Gout* (1779) endorsed his view that chronic disorders demanded attention, originating as they did:

> from some very remote cause, lurking in the constitution long before the disease is developed; which being neglected, the whole constitution becomes gradually, and almost imperceptibly altered: so that many of the chronic diseases are not confined to one organ, or to one humour, but the

whole constitution is affected so much, that they may be called constitutional diseases; and this is the reason why so many of them are hereditary.[149]

Hereditariness and constitutionality were two sides of the same coin: 'for we find', asserted Grant, 'that as the constitutional diseases are often hereditary, so the hereditary diseases are always constitutional'.[150] Cadogan was mistaken as to the source of gout, which had 'its remote cause . . . in the constitution, many years before the formation of a fit'. But, while insisting that gout was constitutional and hereditary, Grant nonetheless believed, rather idiosyncratically, that it was also curable, though 'to cure it' the 'remote cause must be investigated, and then removed'.[151]

With this ambitious plan in mind (seemingly to eliminate a hereditary disorder by rooting it out), Grant proposed to 'ascertain this remote cause'.[152] This required painting the panorama of what we would call the historical sociology of sickness, drawing upon those theories of the paradoxes of progress popular in Scottish Enlightenment circles.[153] Grant's precise intellectual debts are hard to gauge, for his claim was that it was first-hand experience that gave him his leads, teaching him that gout was rare among the rugged and the ragged:

> when I was a young man in the Highlands of Scotland, I hardly ever saw a man able to breed the gout; there is not a word for it in the language of that country. I have known hundreds of strong men there, who have debauched themselves with wine and spirituous liquors daily and regularly for many years together; some have lived to old age; others, by their excesses, have shortened their lives, and contracted a variety of diseases, but never the gout.[154]

Distribution patterns provided plain hints respecting gout's nature and aetiology. The malady was 'very rare' in the 'south and high parts of France', despite the fact that 'they drink wine diluted with water, in prodigious quantities, from morning to night'. It was also 'uncommon' in Spain and Portugal, and on the island of Madeira it was 'confined to the English'. It was 'hardly to be met with' in Russia or the Islamic world; while 'even Egypt and Greece, formerly the seats of empire, arts, and luxury, as well as gout, are now free from all the atrabilious complaints'.[155] Moreover the tropics were free of 'the atrabilious complaints'. A disease of 'people of fashion', it was the great cities of north-western Europe that formed the matrix of gout and kindred bilious diseases.

For this Grant had a pet explanation. Gout was worst 'where people live much on the diseased flesh of pampered animals, fatted in stalls, without air or exercise', whereas, in striking contrast, 'the labouring and common people, even here, are almost exempted', because of their lenten fare.[156] The conclusion was indisputable: 'the gout arises from foul and luxurious eating'.[157]

A conditional reprieve was thus granted to alcohol, despite authorities like Sydenham.[158] In upland areas 'where they all debauch in spirituous liquors', gout was rare. The explanation? – 'their meat is lean, and animal food is not plenty'. Yet alcohol did not get a completely clean bill of health, for though not 'sufficient to produce the gout', yet 'it will assist in the formation of gout, and greatly exasperate a formed gout, unless the excess is worked off by daily hard labour'. On this last point, Grant was of a mind with Buchan and Cadogan.[159] Liquor was thus an accomplice, but over-eating, especially of rich and refined foods, was the prime offender. Gourmandizing was a dire health threat when combined with the indolence ever worsening among civilized society with the 'neglect of going on foot; the encrease of carriages; the high finishing of roads, rooms, and furniture; the softness of beds; the anxiety, vexation, and frequent disappointment introduced amongst us by the encrease of commerce, politics, and gaming' – all contributed to 'the encrease of atrabilious diseases'.[160]

Conviction that dining on stall-fed meat precipitated gout prompted Grant to a profoundly unflattering analogy between animal husbandry and the civilizing process. Poultry-cramming was city living *in parvo*, high society a chicken coop. The consequence of force-feeding was great:

> which will readily appear, by only comparing the *viscera* of fatted with those of lean animals; *e.g.* of two turkies; the one brought up in the natural manner . . . the other shut up in a coop, without light, free air, or exercise, carefully fed and pampered in a warm house.
>
> The first is not so very large, weighing perhaps ten pounds only; his flesh is red and hard; his tendons round, small, and hard; his bones thin, small, and hard; his joints small, and the ligaments thin and smooth; his *alphage*, or crop, small; his gizzard small, thick, tendinous, firm, and wonderfully rough on the inside; his liver firm, and weighing nearly three ounces.
>
> On the contrary, the fed turkey is large and heavy, from sixteen to twenty-six pounds; his flesh is white, soft, and tender; his joints are large, and the ligaments thick, soft, and fleshy . . . his liver is of a prodigious size, weighing from nine to sixteen ounces, and so soft that, when boiled, you may break it down with the back of a spoon, and mix it with your sauce, like chocolate: if suffered to live long, he becomes gouty, and unable to walk.[161]

Urban man was in effect a gobbling, waddling turkey bred in the great metropolitan broiler-house.[162] By contrast, Scottish peasants, like ten-pounders, were the very pictures of health – 'their bodies are light, their motion quick, their wind is good'.[163] Crofters were also long-lived: 'The diseases of such people are few.'[164]

The spry and wiry crofter afforded a complete contrast to the sickly lounger. Grant lingered over the pathology of decadence. 'His chamber is close, his bed soft, his coverings many, his sleep is long, his meals are regular, plentiful, frequent, and full of variety' – that was the pampered young milord. Besides, Grant added, harping on a favourite topic, 'he eats the flesh of animals highly fed, and for the most part diseased, and is tempted to overload his stomach'. You are what you eat, and so Mr Idler turned into a turkey: 'fat, heavy, and bloated; his skin soft, fair, and extended; his muscles soft, smooth, and larded with fat',[165] and the 'whole nervous system easily moved upon slight occasions':[166]

> If he is suffered to remain costive for some length of time . . . he begins to complain of flatulence and indigestion, piles, arthritic pains, or gout; at other times thick wind, suffocation, stuffing in the glands, and even apoplexy; which, if it should not prove fatal, is often succeeded by palsy.[167]

Among such specimens, gout was not only frequent but had assumed a hereditary character. Cadogan might not agree – but Grant claimed the backing of 'experience'.[168] He was thus clarifying the dialectic of Nature and nurture. Like other diseases of civilization, gout was precipitated by environment and habit, but over the generations it would grow hereditary. The upshot was that 'to cure it radically the whole constitution must be altered'.[169]

This had important therapeutic implications. So-called panaceas, specifics and palliatives were quite useless.[170] How could any 'reasonable man' believe such a rooted and intricate disease would yield to any single drug? 'Surely Sydenham could not seriously hope, that such a specific should exist in *rerum natura*, since the destruction of the miraculous tree of life.'[171]

Gout defied specifics and Grant predictably drew attention to the dangers of 'quacking' – the quick-fix folly typical of a lazy civilization: it was then and only then that gout was liable to prove life-threatening.[172] But Grant dissociated himself from the equally lazy doctrine that gout was Nature's safety valve or bodyguard – such self-serving rationalizations merely compounded the crime and undermined health.[173] Far from a blessing, gout was a blight. But if there were no specifics, and quacking was folly, what alternative was there? The answer – here Grant trod in Cadogan's footsteps – lay in prevention.[174]

Echoing Enlightenment opinions, Grant urged readers to harden their children, then atrabilious and other constitutional diseases would wither away.[175] The human condition thus presented a paradox. The Lord had put it into man's power to become the 'most active, most hardy, and, by the same means, the most healthy and long lived of animals':

> if men will abuse the blessings of Providence, if, instead of satisfying the real demands of nature, they will give way to the gratification of a

luxurious and reprobate sense, they have no right to expect the blessings of good health, nor the satisfaction of a numerous, healthy posterity.[176]

The choice was simple. Gout might be hereditary, but that did not mean it was inevitable or irresistible. Hereditary diseases could be *disinherited*, through adopting 'the most proper means of rearing children, so as to give them better constitutions than their parents'.[177]

But was there then no *cure* at all? Growing expansive, Grant conjured up a grand vision of the opportunity presented to civilized man to recuperate his compromised health, by making a fresh start:

He that means to cure the gout radically, and what I call *secundum artem*, must strictly observe the following rules:

1. He must quit the flat, fertile, cultivated plains, during the summer season, every year . . .

2. Learn to amuse himself with country diversions . . .

3. Avoid populous towns and great cities . . .

4. Keep to regular hours of exercise, eating and sleeping; short sleep is best, on hard beds, in the early part of the night.

5. Let his apartments be large, lofty, ill-finished, and well warmed by strong fires.

6. He will soon feel the advantage of frequent bathing, much friction, and warm clothing.

7. His diet must be in proportion to his exercise . . .

8. The best common drink is cold water . . .

9. When he eats heartily at dinner, he ought to eat no supper, but suffer the stomach to be quite empty once in twenty-four hours.

10. He must be well rubbed all over every night and morning . . .

11. When he is quite free from all complaint, sea-bathing, or even cold-bathing, will agree with most people, to restore the strength.

12. But in all situations he must take care to keep his body regular . . .

By such means as these, properly conducted, and steadily prosecuted for a length of time, a man of observation . . . will, in general, radically cure any recent gout, always moderate it, never injure his natural state of health, or shorten his life.[178]

Grant's rules almost coincide with Matthew Bramble's self-imposed therapy for recovery: from the arrival in high Scottish terrains to mild remedies for his own costiveness. Despite this agenda for the recovery of perfect health by going back to Nature, Grant wryly added that he did not 'expect . . . every one of my friends to observe all these directions literally'.[179]

The second half of his book was devoted to the far more critical question of 'Irregular and Complicated Gout'.[180] Its causes were 'improper regimen' and 'improper treatment during the fits';[181] and it came in six varieties.[182] All were characterized by internal lability. While regular gout was barnacle-like, 'in the wandering gout, the pain moves from the extremities to the articulations of the spine, ribs, clavicles, or lower jaw'.[183] Treatment required banishment, 'to divert the fluxion towards the extremities'.[184] There was however a limit to this technique. The joints would finally choke up totally,[185] forcing it inwards and producing 'complicated gout', a grave matter, generally beyond cure.[186]

While not seeing absolutely eye to eye with Cadogan, Grant thus framed gout within the 'diseases of civilization' paradigm, accentuated his critique of modern decadence and called for moral and medical reform. 'Gout did not exist before men had made a considerable progress in luxury.' Once established, however, it was 'hereditary'. This hereditary disposition notwithstanding, 'the gout is curable at a proper time of life, before the disease is become inveterate, or the constitution broken by age or infirmity'. But it could become incurable. Circumspection was essential, for what was truly dangerous was reckless treatment:

> I have seen many gouty people die of apoplexy; I know many who recovered from the apoplexy, and are now paralytic; but still, by strict enquiry, I have been able to discover, that they have brought on those calamities by the wrong treatment of their gout.[187]

Grant thus seized the middle ground, approving of Cadogan's 'country party' stress on simple, healthy living, yet, perhaps because of his Scottish philosophical orientation, stressing the historical and hereditary character of the condition.

Practitioners of a militant tendency in physic or politics enlisted in Cadogan's colours, believing the times were out of joint, and blaming the upsurge of gout upon dissolute patients and deceitful physicians. One such was the radical, anti-Pitt Bristol physician Thomas Beddoes, who epitomized Cadogan by asserting that 'our chronic maladies are of our own creating'.[188] A caustic critic of health faddery and medical jobbery, Beddoes dismissed all the talk about constitutional disorders as cant and obfuscation. 'In attempting to speak of this disorder, one feels as if on *tabooed* ground.' The public had 'unlearned' false opinions with regard to other disorders, but was 'trapped in a superstitious habit of thinking on the subject of the gout'. The orthodox construal of gout as 'a disorder, with which it is impossible to interfere without the most imminent peril – the *noli me tangere* of constitutional affections', was a case of medical obscurantism reinforcing reactionary political dogmas. All stemmed from a 'dread of innocent or effectual remedies', by which Beddoes meant the duty of the affluent to shape up: 'Can it really deserve to be regarded in the favourable light it usually is? Is it reasonable to desire, and wise to cherish, such a complaint?'[189]

He was not alone. In *A Treatise on the Gout* (1792), Thomas Jeans contended that gout was normally 'the painful fruits of our own misconduct'. In the light of this, he twirled the truism on its toes. Far from being constitutional, gout was the 'inimical tyrant of our constitutions' – or, as might have been said, it was unconstitutional. Jeans sought a radical corrective, not because gout attacked the '*fruges consumeri nati*' – why shed tears over them? – but because it afflicted 'the wise, the studious, and the great: – those on whose abilities the progress of letters, the advancement of science, and even the welfare of the state depends'.[190] Jeans therefore backed the radical 'shape up, slim down' Cadogan line. Gout had increased, was increasing and ought to be diminished: any other view was fatalistic and reactionary. 'Gout has generally been deemed an hereditary, periodical, and incurable disease,' he grumbled; 'it has been considered too, by many, as salutary to the constitution, and therefore to be borne, however severe and frequent.' This last notion, with its corollary that 'a fit of the gout is rather a relief than a danger to the constitution', was perverse piffle, offering as it did not 'present relief' but spurious consolation. Such pious fantasies befitted 'only the irresolute and weak', whereas 'the energy of superior minds . . . revolts at the restraint which a torturing malady imposes . . . and willingly offers its agonizing limbs to the salutary intentions of science'.[191] Not to believe gout curable was pusillanimous. Hence, 'if health be this blessing, and disease its opposite evil', it was the nation's duty to face up to a public disgrace.[192] Merely because gout had not been cured it was absurd to pronounce it incurable.[193]

Echoing Cadogan, Jeans denied the hereditary nature of gout and all its quasi-political passive-obedience implications.[194] Such views merely sanctioned laziness. The received view that 'gout is an hereditary disease . . . is by no means to be reconciled to the oeconomy of nature';[195] it was much oftener the 'painful fruits of our own misconduct'.[196] The incurability doctrine was a medical scandal, standing 'at the head of the *Opprobria Medicorum*'.[197] Jeans reminded readers of Sydenham's hint that we might 'expect a future discovery of the means by which Gout may be cured'.[198] Action was essential because if improperly treated it would turn into 'anomalous gout',[199] a condition not to be brushed aside with a jest: 'in what sense to be taken, is that trite observation, that a fit of *the* Gout preserves its sufferers from other, and often more serious diseases – *Diva Podagra Pharmacum amarissimum Naturæ*'.[200]

Thus medical hereditarianism was unmasked as a reactionary ploy, and nowhere more so than in *A Successful Method of Treating the Gout by Blistering* (1779) by William Stevenson, who struck at the idol of inheritance root and branch. Stevenson used his blistering *opus* to speak plain about the dialectics of civilization, sickness and doctoring:

VITA BREVIS, ARS LONGA, is an adage no less just than sarcastic and humiliating. The older men grow, they see the propriety of it the more.

Physic, like other practical sciences, began on simple principles at first. In the progress of society, the cultivation of land, and commercial intercourse among nations, the science of physic underwent material changes, along with the manners of the people; and as these grew more civilized, effeminate, and luxurious, physic became a more intricate, complex, and laborious study, more interesting to society, and more lucrative to its professors.[201]

Progress thus exacted its price, and sickness was nature's sanction against folly, vice and greed: 'Diseases are but constitutional efforts to throw off redundances from the system . . . The multiplication, therefore, of diseases, is in consequence of our multiplying the indulgences of life.'[202] Rather than embracing a sounder philosophy of living, mankind, chid Stevenson, had resigned itself to the melancholy melodrama of mortality.[203]

With some pathos, Stevenson conjured up his new English Dance of Death, with the Grim Reaper harvesting the different classes of men, chiefly from the elite, and thereby illustrating the futile vanity of modern man:

The Philosopher, after having revolved a sublime system of Nature in his thoughts . . . feels himself suddenly seized by a disorder his philosophy at first teaches him to despise . . . Living in his works, in hope, and in the admiration of mankind, he – dies![204]

A similar fate was awaiting the professor 'amid the groves of Science, the retreats of Literature, and walks of the Muses'.[205] His fate was matched by the tragicomic politician, with his stupendous ambitions yet puny vitality. Such a man 'just begins to accommodate his vast acquirements of knowledge and legislation to . . . the high concerns of national virtue, prosperity, and glory', and what happens?

when the latent disease of his constitution . . . becomes too mighty any longer to lie concealed, putting on the alarming form of irregular gout, apoplexy, palsy, cholic, or stone . . . He who had ascended so many glorious steps above the level of humanity, struck off the list of life![206]

The career of the merchant or businessman offered a corresponding scene of infinite ambitions and dramatically limited life – 'he is arrested by some threatening malady, the consequence of long intense application, and corroding anxiety of mind'[207] – and still more pathetic, or ridiculous, was the spectacle of the voluptuary. 'With an effort to live, scarcely amounting to a groan, he expires!'[208]

The twist in Stevenson's tale was that the physician – who might fondly think himself above this black comedy – was an essential actor in it, because he too was part of the coalition of death!

When a patient, therefore, is attacked at the moment, and notwithstanding he has been attended by the most noted of the Faculty, is hurried into the other world, it is justly presumable of ninety cases in a hundred, that the disorder has been mistaken and ignorantly treated.[209]

Nevertheless, despite medicine's lethal role, such was the sway of fashion that the suave but unscrupulous physician had nothing to fear; he could always count on having credulous patients ('particularly female ones') eat out of his hand, so that 'he may kill his thousands when he pleases'.[210] In the light of such facts – frivolity in life, fatalism in death, and all encouraged by the medical profession – Stevenson launched his bruising broadside against medical mumbo-jumbo:

> There is a fashion in physic as well as the cut of our cloaths, or the trim of our hats. How many medicines have been ushered into the world in the most pompous, confident manner, as specifics for certain bodily complaints, and, when tried, have proved as inefficacious as the most despicable news-paper nostrums![211]

Healing had been perverted by the rage for the nostrum, and physic was infested with quacks with their '*never-failing* remedies for all disorders, pub-lished in news-papers under patent royal, and sold in every chymist's, apoth-ecary's, milliner's, bookseller's and grocer's shop'.[212] In this Aesculapian bedlam, one of the most outrageous scandals was the gout:

> Volumes piled on volumes have been written on it, insomuch that a decent library might almost be composed of the treatises published on this disorder singly . . . yet, to the degradation of science, and the disappointment of medical practice, true it is that all these were as accurately known to Hippocrates and Galen, as to any modern writer, not excepting Sydenham himself.[213]

While generally claiming to have pills for every ill, medicine had the audacity to deny that it should have any cures for gout at all.[214]

Gout seemed, no doubt, a mysterious malady, but, Stevenson stressed, the bad physician blamed the disease. The medical tribe had 'plunged into endless theories and hypothetical reasonings, to analyse and describe a disease which is in itself an object of common sense'.[215] The caprice that gout was some unique sort of disease, worthy of a special mystique, was preposterous, because it 'differs not in its properties, liableness to sudden transition, cure, and prevention, from common phlegmons, erysipelatous tumours, chilblains, whitloes, rheumatic swellings, &c.'.[216] That whimsy had created an edifice of error.

The medical world, as well as the world at large, have been unaccountably led to consider the gout as being no less singular in its nature, than impracticable in its cure; as being a sort of original disease, like original sin, entailed upon the species.[217]

Like Cadogan, Grant, Beddoes and Jeans, Stevenson was appalled by the artificial styles of living responsible for the prevalence of gout, 'the misfortune as well as punishment of our species'.[218]

Because gout was triggered by a completely erroneous lifestyle, it was obvious to Stevenson that Cadogan was on the right track in positing that 'the gout only lays hold of the purest and soundest constitutions'. What was essential was to broadcast the, to some, unpalatable truth that:

before people can be cured of the Gout, they must be cured of their *vices*. Intemperance, voluptuousness, and gluttony, by which both mind and body are unqualified for exercise, are the parents of the Gout, as well as of every other disorder. Prevent the one, and you prevent the other.[219]

Gout was actually a relatively simple condition.[220] The gout mystique was thus balderdash, the elaborate talk mere verbal juggling.[221] He would not, unlike conventional physicians, blame constitutions and history, or the atmosphere and the environment, when the real cause lay within. Each individual should take personal responsibility for his body and his state of health – 'the cause proceeds from ourselves'.[222] With characteristic late-Enlightenment radicalism, Stevenson argued that the real evil stemmed from the artificiality of life pursued by the slothful and the greedy.[223]

With expectations rising and life growing daily more unnatural, the frivolous and the thoughtless failed to search their souls; instant cures were all the rage:

we ransack the news-papers for drops, powders, tinctures, balsams, cordials, restoratives, sweeteners, and a long etcetera of *cures*; and when we have *vainly* tried them, with a degree of steadiness we never shewed our best friends, we procure some *celebrated* physician, to get us speedily off his hands, by sending us full of hope and convalescence to Bath, Bristol, Tunbridge, Cheltenham, &c. where, with the *divine waters* gurgling down our throats, (*aqua quietis si non vitae*) we sink into the arms of everlasting rest, with the philosophical consolation that we have not only lived a *fashionable life*, but we have died a *fashionable death*.[224]

The fetishism of medicines had reached grotesque heights, or depths! – 'In the different stages of the Gout, Dr. Shaw recommends no less than *fifty-six* different compound recipes',[225] all of which was quite uncalled for, since 'very few drugs are necessary in the Gout'.[226] Not medicine but a stout constitution would cope: 'in twenty instances of patients recovering happily, the constitution has performed *nineteen* of the cures'.[227] After all a gouty constitution was a good constitution: 'THOSE constitutions that are unable to form the Gout, are, for the most part, liable to scorbutic eruptions of the body, or erysipelatous swellings of the limbs.'[228] Hence certain parallels were to be drawn between gout and the political order: 'If the constitution be of the best kind, gout or rheumatism will carry off from the general circulation the redundant humours in a greater space of time.'[229]

As is evident, Stevenson was well aware of – indeed positively emphasized – the parallels between obfuscatory doctrines on gout and reactionary politics. This he spelt out loud and clear. We have a fondness for 'every thing that is hereditary', he maintained, in an astonishing peroration.

> Hence the tenacious hold of hereditary guilt from Adam, among the orthodox. Hence our dignified estimation of hereditary blood, imbued with which every action is honourable, selling our country, after having first sold our conscience; debauching other men's wives and daughters, and defrauding tradesmen of their bills. – Hence our foibles, defects, oddities, whims, prejudices, and prepossessions, are held to be a sacred part of our sacred selves, approaching very near to beauties and perfections, because they belonged in kind to our fathers or mothers, perhaps, to progenitors higher up, till we arrive at the first parent of all, who, we are told, 'got a son in his own image'. We look upon them as a sort of *antiques*, therefore, industriously keep them in high preservation. And to mention no more ... the deliberate achievement of half our lives, the gout, we strangely consider as being derived to us from hereditary tenure, and a part of our fathers' or grandfathers' last will and testament.[230]

In the last decades of the eighteenth century, debate thus flared over the meaning of gout; the polarization of positions mirrored the political polarization of the times, Old Corruption assailed by reformers, aristocracy threatened by liberalism; indeed, the gout debate is unintelligible unless its politics are foregrounded. As the Cadogan controversy makes clear, the model of gout involved many ramifications: moral, personal, political. Debate was animated, shuttling between the strictly medical and wider cultural politics.

CHAPTER **8**

Change and Continuity, 1790–1850

The happiest man that ever breath'd on earth,
With all the glories of estate and birth,
Has yet some care or pain to make him know
No grandeur is above the reach of woe,
Your lordship feels it in your gouty toe,
But in the keenest agonies of grief,
Content's a cordial that gives some relief.

'To a Man of Quality and Great Riches Confined
by the Gout', *London Magazine* (December 1754), 603.

Gout created powerful intellectual and cultural waves. Meanwhile sufferers
were, of course, seeking relief by any possible means, and practitioners of all
stripes were meeting their demands with advice, regimens, prescriptions and
polychrests. Among regular physicians, however, belief remained strong that
reckless meddling was a dangerous mistake. Richard Mead was informed by
John Freind, George II's physician, that 'notwithstanding all these good
receipts', it was probably best 'not to tamper with it': 'gout is the cure of
gout' was a dictum of Mead's destined endlessly to be quoted by the medical
fraternity. Sydenham's aversion to purging was shared by Mead, although he
would sometimes recommend small doses of Glauber's salt, recently introduced from the Continent. Emphasis upon diet and healthy living remained
the norm. 'Pray, Mr. Abernethy, what is a cure for gout?' – 'Live upon
sixpence a day – and earn it' was that taciturn surgeon's distillation of the
gospel according to Buchan and Cadogan.[1]

Among the more orthodox recourses, taking the waters had many devotees.[2] Mineral-water therapies had been used since Antiquity for joint complaints, acquiring religious rationales in the Middle Ages. Paracelsus had
viewed spas as Nature's laboratories – ocular illustrations of the *vis medicatrix
naturae*. In therapeutic vogue from the seventeenth century, spas grew highly
commercialized in the Georgian age. The thermal waters of Bath became
closely associated with gout, and many gout specialists settled there, including
George Cheyne, William Falconer, John Haygarth and Caleb Parry.[3] Taken

externally and internally, Bath waters often precipitated a short-term aggravation of the condition which allegedly 'cleared the system' and was followed
by lengthy remissions.

In addition to the waters, spa physicians imposed upon their Quality
patients dietary and alcoholic restrictions, together with regular exercise.
William Pitt the Elder was a notable sufferer who rather conspicuously took
the waters and so helped to put Bath on the map.[4] Others were more blasé.
Complaining that Bath – 'the Great National Hospital for Incurables' – bored
him, Horace Walpole quipped that the consolation was that 'Bath is sure of
doing some good. I shall take care of myself for fear of being sent hither
again.'[5]

Many physicians advocated spa treatments, praising the heat or chemical
composition of the waters themselves, combined with change of air and diet.
Others were more cynical. With gouty cases, William Stevenson sardonically
noted, a physician could get rid of a difficult patient by dispatching him to
Bath:[6]

> the merit of the Bath waters consists all in *negatives*. To drink them, you
> must leave the noise, hurry, and perplexity of business; you must leave your
> crapulary debauch, your bottles, your w——; nay more, you must leave
> your affected, hypocritical self, for your best resemblance, the *childhood of
> Nature*, and then drink the waters of life at Bath![7]

Spa treatment found a more measured critic in the renowned William
Heberden. 'I have not been able to observe any good in arthritic cases from
the external use of these waters,' he remarked in his *Commentaries*: 'sea-
bathing has contributed far more to recover the strength of gouty persons.'[8]
He recommended a traditional mixture of abstinence, moderate exercise and
herbal purges, but did not expect radical cure.

Aside from spas, myriad other treatments were in the offing. Numerous
internal medicines and external applications were recommended for forestall-
ing the gouty fit.[9] Books of kitchen physic and domestic medicine proffered
all sorts of remedies and treatments.[10] Some indicated that the recipe was best
served in the very same burgundy and port whose excesses had caused the
gouty attacks in the first place. The operative phrase was 'put in a pint of best
red port'. Like Horace Walpole with his gouty bootikins, individuals developed pet schemes and strategies,[11] and scores of folk and popular remedies
were in circulation. The right foot of a frog, wrapped in a deer's skin, was
said to protect against gout, as were the sinews of a vulture's leg and toes. The
patient, before getting out of bed in the morning, should spit on his hand and
then rub all his sinews, saying 'flee, gout, flee'.[12]

In England the popular *London Magazine* regularly ran clipped columns of
famous persons who had been cured by idiosyncratic remedies, like this one
in 1748:

1. . . . a person of great eminence at the Hague . . . an Indian woman undertook his cure . . . by laying a little quantity of a kind of moss upon the place . . . and then firing it with a little perfumed match . . . after which a clove of bruised garlick bound upon the place with a large plaister of diapalma . . . but if it did not answer the effect . . . proceed on to a second or third burning.

2. Old Prince Maurice of Nassau . . . had a present cure for it . . . boil a large quantity of horse dung . . . of the native white kind . . . in a pail full of water . . . put his leg in it as hot as he could bear it . . . supplying it still with hot for about an hour . . . immediately to bed, to continue the perspiration . . . well by the morning.

3. Governor of Maestricht . . . get abroad and walk as long as he could stand . . . pressing that foot hardest . . . from which he received the pain . . . he made his servants rub it hard some considerable time . . . recovered by morning, or if that failed, he repeated the course next day and was always well . . . indulgence and gentle treatment . . . fasten and exaggerate the symptoms.

4. A Lorrain surgeon . . . [cured] the gout, by whipping the part with a rod of nettles till it appeared blistered . . . The next day the skin appeared stiff . . . but by bathing in oil composed also of nettles, it wrought a cure. He owns what benefit he found from milk diet, avoiding all salt meats . . . decries much the use of wine.

Diverse cures were also advocated by John Wesley in his bestselling work of popular medicine, *Primitive Physick* (1747). 'Regard them not who say', he advised, 'the gout ought not to be cured. They mean, it cannot. I know it cannot by their regular prescriptions. But I have known it cured in many cases, without any ill effects following. I have cured myself several times.' He listed the following for gout in the stomach:

Dissolve two drachms of Venice treacle in a glass of mountain wine. After drinking it go to bed. You will be easier in two hours, and well in sixteen. – *Dr Dover*.

Or, boil a pugil [that is, a pinch] of tansey in a quarter of a pint of mountain wine. Drink it in bed. I believe this never fails.

To prevent its return, dissolve half an ounce of gumguiacum in two ounces of sal volatile. Take a tea-spoonful of this every morning in a glass of spring water.

This helps any sharp pain in the stomach. – *Dr Boerhaave*.

N.B. I knew a gentleman who was cured many times by a large draught of cold water.

Equally, the founder of Methodism was not short of cures for gout in the foot or in the hand.[13]

In the Georgian century, so often called the golden age of quackery, entrepreneurial medicine and consumer-led self-help brought a host of nostrums and quackish cures.[14] Prominent among these was the 'Portland powder'.[15] Its recipe was bought for a great sum by the second Duke of Portland and published by him in gratitude for its benefits. It contained equal parts of birthwort, gentian, germander, ground pine and the tops and leaves of the lesser centaury. One drachm was to be taken every morning, for three months; then $^3/_4$ drachm for a further three months, and so on for the whole year, after which half a drachm was to be taken on alternate mornings for a further year. Sydenham had advocated a similar mixture of herbal bitters. The much touted Portland powder aroused widespread interest and was referred to in popular writings, including the gouty Henry Fielding's *Tom Jones*.[16] Both Cullen and Cadogan deemed it dangerous, but Heberden nevertheless thought it had merit.[17]

Another specific advocated by some leading physicians was Goddard's Drops, the first British patent medicine. Developed by Dr Jonathan Goddard, FRS, Gresham Professor of Physic in London, its composition was sold for a large sum to Charles II 'for the benefit of the Nation':

> Take Humane bones well dryed and broke into bits together with two pounds of viper's flesh. Put them into a retort and distil . . . so will you have a spirit, oyle and volatile salt. Set it in the earth to digest for three months . . . then separate oyle, which keep for use. If you want it for the gout in any particular limb it is better to make it from the bones of that limb. The dose is six to twelve drops in a glass of Canary Wine; but it has an evil scent.[18]

Many other patent and proprietary medicines were also being offered as specifics or salves, as is apparent from newspaper advertisements.[19] Will Atkins, the well-known London quack whom we discuss in Chapter 12, allegedly made a fortune from the sale of 'anodyne' bracelets and rings, and also sold a celebrated 'specific for the gout which contains thirty different drugs, all of which are calculated to ease the complaint. Those who have no faith in it may keep their money – and their disease too.'[20]

Some cures involved beliefs left over from old magical folklore, others derived from the new philosophy. The apparently magical quality of lodestones had long attracted interest, and attempts were made to demonstrate their therapeutic virtue. According to one report, a certain Henry Pelly, Esquire, of Upton, Essex, a lifelong sufferer, 'easily effected a successful cure for his troublesome and painful illness by wearing a very powerful lodestone . . . round his neck next to his skin'.[21]

These anodynes were complemented by a full range of herbal concoctions and vegetable potions that appear to us today as a veritable theatre of the absurd rather than any pharmacopoeia for cure. The same readers of Samuel

Richardson's *Charles Grandison* and Fielding's *Tom Jones* deconstructed prolific passages like this one that appeared in 1753 in the *London Magazine*, detailing a recipe involving the roots of birthwort and gentian and the leaves and tops of germander, ground pine and centaury:

> Take all of these well dry'd, powder'd and sifted . . . mix them well together . . . take one drachm of this of this mixed powder every morning . . . in a cup of wine and water, broth, tea . . . keep fasting for an hour and a half after it, continue this for three months without interuption . . . it will take perhaps two years before you receive any great benefit . . . must not be discouraged . . . so one lives soberly and abstains from those meats and liquors that have always been accounted pernicious in the gout . . .

Such beliefs were both compounded and exploited by one of the most audacious and long-running quack medical enterprises of the eighteenth century, the firm styled by Francis Doherty the 'Anodyne Necklace Company'.[22] Using high-pressure newspaper advertising, this outfit principally marketed a teething necklace, but also a range of nostrums and medical scams, various of which traded upon the supposed virtues of magnets and electricity. In 1713 it advertised *The Practical Scheme of Secret Injuries; and Broken Constitutions; By Fast Living; Former Ill Cures; Salivations, and Mercury. Dedicated to Dr Chamberlen*. The operation of this *Practical Scheme* proved extremely long-lived and included the promoting of *A New System of the GOUT and Rheumatism: Drawn from Reason, Anatomical Observations, & Experience*, together with *A Rational Account of the Cause, Nature, Seat and Cure of Gleets, and Other Such WEAKNESSES, etc. in Either Sex, Usually Attending Persons after Former Cures, Over-Strainings, Self-Abuse, Hard Labours, Miscarriages, etc. Wherein is Fully Explicated the Horrid Nature, and Most Miserable Consequences of Self-Abuse in Particular, the Ruin and Bane of the More Flourishing part of Mankind, Punished in the Person of Onan*. For a generation, gout and venereal cures were linked in the company's advertising, presumably because of the familiar idea of 'broken constitutions' and because both were disorders of the affluent middle-aged males likely to be reading the newspapers and forking out on patent medicines.[23]

Not all gadgets were so brazen. By the close of the eighteenth century, the new technology typical of the industrial era was making itself felt, with patent hot baths, steam-jets, atmospheric chambers and electrical machines. Mead himself – the great luminary of the London medical establishment in his generation – had been the recipient of a letter recommending a type of Finnish sauna. Reprinted in several of the most popular mid-century magazines, as in the *Gentleman's Magazine* for January 1752, it described a man suffering from the 'seratic gout' for three years who could not move without pain. The correspondent assured Mead that the patient was cured by the

'Indian method'. This prescribed the making of an 'arbour four feet high and four feet wide' of 'young trees'. The idea was to plant them 'near a river, cover them with blankets; heat stones and put in this sweat-house', as if constructing a sauna. Then 'to enter naked, pour water over stones and sit until sweating'. This followed by jumping into the close-by river for no more than a few minutes, succeeded by retreating back into the 'sweat-house' until the 'pores are well-opened'. The user—patient then dried off and got dressed, as in the modern versions of sauna cure. Mead's correspondent assured him that this therapy had cured the 'flying gout' of a man over seventy.

Technology and the gout continued to be imaginatively yoked in the eighteenth and nineteenth centuries, in all sorts of instruments and gadgets used in the flourishing spas. One such piece of equipment was marketed by Ralph Blegborough, a London surgeon. His *Facts and Observations Respecting the Air-Pump Vapour-Bath in Gout, Rheumatism, Palsy and Other Diseases* (1803) was designed to promote apparatus for a physical cure, and was, not surprisingly, dismissive of the absurd incurability doctrines. 'In Germany it is not unusual for one, who is known to have been attacked with the piles, to have the earnest congratulations of his neighbours,' he observed; in England, that was so with gout. 'They are equally ridiculous.'[24] Blegborough's aetiological views were in the Cadogan mould, though with an unusual, anxiety-making accentuation of the sexual factor: 'The state of collapse *post coitum* also peculiarly predisposes to it; and its severest paroxysms often immediately succeed immoderate exertions of this nature.'[25]

Electricity was also being widely touted for all manner of physical and mental maladies, and Blegborough thought it promising in gouty cases 'by taking sparks from the parts affected'.[26] But, while sympathetic to electricity, he distanced himself from popular frauds which all too often depended 'on the influence of the imagination' or on the 'mystical deceptions of the tractors' or even on 'the magical delusions of animal magnetism'. His, by contrast, was 'founded on the unerring principles of nature', and it had made its way in the world 'without finesse or chicanery'.[27] His device was fully scientific, 'a machine for conveying a vapour-bath to diseased limbs, and for taking off the pressure of the atmosphere':

> I have little doubt but it will rank among the first of the modern improvements in our art; and that under the superintendence of professional men, it will prove a powerful means not only of alleviating, but frequently of removing, many diseases which have been hitherto considered as incurable.[28]

The rationale of the coffin-like contraption lay in using an air-pump to exhaust the atmosphere around a limb, thereby relieving pressure on it. Doubtless to dissuade rivals, Blegborough abstained from describing the apparatus in detail, but he festooned his book with:

a few cases out of a great number which have occurred to me lately, selecting those of such persons as are least difficult of access; and first, that of Mr Seares, surgeon, of Half-Moon Street, Piccadilly, to whom I am indebted or [sic] the following statement, which I shall give in his own words.

The gouty surgeon's letter stated that on reading in the *Medical and Physical Journal* Blegborough's description of his machine, he had felt moved to write giving his 'testimony of its beneficial effects in gout', having 'experienced such relief from it myself'. He had been stricken 'in the winter of 1799, by being thrown out of my chaise'. A further attack 'with increased violence' had occurred in the following winter. But he had been lucky, since he had heard 'that a gentleman at Pimlico, whom I knew, had received the greatest benefit from the application of the machine' – Blegborough's apparatus 'succeeded beyond my most sanguine expectations'. On the evening previous to its application, 'I could not bear my feet to touch the ground'; but, once 'the machine had been applied, I could press on them without pain'. It worked even better on the second occasion: 'I was enabled in a day or two to attend to business.' Gratitude had obliged him to write in hopes that 'this, with other documents, will tend to make the machine more generally known, and I trust approved'.[29] Blegborough offered a follow-up report, which stressed that, after treatment, Seares 'enjoyed an uninterrupted state of good health' for two years. Succumbing to a further attack:

> He immediately had recourse to the machine; four applications of which were made on the 25th, the 26th, the 28th, and the 30th. After the 3d application, he was enabled to resume, and has since continued, his usual activity in his profession. He is now entirely free from all appearance of the complaint.[30]

Alongside such technological gewgaws, two post-1750 developments were of major scientific and therapeutic importance. One was the reinstatement of colchicum.[31] Well known to Antiquity, hermodactyl had been extracted by Alexander of Tralles from the corm of a species of colchicum similar to the more effective *Colchicum autumnale*, so named because it grew in Colchis in Asia Minor. Alexander graphically described the immense relief from joint pain and swelling rapidly experienced by many of his patients. Aetius too advocated its use, while taking note of its side-effects:

> hermodactyl is bad for the stomach, producing nausea and anorexia, and ought therefore only to be used in the case of those who are pressed for time by urgent affairs of business, for it does remove the disease quickly, after two days at most, so that they are enabled to resume. For this reason some do call it *anima articulorum* – the soul of the joints.[32]

Colchicum was studied by Islamic physicians and its properties taught at the first European medical school in Salerno: 'it helpeth the arthritic gout', states the Salernitan *Regimen*. Medieval pharmacopoeias like the *Antidotary* of Nicholas mention hermodactyl as a constituent of an arthritic pill. In 1282 it was contained in a prescription for the Byzantine Emperor Michael Paleologus VIII by his private physician – with the pious and precautionary message: 'This will cure you provided we have assistance of Heaven, the intercession of the Blessed Virgin Mother, and the help of God.'[33] But its reputation as a poison, emphasized by Dioscordes and Pliny, limited its popularity: Hildegard of Bingen forbade its use as 'a deadly poison'. There-after colchicum fell into disuse,[34] and Renaissance physicians widely dismissed it as a fearsome purgative. William Turner, the leading Tudor botanist, wrote in *The Names of Herbes* (1548) that colchicum – which 'hath leaves and seedes in Sommer, and flowres lyke saffron aboute Mihelmesse' – should not be used.[35] William Bullein agreed in his *Booke of Simples* (1579).[36]

The herbalist and apothecary John Gerard believed that though 'it could 'be very hurtfull to the stomach', it could prove efficacious for joint pains 'when mixed with white of eggs, barley meal and crumbs of bread and applied plaister-wise' – or if the corm were worn round the neck or hidden in the pocket.[37] But broadly speaking its reputation sank. Jacques Grévin, a Paris physician, observed in his *Deux Livres des Venins* (1568), 'ce poison est ennemy de la nature de l'homme en tour et par tout'; Rembert called it 'perniciosum'; while, in his translation of Rembert, Henry Lyte judged 'Medow or Wilde Saffron is corrupt and venemous, therefore not to be used in medicine'.[38] Colchicum is among the simples listed in the first edition of the *Pharmacopoeia Londinensis* (1618); it also appears in the editions of 1627, 1632 and 1639; but it was omitted from that of 1650, not appearing again until 1788,[39] possibly because Sydenham condemned purgative treatments for gout.[40]

Modern use resumed with Anton Stoerck of Vienna.[41] He described *Colchicum autumnale* (meadow saffron) as a diuretic, useful in dropsy, ascites and anasarca, testing distillations of the root on himself, and finding they increased urine flow. The whole root, however, gave him abdominal pain and diarrhoea, while, administered to a dog, it killed the animal after thirteen hours of intense vomiting and diarrhoea. He finally used a vinegar extract of the plant, sweetened by honey (an oxymel), and treated thirteen dropsical patients with it. All, including several who had not responded to extracts of squill, had strong diarrhoea.

Stoerck did not, however, use colchicum for gout but rather for dropsy, for which it was highly effective.[42] For gout, it was reintroduced by Nicolas Husson, a French army officer, who in the 1770s concocted a panacea which he called *Eau médicinale*. Its formula a closely guarded secret, it had a great vogue, and for many years its ingredients were the subject of fierce contro-versy.[43] Husson promoted his nostrum as a polychrest – it would cure gout along with sciatica, rheumatism, madness, apoplexy, lethargy, catalepsy, paralysis and epilepsy, while also being recommended for constipation, dysentery, worms, gastric and intestinal colic, indigestion and mercury and lead poisoning; it would relieve scrofula, venereal diseases, smallpox, putrid inflammatory fevers and cholera; help in the treatment of rashes, scurvy, cancer, hydrops, asthma and gravel; and also relieve childbirth pains. It strengthened the tired patient, the convalescent, those with weakness, nervous affections and the infirmities of old age. In fact, according to Husson, the *Eau médicinale* was effective in all diseases – except pulmonary disorders, paralyses and tumours. The compound met much opposition, however, and in 1778 its sale was suppressed in Paris by police order, a prohibition soon removed but sporadically reapplied.

The *Eau médicinale* was introduced into England in 1808 by Edwin Godden Jones and was tried on a certain Mr John Crawford, who experienced benefit. Jones then wrote *An Account of the Remarkable Effects of the Eau Médicinale d'Husson in the Gout* (1810), dedicated to the Prince Regent's physician, Sir Walter Farquhar, who declined, however, to use it on the gouty Prince.[44] The courtly physician Henry Halford became interested: by early 1810 he had given it to twelve patients.[45]

Another gouty eminence who became involved in the *Eau médicinale* affair was Sir Joseph Banks, the naturalist and President of the Royal Society, who had been suffering from the disorder since 1787.[46] On 14 December 1809 he could write to Thomas Andrew Knight, 'I am at present free from the Gout; I feel better than I have done for some years, & begin to hope that my abstemious diet begins to produce an effect in my condition.' But another attack ensued, precipitating the climax in Banks's clinical history. On Saturday morning, 17 February 1810, Lady Spencer sent to Soho Square a bottle of Dr Husson's *Eau médicinale*, with Sir Henry Halford's instructions. Banks agreed to try it. Some hours later, Everard Home, his regular physician, visited. Without telling Home of his intentions, he obtained a detailed clinical description of his present state and a gloomy prognosis of an attack liable to last a month. Banks succumbed and took his first dose of the *Eau médicinale* – half a bottle by one account, two teaspoonsful by Banks's testimony. Next day, Home found Banks 'in a very extraordinary state'. 'How? What's the matter?' he asked. 'Why,' replied Banks, 'I have taken a quack medicine,' being then chid by Home for being so stupid. The soothing effects were, however, clear as Home discovered much to his astonishment – the pulse had dropped to 62 and the joint pains had dwindled. On Monday, a second dose was taken, and five bowel motions followed. A slight nausea was the only side-effect and on Wednesday Lord Spencer found Banks free from all gouty pains.

Banks now entered the pages of British medicine in John Ring's *Treatise of the Gout . . . and Observations on the Eau Médicinale* (1811) and the surprised Home began a study of its properties, coming up with his own recipe, extracting two pounds of macerated roots of colchicum with gentle heat in twenty-four ounces of sherry for six days. There were also imitations, such as 'Wilson's tincture' and 'Reynolds specific'.[47] Banks too investigated the origins of the decoction whose composition Husson had kept a close secret, though its relation to extracts from Colchicum plants had long been suspected. Through correspondence with his kinswoman Lady Hester Stanhope, living in Syria, Banks pursued the mystery of the hermodactyl plant as used by the Ancients. She sent him roots, and French translations from Arabic texts, though he was already convinced that the genus *Colchicum* harboured an active principle with effects similar to Husson's medicine.

Meanwhile the new medicine was creating a stir in lay and medical circles alike. On 9 February 1811, the artist and gossip Joseph Farington mentioned the *Eau médicinale*. His physician friend Hayes identified it as the 'celebrated medicine which in gouty complaints produces extraordinary effects'.[48] 'He said', noted the diarist, 'it has not been yet ascertained what this medicine consists of, but it has no mineral in it, & its quality is of a vegetable nature.' Here further medical opinion weighed in, heightening the mixture's mystique:

> Dr Clarke informed Hayes that Sir Henry Halford had assured Him that He had given it in 18 instances in each of which it was successful. Hayes gave it to a patient lame with the gout on whom it operated so quickly that in three Hours he was able to run up stairs.[49]

(Echoes of quack puffery here!) But if the *Eau* was clearly hot stuff, physicians were anxious to dissociate themselves from its possibly mountebankish abuses:

> When further experience of it has been had Hayes thinks it may become a medicine of very great value; at present, as no medicine will suit all constitutions, objections have been made to it on acct. of unfavourable effects having been produced in some instances: but He observed that similar objections might be made to that most valuable medicine *Opium* & to the no less Soveriagn remedy *Mercury*, when injudiciously given.[50]

In 1814 John Want reported the successful use of an extract of *Colchicum autumnale* in the treatment of rheumatism. Having discovered that the basic ingredient of the *Eau* was extract of the corm of the *Colchicum autumnale*, Want published a formula for preparing a tincture as an alternative to Husson's medicine. Once the active ingredient of the *Eau* had been identified, colchicum gradually replaced it.[51]

Use spread. Though patients loved it, physicians initially disapproved. Wilson's tincture enjoyed considerable notoriety, and its discoverer presented some bottles to the Prince Regent, which Sir Henry Halford sternly forbade him to take. By that time, however, everybody was interested and the market was flooded with *Eau médicinale* lookalikes. A patriotic element of course figured in this rush for a cure – why take a French medicine, Edward Jenner asked 'John Bull':

> Oh John, thou art surely the greatest of Ninnies,
> Why load the French shores with such heaps of thy guineas?
> Do prithee thy senses recall.
> Knows't thou not, honest John, that all curable ills
> Are soon wash'd away by fair Chelta's bright rills?
> Come John, then, and try
> And thou wilt not deny
> That here's the Eau Médicinale.[52]

The Prince Regent finally became aware of the value of colchicum, and is recorded in 1817 – when he was swallowing 1,200 drops of laudanum daily without pain relief – as telling his doctors he would abandon their 'half measures' for the quack remedy.[53] It helped him greatly – and with its aid the gouty Bourbon Prince Louis had also recovered his health sufficiently to be restored in 1815 from his sedentary Richmond existence to the throne of France as Louis XVIII.[54]

Such successes initiated a spate of proprietary specifics, one of which was 'Moore's Wine of White Hellebore and Laudanum'; of this Charles Scudamore wrote: 'I am well persuaded that in any form or combination it should be entirely deprecated as a remedy for the gout.'[55] Other proprietary medicines cashing in on Husson's evident success included one developed by Anthony Welles and advertised in *An Account of the Discovery and Operation of a New Medicine for Gout* (1803).[56] In 1820, Edward Haden published a monograph on colchicum in acute and chronic inflammatory diseases. His father had begun to use colchicum in gout after Want's report, and had 'then extended the use of the remedy from gout to rheumatism, and from the latter to the treatment of cases of inflammation in general'. He praised its benefits in rheumatic inflammatory fevers, lung inflammations, catarrhs, influenza and puerperal fever. During a fortnight in October 1820, he successfully treated twenty-nine non-gouty patients with colchicum. He also gave it to his three children for colds and severe sore throat: all improved.[57] By around 1820, colchicum had become thoroughly accepted. Sydney Smith's daughter, Lady Holland, related that on one occasion, on observing some of his autumn crocuses in flower, her father had stopped. 'There,' he said, 'who would guess the virtue of that little plant? But I find the power of *Colchicum* so great that if I feel a little gout coming on, I go into the garden and hold out my toe to that plant, and it gets well immediately.'[58]

The illustrious Trousseau, however, held out against it, thinking the side-effects too serious to justify its use.[59] Many physicians suspected that, although colchicum was useful in dealing with acute gout, it aggravated the underlying disease, increased the frequency of the attacks and in no sense represented a cure.[60] In time, the chemistry of colchicum was better understood. By 1820 its active principle, the alkaloid colchicine, was discovered by Pellétier and Caventou. Produced in crystalline form in 1884, this replaced the time-honoured tinctures, extracts and other Galenical preparations of colchicum, as it was stable, reliable and easy to take in exact dosage, and its effective and rapid control of pain in acute gout remained unrivalled.[61]

Independently of the re-entry of colchicum, if in certain respects paralleling it, was the elucidation of the pathology of gout. A key breakthrough came with the analysis in 1776 by Carl Wilhelm Scheele of urinary concretions (*acidum concretum*), his findings being published in the *Transactions* of the Stockholm Academy of Sciences. The Swedish apothecary and chemist found a new acid substance with specific chemical reactions, later called lithic acid. He described its chemical characteristics but did not draw any connection with gout.[62] In the same year his countryman Tobern Bergman analysed a bladder stone and found it contained the same acid.[63] The Scottish physician Murray Forbes held in his *A Treatise upon Gravel and upon Gout* (1793) that, as urine contained uric acid, it was probable that the blood did too.[64] Were that so, he believed it might become precipitated in various parts of the body, explaining the appearances in acute gout of tophi.[65]

The key paper in this respect was published by William Hyde Wollaston in 1797; he was apparently the first (since Leeuwenhoek) to examine a tophus.[66] He isolated uric acid from both the gouty and urinary concretions, establishing that the substance extruded from gouty tophi was the same as the uric acid Scheele had identified in urinary concretions. 'Gouty matter', Wollaston concluded, 'is lithiated soda.' Forbes's shrewd clinical guess had been chemically vindicated.

The chemistry of the urinary system was being explored more systematically. In 1800 the pharmacologist John Bostock found that the red sediment in the urine of gouty patients was crystalline sodium urate.[67] A new breed of chemical physicians followed, above all Justus von Liebig (1803–73) of Giessen, who without much anachronism may be said to have founded modern organic chemistry. He considered that the physiological basis of both gout and renal calculus lay in a lack of effective oxidation of the normal products of metabolism. His remedies, however, were familiar: abstinence, bitter herbal infusions and exercise to stimulate the inhalation of pure air.

In England Liebig's disciples included Henry Bence Jones, who advocated hydrotherapy as the best application of Liebig's oxygenating principle.[68] In 1844, Alexander Ure of St Mary's Hospital recommended the taking of benzoate of soda internally, with naphtha applications externally, a combination which, he said, had Liebig's approval.[69] He also advocated excising tophi before they hardened: thus treated, they seldom recurred. The murexide test was first described by William Prout, who showed that neutralizing the colourless nitric acid solution of uric acid with ammoniac brought out the ammonium salt of purpuric acid – a test shortly to be taken for granted by Alfred Garrod.[70] Laboratory science was thus giving a new look to clinical medicine, but research into gout progressed only by small steps in Britain in the first half of the nineteenth century. At the Royal College of Physicians, one Goulstonian lecture (1826) and two Croonian lectures (1827 and 1843) touched on the subject, while in 1833, in the first written medical examination held in the University of London, candidates were asked: 'What are the chief remedies of rheumatism; the circumstances in directing the use of each; and the mode of employing them?'[71]

The Cadogan controversy subsided and among clinicians a consensus emerged. Received opinion was digested for lay readers in Richard Reece's *Domestic Medical Guide* (1803).[72] There were two basic sorts of gout, he declared: regular and irregular. Irregular gout could be further divided into three kinds:

> 1st, *Atonic.* – When there is not power in the nervous system to produce a sufficient degree of inflammation in the extremities; in this case, the organs of digestion are impaired, and the general health variously affected.
> 2dly, *Retrocedent.* – When the inflammation in the joints is light, and suddenly abates, and occurs in an internal part. And,
> 3rdly, *Misplaced.* – When it takes place in any of the internal parts.[73]

Regular gout had as its causes a 'sedentary indolent manner of life, full diet, especially of animal food, and the excessive use of weak or light acid wine and spirituous liquors'. In general, Reece recommended opening medicines, and, in the case of 'a healthy constitution' with 'no strong hereditary predisposition', the 'immersion of the extremity in cold water for ten minutes, as recommended by Dr Kinglake'.[74] Reece took note of the *Eau médicinale* but concluded it dangerous.[75] Irregular gout was more difficult to handle. With retrocedent gout, 'relief is to be attempted without delay, by the free exhibition of warm brandy and water . . . A dessert-spoonful of either has, in this case, answered very well.' Misplaced gout was a mystery.[76]

Though home treatments for regular gout were fairly safe, Reece warned against self-help in case of misplaced gout. Overall, combining traditional holistic humoralism with the new theories of Cullen, he argued that 'it appears that the paroxysm is an operation of nature to restore the nervous system, impaired by abuse of spirits, stimulating diet, and excesses, to vigour and health; and, therefore, topical applications to disperse the inflammation, and remedies to weaken the system, are dangerous'.[77] Prevention was better than cure, however, and 'the best preventive treatment is, to attend to the state of the digestive organs'.[78]

Reece's account represents a digest of views around 1800. How far did these change in the next half-century? Three authors will be examined. First James Parkinson, a polymathic doctor with interests in geology and politics as well as in medicine and most famous for his *Essay on the Shaking Palsy* (1817).[79] Parkinson's *Observations on the Nature and Cure of Gout* (1805) gave a familiar outline of the aetiology and pathology of the malady, but is mainly memorable for its vivid account of the symptomatology, culled from intimate experience. Not only had his father been a sufferer, but 'nearly fifteen years ago', he stated in his Preface, 'I experienced the mortification of finding that I was also under the influence of this tormenting malady.'[80] Not surprisingly, he stressed that his book had practical and humane aims, the 'hope also of rendering an essential benefit to the labouring part of the people'.[81] He detailed his father's plight:

> Case J. P. was of a sanguine temperament, and born of parents who had not been subject to either the gravel or the gout. His food was generally plain, and his convivial indulgences were by no means frequent, but wine, or some other fermented liquor, was at times generally employed. Until nearly forty years of age he had enjoyed almost uninterrupted health; but at this period he was first attacked by gout in the foot; the fit being uncommonly severe. During the succeeding six or seven years, he was subject to very violent paroxysms, which during the latter three years, occurred twice every year, and confined him at least a month or six weeks each time.[82]

Parkinson explained the kinds of treatment his father had received. Black Lixivium (a solution of pure fixed alkali) proved effective, when combined with abstinence from alcohol. But, when he started drinking again, 'an acute pain took place immediately beneath the pubis, which did not abate of its excruciating violence until two hundred drops of laudanum were injected, mixed with a proper fluid into the rectum'.[83] Having discussed his father's exceedingly melancholy case, Parkinson proceeded to his own affliction, which he had borne for many years while going about his business as a surgeon and writing works of popular science:

> J. P. whose father was much afflicted with gout, is evidently of that temperament which is supposed to be most prone to that disease, and always possessed a peculiar idiosyncrasy in consequence of which the taking of any acid, or even acidulous matter, into the stomach, occasioned in a few minutes, a considerable glow of heat in the face and in the extremities. In youth, chilblains, with cramps in the calves of the legs; and through life, coldness, particularly in the evenings, with dryness of the feet, have seemed to point out a languid circulation in the lower extremities.[84]

Parkinson experienced his first attack in 'the ball of the right foot' at the age of thirty-eight. It was 'slight' and caused no more than 'a week's inconvenience'. Two years later, 'an attack of more violence and of longer duration was suffered in the left hand, the pain and swelling lasting about ten days'. The next year, after drinking 'nearly a pint of wine, and being exposed to a heavy rain', he had awoken 'about three o'clock in the morning in such severe pain in the instep of the right foot, as excluded all hopes of regaining sleep':

> Convinced of its being a gout affection, and wishing to induce perspiration in the part, he quitted his bed, but found himself entirely incapable of standing on that foot: he, however, drew on a woollen stocking, and regained the bed. The pain now soon became so exceedingly acute as to be almost beyond endurance. Recollecting the case of Mr Alexander Small, related in the sixth volume of the *Medical Observations and Inquiries*, in which great relief was obtained by lessening the temperature of the part, he now stripped off the stocking, and laid with it, about ten minutes, on the outside of the bedclothes, exposed to the open air. The swellings on the finger joints now being considerable, and that on the third finger of the left hand manifesting a disposition to inflammation, a leech was applied to it, and the bleeding promoted as much as possible. Almost directly after the bleeding from this joint, the stinging burning sensation began to abate, and was in two or three days removed.[85]

Parkinson maintained that 'indulgence in acids is a frequent cause of gout'.[86] Respecting treatment, he took issue with the views expressed by Robert Kinglake in his *A Dissertation on Gout* (1804).[87] Kinglake, who believed gout was essentially a local disease, was the originator of the 'refrigeration treatment', which consisted of the application to the affected parts of cloths soaked in a solution of equal parts of cold water and ammonia. When Parkinson criticized this theory,[88] Kinglake responded with *Strictures on Mr Parkinson's Observations* (1807), and then *Additional Cases of Gout* (1807).[89]

The Parkinson–Kinglake controversy was not merely about treatments but about aetiology. Parkinson conjectured that the 'proximate' cause of gout was 'a peculiar saline acrimony, existing in the blood'. This he supposed to be 'the acidifiable base of the uric acid'.[90] Kinglake by contrast believed that gout was the product of inflammation and not of acids.[91]

The opening chapters of Parkinson's *Observations on the Nature and Cure of Gout* were devoted to pathology and aetiology. Proposing a constitutional tendency for the most part hereditary, he mentioned intemperance and intense application to study or business. Against most medical opinion at the time he believed that 'nodosity of joints' could be found among the poor no less than among the wealthy sufferers.[92]

Turning to treatments, two cases were described. One, 'a gentleman of considerable respectability in the City, about forty years of age', who was cured following a 'a regimen' (abstinence from alcohol, a liberal supply of vegetables and ample exercise) and fifteen grains of sodium bicarbonate a day.

The other case, a gentleman about fifty years of age, 'who had indulged freely in the pleasures of the table', was described, but his treatment was less successful.[93]

The final chapter dealt with 'retrocedent gout'; here he condemned Kinglake's cooling treatment as making bad worse. 'The process being suddenly checked in the extremities', he argued in the orthodox manner, 'is liable to be taken up by some other part; whose healthful state is much more important to the preservation of life.'[94]

Overall, Parkinson showed clinical acumen but did not develop any of the new scientific discoveries. The same may be said for Sir Charles Scudamore (1779–1849), himself, like Parkinson, a gout sufferer,[95] though whereas Parkinson treated London tradesmen, Scudamore became one of the great society physicians of the age. Born in 1779 into an old Herefordshire family, Scudamore served as an apprentice to his father and practised without any further qualifications for ten years before obtaining his degree in medicine from Glasgow in 1814. In 1820 he was appointed physician to Prince Leopold and was knighted by the Duke of Northumberland in 1829. His *A Treatise on the Nature and Cure of the Gout with Some Observations on Rheumatism* (1816), dedicated to Matthew Baillie, John Hunter's nephew, was a systematic survey of the subject.[96] Based on personal observation of about one hundred patients, it proved such a success that a fourth edition had appeared by 1825.[97]

Stimulated by John Hunter, Scudamore performed experiments on dogs, and although his outlook remained clinical he made use of those ancillary chemical aids becoming available to scientific physicians, if sceptical of the importance of their findings. 'We have no actual proof', he wrote, 'even of the existence of uric acid in the body . . . or if present there is no apparent cause why it should not be excreted by the kidneys, the glands obviously designed to separate and excrete saline matter.'[98]

He believed previous writers had over-elaborated.[99] Three categories were sufficient, namely acute, chronic and retrocedent. A protagonist of the visceral conception of gout, he maintained that 'the inflammatory process will seldom be confined to the joints, but will affect all tissues which are subservient to the function of the joints'. Not all dyspeptic states, however, were indicative of gouty dispositions: 'We cannot boast that our knowledge of the intimate nature of disease is sufficient to authorise such conclusions.'[100]

Nor did Scudamore believe gout was invariably hereditary. In an analysis of 523 of his own patients he found an hereditary disposition in 309.[101] An additional precipitating factor was also necessary, such as 'mental stress'. 'The late Mr Pitt and his father both suffered with the gout at an early period of life,' he commented: 'The father was a votary of Bacchus; of the son this could not strictly be said; but he was an ardent student.'[102] The younger Pitt was in fact a prodigious drinker. Commenting upon the well-observed fact that the initial attack of gout occurred most frequently in the big toe, he reported that in a series of 516 patients this had been so on 341 occasions.[103]

Scudamore spent some weeks each year at Buxton, analysing the medicinal waters.[104] He was suspicious of the notion of 'misplaced' gout, in which the gouty lesion was internal from the beginning: it gave unbounded latitude to call every disease occurring in a gouty individual '*disguised gout* arising out of this'.[105]

Scudamore was a consummate clinician, suspicious both of theory and of science. The other eminent gout doctor of the age was of the same cast of mind. William Gairdner (1793–1867) was an Edinburgh graduate who spent most of his career in private practice in London. His *On Gout: Its History, its Causes and its Cure* (1849) proved successful, reaching its fourth edition by 1860.[106] With Scudamore, Gairdner was the last of the old-school bedside doctors, regarding the malady in a holistic manner as a consequence of a very particular discrasia of the atypical individual. He stressed disordered blood as the prime site – 'in the disturbance of sanguification', he wrote, 'gout may be said to take its rise' – though, in the Scottish manner, he also stressed the key role played by the nervous system in atonic gout, producing migraine and neuralgia.[107] Above all, he judged each case of gout unique, its symptoms protean. Having a 'gouty diathesis' was fully consistent with never experiencing an actual attack – the diathesis would manifest itself in what Cullen had called 'atonic gout' or other sickness symptoms and could be, therefore, all the more dangerous.[108] The physician should thus not merely be a good pathologist in the modern manner; for 'nothing indeed more amply requites the labour of a physician than the study of the constitutional origin of disease'.[109] A traditionalist, Gairdner was quite convinced that gout was a hereditary disorder:

> The experience of physicians in every age, indeed the common observation of mankind, has sufficiently established the fact of the hereditary nature of gout. It does not always descend from father to son in uninterrupted succession, but often passes over a generation or two, though freely exposed to its exciting causes. It rarely, however, fails to resume its dominion, even in a third or fourth generation.[110]

Gout formed an exclusive sociobiological club. When Lord Grey, the English Prime Minister associated with the Great Reform Acts of 1832, was taken gravely ill in 1841, at the age of almost eighty, the immediate diagnosis was gout.[111] No doubt lingered in the minds of his physicians. The medical evidence for this diagnosis was scant, but gout was privileged over its competitors for reasons discussed in this chapter. Gout was the only candidate in view of Grey's social stature, political sway and lifestyle – but none of these *consciously* figured into the doctors' diagnosis. It was rather that the gout verdict itself, like the lifestyle it assumed, had become ingrained. The parallel with AIDS and its homosexual patients requires no comment. Lord Grey's circulation problems were the result of, not the cause of, his swollen legs, but this hardly mattered: the doctors claimed gout and it was not until shortly before his death that they changed their minds.

It was therefore hardly surprising that lesser figures than England's Prime Minister should also have been diagnosed as gouty and Gairdner's gout diagnosis validated merely by the sheer *numbers* of examples he produced. Gairdner's book is essentially a succession of cases designed to demonstrate his clinical acuity. He would discern that all manner of symptoms were truly gouty; he would be alert to perceive the transformations of regular gout into its irregular forms; he would prevent gout metastasizing to the head. This was the role of the good physician: 'let no practitioner neglect the slightest warnings of these aberrations of gout'.[112]

In his view, his most useful service was gently but firmly to disabuse patients of any simple idea that gout was a cure as well as a disease; contrary to genteel folklore, the gouty attack by no means necessarily provided relief. With some echo of Cadogan, Gairdner suggested that this theory was a form of self-deception: 'patients, too, have aided in spreading the convenient belief. It is flattering to their conceit and pride to attribute their sufferings rather to a constitutional peculiarity than to self-indulgence and ill-regulated appetite.'[113] Gairdner nevertheless was insistent that a grasp of gout could not be boiled down to test-tube demonstrations. It was not merely a matter of acids but 'a condition of the constitution'; disorders of uric acid were therefore 'symptoms' not causes.[114]

As to therapies, no universal cures were to be expected, and different patients, helped by sympathetic practitioners, had found their own ways of coping – not least an eighty-five-year-old gentleman whose regular response to gout was to say: 'I'll walk it off.'[115] But, while stressing the hereditary dimension, Gairdner was insistent that excess was the key precipitant and dietary restraint the best remedy.[116] Certain medicines were also effective; and, despite folklore and the views of eminences like Sydenham, he believed in the efficacy of both bloodletting and purging, if carried out prudently.[117]

Not least, he insisted the heart was often affected by gout, a view which came to prominence during his lifetime.[118] James Wardrop, one-time surgeon to George IV, wrote a treatise *On the Nature and Treatment of the Diseases of the Heart, etc.* (1837), which focused attention on gouty heart.[119] Wardrop believed that gout was translated to the heart when the arthritic inflammation subsided. Called to the King during his last illness when he was being treated by Sir Henry Halford for inflammation of the lungs, he diagnosed gouty heart disease. Such views seem to register genuine developments in clinical observation combined with a somewhat myth-making insistence that the exclusive gouty complaints of gentlemen must involve what could be called the heart of the matter.[120]

CHAPTER 9

Indian Summer: Romantic and Victorian Gout

'In English, gout?'
'Not gout in the conscience, I trust,' said my father.
'Oh! that's curable,' laughed the captain.

George Meredith, *The Adventures of Harry Richmond* rev. edn
(New York: Scribner's, 1906), ch. 21, p. 198

The age of Walpole, Johnson and Gibbon is popularly regarded as the high noon of gout, but there is no reason to believe its incidence, in reality and in representation, diminished until deep into the Victorian era. After all, insofar as gout was the product of the high living of landed society, such lifestyles underwent little change, at least before aristocratic hegemony began to be challenged in the latter half of the Victorian era. The diet of the rich remained rich. In 1825, there were 40,277 tuns of port imported, which Henry Halford not altogether jocularly estimated to be the equivalent of forty thousand cases of gout.[1] Smollett's Matt Bramble had been the virtual embodiment of the great gout narratives – the notion that it had fatally, if comically, insulated its heroes and guaranteed them longevity – but literary representations hardly died out after 1771. They continued for a long time, for at least a century, slowly losing force, to be sure, but not without a demise worthy of narrating for various reasons. For one thing, the literary heritage reveals a great deal about the cultural perception of the disease and what it had become by the late eighteenth century. For another, the mere fact that all sorts of writers – novelists, poets, diarists, dramatists – incorporated gout into their image of excess and corruption, says much about the stresses on gender and sexual relations in the early modern period, about which so much has been written in our generation, oddly though without the slightest mention of this most male of all masculine medical maladies. Finally, the literary tradition, more than any other, demonstrates how gout became the emblem of an upper social class – the virtual insignia of a ruling patriarchy. Think what one did of this upper class, gout was its crest and credo. No sense could be had – the myth continued – of this landed class without its chief signs: country and city houses, manners and morals and breeding, and the one illness resulting from vice and excess. Gout was in this sense a national disease as well: the very living proof of the island nation.

Not to understand how this myth crystallized, how its male members not merely succumbed to its gripping stranglehold, but cultivated the gout as an insulating and protective shield is to overlook perhaps its signal message for the nation. Its comic elements held a main role in this crystallization. The jokes in *Punch* by the late nineteenth century had their origin much earlier, in the grand narratives dramatized comically in the tradition of the novel from Smollett and Scott and Dickens through George Eliot and down through the twentieth-century novelists. It must never be forgotten that no less a novel than *Middlemarch* – the very mirror of high Victorian society – ends with Dr Tertius Lydgate composing a treatise on the gout. More will be said about this important ending of George Eliot's masterpiece later on. For now it is important only to comment that the literary heritage is vital to understand the burgeoning of gout as a cultural energy as well as medical condition.

Writers, then as now, wrote out of personal risk and gain. Smollett and Walpole, like Hill and Cheyne and the great gout doctors, all suffered from the condition. Indeed there were so many male victims that one inquires what gout was if it afflicted men in these numbers – moreover, what was masculinity itself it if had to be mythologized in this painful way? At what price was masculinity to go the way of all flesh in this manner? The malady, of course had always been entirely genderized, but the pattern became so steadfast by then that there is not a single *extended* description of the condition by a woman at the length of an entire narratives. Milady this or that suffered of course and her case was described, as by Lady Mary Wortley Montagu who documents 'Lady Fanny's gout':

> I am extremely sorry for dear Lady Fanny's disorder. I could repeat to her many wise sayings of Ancients and Moderns, which would be of as much service to her as a present of embroidered slippers to you when you have a fit of the gout. I have seen so much of hysterical complaints, tho' Heaven be praised I never felt them, I know it is an obstinate and very uneasy distemper, tho' never fatal unless when Quacks undertake to cure it. I have even observed that those who are troubled with it commonly live to old age. Lady Stair is one instance; I remember her screaming and crying when Miss Primrose, my selfe, and other girls were dancing 2 rooms distant.

But there is no description even mildly comparable to the great extended self-narratives or autobiographies such as we have seen written by Walpole, Gibbon, Cadogan and dozens of other men. The authors of this book used to jest among themselves that they would have given much for just one lengthy self-analysis in the manner of these victims of the insulating disease.

Jane Austen may be unrepresentative in that she herself is not known ever to have had a touch of the gout, nor was anyone in her immediate family, but she remains consistent with the comic portraiture of the novel as it developed in the aftermath of Smollett – that is, the avoidance of the condition in any major protagonist. Indeed, gouty males are non-existent in her fiction. Emma's father, the notoriously hypochondriacal Mr Woodhouse, is a splendid candidate, except that he is not gouty. Melancholic, nervous, forever fearful for his health, to the extent of harbouring phobias about winds around corridors and the weather in general, he has even visited Bath, to no avail. While there, he did not consult the gout doctors, though the tribe of gout doctors we discussed in the last chapter swarmed all over the place.

John Wiltshire has shown to what degree Austen, contrary to prior belief, was preoccupied with matters of health, physical and mental, as well as the normal and pathological states of her body.[2] And when she grew ill of Addison's disease at the end of her life and quickly decayed, with the by now legendary 'pain in her face', she grew fastidious to document her own demise. Bath waters repelled her most of her life, as any reader might know from the negative symbolic value she endows on that place in her novels, preferring the more genteel Regency Cheltenham. But there is no major male figure in her *œuvre* for whom the gout is an ongoing preoccupation, as it had been in Smollett, entirely comic though her treatment of it remains: an illness emblematic of rank and class, leisure and vacancy, and the inevitable eccentricity accompanying these modalities of life.

In *Sense and Sensibility* – like *Emma* another likely candidate for gout, in view of its preoccupation with a nervous breakdown as part of its main action – Mrs Jennings remembers that she has some fine old 'Constantia wine', a well-known gout remedy. She brings a glass for the hysterical Marianne Dashwood, nostalgically exclaiming 'My poor husband! how fond he was of it! Whenever he had a touch of his old cholicky gout, he said it did him more good than anything else in the world. Do take it to your sister,' she implores Elinor. Elinor smiles at the absurdity of the notion that a gout remedy – 'Constantia wine' no less – would revive her hysterical sister, whose malady of lovesickness lies as far from the gout as possible. Instead Elinor administers hartshorn and lavender drops, as well as glasses of wine, remedies – ironically – often given to the gouty. The point is that there is no male in Austen of any great interest for our purposes, a fact that needs to be established rather than merely stated.[3]

This development is not surprising. Even if Austen's comic talent was cut of the cloth of Richardson and Samuel Johnson, and drenched in the dye of moral value, she understood women and their bodies better than men. Why then should she have permitted gout to stand for anything – as a metonymy – other than the trivial peculiarities that afflict the Mr Woodhouses of this world? Wind is the element to which the decrepit and peculiar Woodhouse objects, almost more than anything, and wind – draughts and corners – had been the gouty man's constant complaint from the seventeenth century if not earlier. Still, the legacy of a comic, insulating condition in her fiction is beside the point: it is rather the absence of the possibility of Matt Bramble. For with Smollett and the disappearance of his imagined world, something began to decline in the cultural conception of gout, although it would take another century before this slow decline amounted to demise.

Austen can be compared profitably to the representations of two very different writers, the young Benjamin Disraeli and Sir Walter Scott, very nearly contemporaries of hers even if male writers both, to see what had changed from the world of Smollett. Benjamin Disraeli is a particularly useful patrician writer to exemplify the point about a grand comic legacy because he fictionalized gout when young and later acquired it himself.[4] The son of the prolific author Isaac, who wrote so many scenes of popular life at the end of the eighteenth century, Disraeli was born into a wealthy Jewish family in Bloomsbury, London, eventually to become the first and only Jewish Prime Minister of England. As a youth Disraeli wrote fiction in the form of social commentary, encouraged by a Bloomsbury neighbour, Sara Austen (no relation to Jane). Austen served as an informal adviser to the local publisher Henry Colburn, on whose advice anonymous novels were often published.[5]

The post-adolescent Disraeli fantasized about a *beau monde* he himself did not yet know first hand (he would later on), and during the mid-1820s wrote a five-volume novel entitled *Vivian Grey*, an anatomy of Regency society and one of the earliest of the 'Silver Fork' novels, as they would later become known, dealing with the manners and mores of the rich and influential.[6] Keys to the identity of Disraeli's figures were published within weeks, and the work became a bestseller. London's salons bristled with table talk about it, and socialites like the well-connected Helen Salina Blackwood were quoted as spouting entire pages by heart. Disraeli himself feared accusations of 'Gallomania' on grounds of the severity of the criticism. In faraway Germany, Goethe read it and said it was one of his favourite English books.[7] *Vivian Grey* demonstrates, simultaneously, Smollett's satiric legacy of the patrician gouty gentleman and the drastic shift in the writer's sense of novelty that had occurred in a mere two generations.

In youth, Disraeli himself was hardly healthy or ruddy as he wrote. He never enjoyed solid good health, according to his letters or his biographers. His correspondence, like Pope's and Walpole's in the previous century, is littered with doubts about his health and ejaculations about his lifelong fear of the east wind. His male figures, like himself, are racked with minor illnesses, several of them gouty and appropriately insulated from more life-threatening diseases. Vivian Grey, probably modelled on the hero of Robert Plumer Ward's *Tremaine, or the Man of Refinement* (1825), a young aristocrat, is the protagonist.[8] There is the Countess Zavadouska, claiming to be the 'author of *Vivian Grey*', who dotes on young, rich, consumptive types like Vivian, 'ailing knights' in the Keatsian sense. And there is the frail 'Lord Grandgoût', based on the very well-known Marquess of Hertford, whose legendary decadence contributed to his notorious reputation in England and, in the late 1830s, if indirectly, to the demise of the Silver Fork Society. Even Grandgoût's name provides clues to his stereotype of portly excess and delusions of grandeur, as in the old humoral characters comically portrayed in Smollett's fiction.[9] Grandgoût appears in an epistolary section of the novel when the Honourable 'Cynthia Courtown' – another humoral creation – writes to him that 'The Marquess of Grandgoût arrived here last week with a most delicious party,' including 'all the men who write "John Bull" '.[10] Courtown then relates her disappointment 'at the first sight of Stanislaus Hoax' before noting, 'I like the Marquess of Grandgoût so much! I hope he will be elevated to the peerage: he looks as if he wanted it so! Poor dear man!'

Grandgoût's patrician infirmity was construed by a community of readers then well versed in the Marquess of Hertford's dissipations.[11] He had been the subject of abundant abuse, verbal and visual, and Disraeli committed no assault on his character in *Vivian Grey* by capturing him comically as a type of post-Smollettian Bramble. The name, as well as the malady – if malady is what 'grand-gout' was – signalled a type of promiscuous, almost extravagant, male requiring no further amplification to a readership composed very heavily of women. Fifty years earlier, Smollett's incorporation of Bramble's patronymic gout into a complex set of psychological antitheses – sensibility–irritability; benevolence–misanthropy; regeneration–demise; country–city – was necessary to explain how Bramble had become what he was.[12] Now, in the Regency, such amplification was supererogatory because the type had already been so precisely depicted: as dissipate, dandy, patron, keeper – in every excess imaginable. Gout had not at all diminished as a region of the imaginative mind in the 1820s. Historically and culturally it is rather that there was no longer any need to narrate at length its versions of comic insulation and masculine excess. That had been accomplished by Smollett and his contemporaries. Even so – and the main point needs reiterating – Grandgoût is only *one* character among many in Disraeli's five volumes, and hardly a main figure at that. Something fundamental in the representation of the upper-class male had altered, which must be captured in this chapter.

Years later, Disraeli himself contracted gout, and the irony of his earlier depiction of the very condition he himself would acquire must have struck him as curious, although there appears to be no record of the irony in his letters. His own gout was compared in the 1860s to Lord Derby's, whom he succeeded as Prime Minister. And like Emma's father, Mr Woodhouse, the historical Disraeli feared the northern and eastern winds to the end of his life, as he became increasingly racked by gout. In old age Disraeli approximated the exemplum of a Georgian Cheyneite, curbing his penchant for good food and drink, minding his abstinences, encouraged by his even more abstemious wife Mary Ann.[13] The dissimilarities between the fictive Lord Grandgoût and the historical Lord Beaconsfield are thus paramount: both gouty and frail, but the fictive one far more comic in his excesses than the abstemious British statesman nursed by his wife. Here was life again in its paradoxical mode, delimiting a comic strain the real Disraeli had narrated forty years earlier in the 1820s.

Walter Scott's biographical situation was dissimilar, his politics also different from Disraeli's 'Vivian Grey', but his fictive representations of the comic gouty type seemed equally reminiscent of types perfected in the last century by Smollett. Smollett had been Scott's favourite novelist, *Peregrine Pickle* (1751) his favourite among favourites. Scott even based one of his own fictional characters – Touchwood in *St Ronan's Well* – on a Smollettian original, the rambunctious and ludic Peregrine. Scott elevated Smollett above Fielding when writing the lives of the English novelists for Ballantyne, preferring Smollett's swashbuckling stories to the more sentimental ones of Richardson and Sterne. One among seven siblings, he himself had been remarkably healthy, although what we would call polio in the right foot caused him to be lame, but not gouty. A deeply well-read man, he eventually amassed a library of approximately 20,000 volumes containing a fair proportion of medicine.[14]

Among his favourite books was Sir John Sinclair's four-volume *Code of Health and Longevity* published in 1807.[15] Scott rummaged in it as well as freely lifted from its contents. Its pages are permeated with advice in the manner of Cheyne about the healthy life and temperate regimen: curbed diet, low intake of alcohol, plenty of exercise, and – sexually speaking – as little in the venereal way as possible. Whether this early-nineteenth-century pragmatism or puritanism (Cheyne had been most careful not to appear a prude in an age when genital sex was less policed) had any Scottish basis or medical underside is difficult to say. The point is that Scott inherited one mind-set about gout as man's grand comic insulating condition from his favourite novelist; and inherited another based on caution and care of the body from the medical books he read and from the assimilations of his own culture. They were not mutually exclusive, although at times incommensurate.

Scott wrote no fewer than twenty-three historical novels and tales in his lifetime, only three of which are likely candidates for inclusion in our narrative about gout. His male characters reveal little, if any, interest in the malady. How can this be? Our point in delving into their contents extends beyond any empirical proof that something important had changed culturally in the space of two generations. The matter is rather that, at least in literature, the time for a grand narrative based on a major gouty type (like Matt Bramble) had passed: a departure reflecting an attack on the stereotype of the male. All of Scott's *historical* novels take place in a prior age: in the Renaissance, in the period of the English Revolution, in the eighteenth century, when one would expect a plethora of gouty characters if for no other reason than realism and historical fidelity.[16] *Kenilworth* is set in the 1570s; it contains no gout. *The Antiquary* is situated in 1794, its protagonist a classic sedentary type who should be racked with gout if eighteenth-century medical theory retained any validity. Two of the characters – Oldbuck and Wardour – are inherently gouty. *St Ronan's Well* takes place during the years 1809–12, as Wellington was fighting the Peninsular Wars against the French and before he had deterred Napoleon – it contains no trace of gout. The rest of Scott's fiction is, loosely speaking, romantic rather than historical, a less likely source for such insignia based on medical theory of any type.

Sinclair's *Code to Health and Longevity* informs both *St Ronan's Well* and *The Antiquary*, as any attentive reader then would have expected, given the former's setting in a contemporary British spa. The German quack Dousterswivel, in the latter, somewhat reminiscent of Smollett's Dr Linden in *Humphry Clinker* who makes his histrionic appearance at Bath, espouses Sinclair's paradigms for lean living.[17] Baron Rasp absorbs these 'principles of health' and sets them into practice. In *The Antiquary*, Wardour and Littlejohn are both gouty, in ways one might not expect for an ardent devotee of Smollett. Scott's more likely candidates in this novel are Oldbuck and Ochiltree: the first seemingly a Scottian correlative of Squire Bramble, similar in age (about fifty-five), also a bachelor, crusty and generous in equal parts, energetic, aggressive, corpulent, an elder in the Church of Scotland, the sort of figure the most popular novelist of the early nineteenth century might have endowed with an all-encompassing and insulating gout, at once heroic and comic; the second, Ochiltree, is more romantic if more problematic a figure. Oldbuck's stories are bawdy, revealing an inner prurience, but his penchant for the lewd has apparently not given way to the excesses said to result in the insulating and comic condition – gout. Nor has it in the case of beggar Ochiltree, similarly aged to Oldbuck, the pair constituting something of a set of romantic quixotic variations on the squire and his man, as had Bramble and his pink-skinned Humphry. Neither of Scott's Cervantic couple has a trace of the gout; Sir Arthur Wardour and Baillie Littlejohn – both minor figures observed by the major ones – do and both have strong military ties.

Sir Arthur, a magistrate, conceives of himself as first and foremost a military man, a loyalist who had served his country. The extremely corpulent Littlejohn is a shopkeeper who also fancies himself a soldier before all else, though his indolence and inactivity are his most noteworthy attributes. Both characters come in for Scott's proverbial ridicule – genial and generous, but cutting to the heart of the matter about gout having been the sign of an old world we had lost. Littlejohn 'was a zealous loyalist of that zealous time, somewhat rigorous and peremptory in the execution of his duty, and a good deal inflated with the sense of his own power and importance, otherwise an honest, well-meaning, and useful citizen'.[18] Thus 1798 has turned nostalgic for Scott and his readers through the devices of war: always a zone of nostalgia. But Scott's rotund Littlejohn is also Rowlandsonian, from whose watercolour sketches he could have stepped forward: 'my gouty chair . . . for I am scarce fit for drill yet – A slight touch of our old acquaintance *podagra* – I can keep my feet, however, while our sergeant puts me through the manual.'[19] Gout, more than anything else, seems to be the would-be-sergeant's constant companion, its comic treats captured by Scott in the mouthpiece of the upper-class Oldbuck, who comprehends these matters residual from a prior age:

> And so exit the martial magistrate [Sir Arthur], with his maid behind him bearing his weapons.
>
> 'A good squire that wench for a gouty champion,' observed Oldbuck. – 'Hector, my lad, hook on, hook on – Go with him, boy. – keep him employed, man, for half an hour or so – butter him with some warlike terms – praise his dress and address . . .
>
> Captain M'Intyre, who, like many of his profession, looked down with infinite scorn on those citizen soldiers, who had assumed arms without any professional title to bear them, rose with great reluctance, observing that he could not know what to say to Mr Littlejohn; and that to see an old gouty shopkeeper attempting the exercise and duties of a private soldier, was really too ridiculous.[20]

Ridiculous these ludic prancings may have appeared to Scott's most modern readers, but these gestures had embodied the masculine temperament in the *ancien régime* viewed through the eyes of 'old-buckle' himself. These were the gouty types of the last generation, it seemed in the 1820s; so unequivocal that novelists like Scott could depict them with just a few strokes of the pen. These military buffoons, the comic heirs perhaps of Commodore Trunnion in Smollett's hilarious 'garrison' in *Peregrine Pickle* and the Uncle Toby–Captain Trim mock military axis in *Tristram Shandy*, differ, however, from Austen's Mr Woodhouse. They diverge again, from Disraeli's Regency dandies and silver-lined salonistes. All are 'gouty'. All share a masculinity now very much having come under the gun of new interrogation about class and rank and moral worth. But the gout insignia was a disparate signification: denoting myriad forms of a world some thought well worth having lost. The varieties of these gouty types are surely more diverse than we give out here: not uniform, even if monolithically comic and often grotesque in the Smollettian sense. Their versions beckon us to retrieve a cultural history embedded in the novel from Smollett and Scott to Dickens and the Victorian novelists, one whose centrepiece down through the nineteenth century remains the definition of manliness and masculinity.[21]

As Emma Bovary discovered in a period chronologically proximate to Scott and Disraeli, illness, especially sickness leading to death, is the most predictable validator of human worth. There was nothing unique to gout in this capacity of measuring the pulse of character. But gout had been more than just another disease. It was the grand comic insulator; the monarch of disease because it afflicted the great and famous, yet was itself inexplicable in its ability to shield its victims from life-threatening calamity. Thackeray and Trollope also exemplify these points as the two Victorian novelists closest to the century in which gout had so rampantly flourished – the eighteenth.

The signal fact is that not a single major character in their vast novelistic *oeuvre* has gout, not in the ten novels Thackeray wrote or the approximately fifty volumes constituting that encyclopedia of the human heart, the 'Waverley Novels'. The most likely places yield nothing. We would think Jos Sedley and Lord Steyne to be prime candidates in *Vanity Fair*, or the many upper-class males in *The Adventure of Major Gahagan* or *Barry Lyndon*. Gahagan is a military man who had gone out to India and remains forever boastful of his cast and lineage. Yet here is no hint of the gouty conceit despite all sorts of real and pretended pedigree. *Barry Lindon* is set on a country estate in the heart of eighteenth-century Ireland, the natural environment, we would have thought, for gouty figures and their conceits of caste, but not so. Steyne (readers never missed the pun) is Thackeray's antidote in *Vanity Fair* to Dickens's Sir Leicester in *Bleak House*: the right age, steeped in claret and port, eating himself into the grave, vast and corpulent, sexually interested in Becky Sharp, with a taint of madness in his character but not of gout. The most likely candidate of all, surely, is Major Pendennis himself, the ageing dandy in *Pendennis*, written after Dickens had presented the gouty Sir Leicester to the literate world. But here too there is no mention until the Major is described as emerging from an evening party, feeling his age: he 'had two or three twinges of the gout in the country house where he had been staying'. Then the matter is entirely dropped, as if requiring no further amplification, certainly no clue to inner selfhood or moral worth.

One of Major Pendennis's friends is delightfully named Viscount Colchicum, as if he were some homoeopathic aristocrat, described as a 'pillar of the state' drenched in caste and claret who has a tinge of the gout. He functions similarly to the first Duke of Omnium in Trollope's Palliser novels, a version of the 'great man' derived from the earlier Lord Steyne. Omnium dies – of course not from gout – and is replaced by a new duke by the time *The Prime Minister* is published in 1876. Trollope's description of Colchicum is so proverbial of the gouty type that it is worth citing:

My Lord Colchicum, though stricken in years, bald of head and enfeebled in person, was still indefatigable in the pursuit of enjoyment, and it was the venerable Viscount's boast that he could drink as much claret as the youngest member of the society which he frequented. He lived with the youth about town: he gave them countless dinners at Richmond and Greenwich: an enlightened patron of the drama in all languages and of the Terpsichorean art, he received dramatic professors of all nations at his banquets – English from the Covent Garden and Strand houses, Italians from the Haymarket, French from their own pretty little theatre, or the boards of the Opera where they danced. And at his villa on the Thames, this pillar of the state gave sumptuous entertainments to scores of young men of fashion, who very affably consorted with the ladies and gentlemen of the green-room – with the former chiefly, for Viscount Colchicum preferred their society as more polished and gay than that of their male brethren.[22]

In 1841 Thackeray founded *Punch*, the source of dozens of cartoons about gouty men.[23] We discuss them in Chapter 12 below, and merely note here that word and image are in accord in regard to the pedigree conceit. Later on, in 1860, Lord Ringwood, the hero's great-uncle in *The Adventure of Philip*, is described as having the gout. His characterization covers the predictable zones of class, rank, pedigree, education and place in the military, but tells us nothing about moral character or assumed inner worth. Generation thus passes to generation the chief conceits of its pedigree, but for more specificity than this, the artifice is silent. In Trollope there is surprisingly even less. Here the gouty conceit seems reserved for the least sympathetic of elderly characters, for a few minor figures such as Earl De Courcy in *The Small House at Allington* and Sir Anthony Aylmer in *The Belton Estate*: 'a heavy man, over seventy years of age, much afflicted with gout'. Gone was the comic emblem of a Georgian generation. Smollett's sense that gout could be the key to unlock the mysteries of mind and body, as it was with Bramble, was irretrievably lost.

None of these literary figures is a martyr to gout, certainly not in the way real-life figures had been. Perhaps the pose was too sentimental or, alternatively, too artificially heroic for a Victorian milieu sceptical of all martyrdom. Life had changed since the days when gout could form the basement – the brick and mortar – of Bramble's daily routine, determining when he would rise or sit, when imbibe or evacuate. We noted in the previous chapter that clinicians like William Gairdner, highly influential in the mid-nineteenth century, were propagating a paradigm of the disease which posited it as the centre of a spider's web of symptoms.[24] And the old gout rigmaroles, however played out in the novel, nevertheless continued to circulate in nineteenth-century magazines and the popular press. One is worth citing at some length:

'That pain which you feel in the joint of your great toe,' quoth Monsieur Gout, 'has, you flatter yourself, become rather less since 8 o'clock, when you took your last dose of colchicum. Quite a mistake, my dear sir! The member is, if anything, more swollen and inflamed than before. Observe now – I shall take the liberty of inserting this little awl, just by the way of probe. Aha! it makes you wince! A very good sign that, however, since it proves that there is no grounding for apprehending immediate mortification. Now, do you know why it is that your toe is so singularly sensitive? I'll tell you. You remember, three years ago, ordering a batch of burgundy!

Previous to that time you had been in very good health, for you had plenty of occupation and little leisure for gluttony or wine-bibbing; your means were limited, and during the holy-days you took a sufficiency of pedestrian exercise. Really, in those days I never expected to have the pleasure of making your acquaintance. I considered you just the kind of fellow likely to come an ornament of the Alpine Club. But your estimable uncle, old Jones, the stockbroker – bless you, I knew him very well indeed! many a time have I chatted to him when he was roaring like an aggravated bullock – your old Uncle Jones, I say, died and left you his money – you are not going to sleep, are you? Well, I call that rather unhandsome treatment, considering that I have taken the pains to come here and bear you company. A slight touch of the pincers may, however – aha! all's right again; you are as lively as a snapping turtle! Whereabouts was I? Oh, I remember, Old Jones left you his money, and you determined to take your ease. No one can blame you for that. What's the use of fagging to make more when you are in a possession of a cool 4,000*l.* a year, and may indulge in a shooting box and hunters? But you could never make up a respectable bag on the moors, and on horseback you were anything but a Ducrow. You preferred living in town, took chambers in the Albany, gave nice little *recherché* dinners, and laid in that stock of burgundy to which I have already alluded. It was of a fine vintage, strong and heady, and made the blood circulate in the veins like lightning. To it I attribute the honour of our first introduction, though port and claret, not to mention sundry kinds of delicious *entremets*, did undoubtedly contribute to lessen the distance between us. Then you took to late hours, hot rooms, and *écarté*, almost justly included in the catalogue of fashionable pleasures; and our acquaintance, at first only slight, has now ripened into permanent friend-ship. But I really must not allow my feelings to divert me from the scientific purpose for which I have visited you to-night, Don't be afraid! I shall lay aside awl and pincers, and vary the experiment by injecting a few drops of molten lead between the flesh and the bone. Ha! what an enviable yell! Your lungs, I can assure you, are in a perfectly healthy state, and may last you for the next twenty years, if you don't force me to get into your stomach. By the way, what a silly proverb that is against pushing things to an extremity. It is with the extremities I always make a point of dealing in the first instance, and I take it that very few people would wish me to depart from the practice. What is that you say? You wish that I would go to the devil. Pardon me for hinting in reply that you are both rude and unreasonable. I am here, as you well know, in consequence of your indiscretions.'[25]

Extended passages like this could no longer be admitted into the novel, neither English nor French, as in the eighteenth century, but nineteenth-century essayists and anecdotalists carried on retailing stories that included gouty tipplers and beflannelled sufferers. The traditional connotations of the condition were still taken for granted. Dickens, like Disraeli and Scott before him, and like Meredith and Collins after him, made subtle use of the malady. The 'pedigree of podagra' conceit is quite central in *Bleak House*, as we have suggested, where Dickens's old county baronet, Sir Leicester Dedlock, immobilized for long periods in the ancient oak bedchamber at Chesney Wold, reflected that 'all the Dedlocks in the direct male line through a course of time during and beyond which the memory of man goeth not to the contrary', had had the gout. The gouty paralysis served as an emblem for the dead-weight of tradition.[26] Gouty limbs had descended since the Conquest with the family plate, seat and portraits. In a more light-hearted exchange in *Pickwick Papers*, Sam Weller warned his father against excessive brandy-drinking, lest it brought on his old complaint:

> 'I've found a sov'rin cure for that, Sammy,' said Mr Weller, setting down the glass.
> 'A sovereign cure for the gout,' said Mr Pickwick, hastily producing his note-book – 'what is it?'
> 'The gout, sir,' replied Mr Weller, 'the gout is a complaint as arises from too much ease and comfort. 'If you're ever attacked with the gout, sir, jist you marry a widder as has got a good loud woice, with a decent notion of usin' it, and you'll never have the gout again. It's a capital prescription, sir. I takes it reg'lar and I can warrent it to drive away any illness as is caused by too much jollity.'[27]

There is more to gout in Dickens than this. Gout, like mesmerism or consumption, captured his imagination in a number of ways, particularly as a topic of contemporary popular interest, but never violates the truth that Bramble is the last gouty protagonist in any canonical work of British literature. 'Other men's fathers may have died of rheumatism,' Dickens narrates at the opening of the famous Chapter 16 of *Bleak House*, 'or may have taken base contagion from the tainted blood of the vulgar sick, but the Dedlock family have communicated something exclusive, even to the levelling process of dying, by dying of their own family gout.'[28] Something exclusive indeed! – something which no degree of imitation, theft or purchase can remove, so innate are its acquisitions, hence the grand theory of acquired gout. Marxist approaches to these 'levelling processes' can run wild with excesses of interpretation, but cannot invalidate the reasons for the acquisition theories of the doctors.

The deceased 'Mr F' in *Little Dorrit*, nephew of the draconian 'Mr F's Aunt' who is never more specifically named than this, is another such spectacular specimen. Dickens paints him indelibly as a member of the gouty tribe, speaking through the breathless and unpunctuated Flora:

I will draw a veil over that dreamy life, Mr F was in good spirits his appetite was good he liked the cookery he considered the wine weak but palatable and all was well, we returned to the immediate neighbourhood of Number Thirty Little Gosling Street London Docks and settled down, ere we had yet fully detected the housemaid in selling the feathers out of the spare bed Gout flying upwards soared with Mr F to another sphere.[29]

Such 'Gout flying upwards' is a mordant variation of the gout of dynasties, something indelible and constant throughout the generations, but a lesser gout, like that of Tite Barnacle in the same novel:

The Mr Tite Barnacle who at the period now in question usually coached or crammed the statesman at the head of the Circumlocution Office, when that noble or right honourable individual sat a little uneasily in his saddle, by reason of some vagabond making a tilt at him in a newspaper, was more flush of blood than money . . . If a gentlemanly residence coming strictly within this narrow margin, had not been essential to the blood of the Barnacles, this particular branch would have had a pretty wide selection among let us say ten thousand houses, offering fifty times the accommodation for a third of the money.[30]

Here again, blood as rank, gout as proof. There was something risible in the formulaic application of these old truths, as if do what one will they could not die, but the tropes continued to be applied again and again in Dickens, even if he could not resuscitate the likes of a Matt Bramble.[31] At the heart of the matter was the notion of a gentleman: what it was, how it functioned, its living proofs. Nothing could replace gout here. Nothing less than blood would tell the truth.[32]

It is therefore not surprising that in real life there were many notable nineteenth-century martyrs to classic articular gout. Thanks to the 'diagnostic creep' of the disease label countenanced by physicians like Scudamore and Gairdner, who were inclined to identify as 'gouty' a host of non-specific internal pains and complaints, there were also innumerable sufferers who claimed to have types of suppressed, retrocedent or atonic gout. These, especially the atonic variety, were convenient devices for covering medical ignorance with a diagnostic figleaf while conferring upon the patient a prestigious diagnosis. A good instance is offered by Samuel Taylor Coleridge. It may be disputed, of course, whether Coleridge presents a true case of gout; he believed himself to be afflicted by it, however, and he was one of the century's most eloquent sufferers.[33]

During the 1790s, Coleridge, in his late teens, began to experience a constellation of complaints – rheumatic fever, neuralgias and so forth. It would be misguided to attempt to distinguish which were organic, which psychosomatic and which iatrogenic – that is, the consequence of (initially) medically prescribed opium-taking. Partly to quell the pains, he started to consume opiates on a regular basis in large quantities. He grew hypersensitive to his sufferings, we might say a hypochondriac. The flexible terminology of gout proved useful to him as a way of expressing his almost kinaesthetic bodily experiences.

In the summer of 1803, he concluded that the only solution for his ailments was a long journey, preferably to some warm climate, or, failing that, in some romantic region like Scotland. He had come to this resolve in view of the fact, as he informed his friend Robert Southey, that he had been 'very ill, & in serious dread of a paralytic Stroke in my whole left Side'. As a voracious medical reader (the perfect susceptible for hypochondriasis!), he now had 'no Shade of Doubt' as to the disease from which he was suffering: 'it is a compleat & almost heartless Case of Atonic Gout'. In typically Coleridgean manner, he gave chapter and verse: 'If you would look into the Article Medicine, in the Encyc. Britt. Vol. XI. Part I. – No. 213. – p. 181. – & the first 5 paragraphs of the second Column / you will read almost the very words, in which, before I had seen this Article, I had described my case to Wordsworth.'[34]

So what was to be done? He had conceded the 'possibility or propriety' of a tour into Scotland. Mr Edmondson, a surgeon–apothecary known to Coleridge, recommended it: the 'Exercise & the Excitement' would be of 'so much service as to outweigh the chances of Injury from Wet or Cold'. Hence he had decided to go. At the same time he had resolved to give a try to a new gout medicine, recommended by Coleridge's friend and physician Thomas Beddoes. As the continuation of the letter to Southey makes clear, Coleridge had been engaged in a considerable medical conflict with Beddoes, and hoped to use Southey as a go-between:

> whatever the expence be, I will give it one Trial – & should be very greatly obliged to Dr Beddoes if *he* would desire Mr Wells to send down a sufficient Quantity of the Medicine, if he think it likely to be serviceable in a clear Case of atonic Gout / a case of capricious Appetite – indigestion / costiveness that makes my evacuations at times approach in all the symptoms to the pains of Labor – viz – distortion of Body from agony, profuse and streaming Sweats, & fainting – at other times, looseness with griping – frightful Dreams with screaming – *breezes* of Terror blowing from the Stomach up thro' the Brain / always when I am awakened, I find myself stifled with wind / & the wind the manifest cause of the Dream / frequent paralytic Feelings – sometimes approaches to Convulsion fit – three times I have wakened out of these frightful Dreams, & found my legs so *locked* into each other as to have *left* a bruise – / Sometimes I am a little giddy; but very seldom have the Headach / And on the whole my Head

is wonderfully *clear*, considering – tho' less so than in an earlier Stage of the Disease / & this being the strongest part of my Constitution, when that goes, all goes – / My hands & fingers occasionally swell – my feet are often inflamed / with pulsations in the Toes – & twice last week I was lame in my Left Leg, & the ancle was swoln / but these inflammatory Symptoms soon go off. My Mouth is endlessly full of water – itself no small Persecution – but above all, the *asthmatic Stuffing* – which forms a true suspension of the Habeas Corpus Act. – I live very temperately – drinking only one tumbler of Brandy & Water in the 24 hours . . .

What I want is to have a quantity of the Gout Medicine sent to Greta Hall, Keswick, Cumberland – by the waggon either from London or Bristol – so that on my return from Scotland I may find it here.[35]

The new medicine to which Coleridge was referring was not Husson's *Eau médicinale* but Welles's gout remedy, at that time being touted by the scientifically minded Bristol physician Thomas Beddoes. Beddoes was resisting Coleridge's conviction that a few months in the sun would be highly medicinal; one imagines that in Coleridge's case he regarded it as psychological escapism.[36]

Gout cures competed in Coleridge's head. Gout was the affliction *sine qua non*: the rich and influential, and even the not-so-rich, could live neither with nor without it. The only dilemma was that almost everyone capable of understanding its cultural components also bought into its mythologies: patients and doctors alike, and not merely the Coleridges and other martyrs to the cause, but also those who could have known better: for example, Isaac Milner, one of Coleridge's early group, a prominent natural philosopher in Cambridge who held the first endowed chair in the subject.[37] Milner was a mathematician with no known medical interests. His chair's benefactor, the Revd Richard Jackson, suffered from gout himself and sought cure.[38] His stipulation in making the bequest was that its holders would apply themselves as part of their remit to the search for a cure. Milner accepted the condition and spent his first few years searching. The experiments, if Milner performed experiments, remain undocumented, but it would be interesting to know if there were other chaired professorships with these stipulated remits. The Continental universities are unlikely to have been sites because gout was first and foremost an English malady by the nineteenth century. Still, the natural and social historian of gout wonders what a thorough search – which we have not performed – would reveal.

Milner's patron, the Revd Richard Jackson, suffered acute pain and is not known to have travelled to sunny climates for repair. But the thirty-three-year-old Coleridge, together with William and Dorothy Wordsworth, embarked upon his regenerative Scottish jaunt, hoping to reach the Mull of Kintyre, and he continued the wail of pain begun in his outpourings to

Southey in letters to his wife. 'My dear Sara,' he wrote on 2 September 1803, having just been trudging through the Trossachs:

> We returned to E[ast] Tarbet, I with the rheumatism in my head I burnt my shoes in drying them at the Boatman's Hovel on Loch Ketterin / and I have by this means hurt my heel – likewise my Left Leg is a little inflamed / & the Rheumatism in the right of my head afflicts me sorely when I begin to grow warm in my bed, chiefly, my right eye, ear, cheek, & the three Teeth / but nevertheless, I am enjoying myself.[39]

The tale of woe continued the next day in a further letter to her complaining of 'Gout in my Stomach'.[40] Around the same time he wrote to his friend and protégé Tom Wedgwood, promising 'I will not trouble you with the gloomy Tale of my Health,' before launching into just that:

> I am grown hysterical. – Meantime my Looks & Strength have improved. I myself fully believe it to be either atonic, hypochondriacal Gout, or a scrophulous affection of the mesenteric Glands. In the hope of driving the Gout, if Gout it should be, into the feet, I walked, previously to my getting into the Coach at Perth, 268 miles in eight Days, with no unpleasant fatigue: & if I could do you any service by coming to town, & there were no Coaches, I would undertake to be with you, on foot, in 7 days. – I must have strength somewhere / My head is indefatigably strong, my limbs too are strong – but acid or not acid, Gout or Scrofula, Something there is [in] my stomach or Guts that transubstantiates my Bread & Wine into the Body & Blood of the Devil – Meat & Drink I should say – for I eat but little bread, & take nothing, in any form, spirituous or narcotic, stronger than Table Beer. – I am about to try the new Gout Medicine / & if it cures me, I will turn Preacher, form a new Sect in honor of the Discoverer, & make a greater clamour in his Favor, as the Anti-podagra, 'that was to come & is already in the world', than ever the Puritans did *against* the poor Pope, as Anti-christ.

> *Epitaph*
> Here sleeps at length poor Col, & without Screaming,
> Who died, as he had always liv'd, a dreaming:
> Shot dead, while sleeping, by the Gout within,
> Alone, and all unknown, at E'nbro' in an Inn.[41]

As may be seen, Coleridge was essaying the most orthodox of strategies – to drive atonic gout from his innards to the extremities – through the most unorthodox of means, walking over 250 miles in a week (there cannot have been many 'gouty' folks who put themselves through such therapeutic walking tours). His attempts did not seem to bear much fruit, as he explained later that month to Sir George and Lady Beaumont:

The attacks of the Gout, now no longer doubtful, have become formidable in the stomach, & my nature is making continual tho' hitherto alas! fruitless efforts to throw the Disease into the Extremities / and as it never rains but it pours I have an intermittent Fever with severe Hemicrania, which returns every evening at $^1/_2$ past 5, & has hitherto baffled the use of Bark.
    – To morrow I expect to receive the new Gout medicine from Welles.[42]

Later that year, he noted to Matthew Coates, a Bristol friend, his continued jointy swellings, seemingly drawing an unconscious parallel between the torments of gout and of guilt:

After a time of Sufferings great, as mere bodily Afflictions can well be conceived to be, and which the Horrors of my Sleep, and Night-screams (so loud & so frequent as to make me almost a Nuisance in my own house[)] seemed to carry beyond mere Body – counterfeiting, as it were, the Tortures of Guilt, and what we are told of the Punishments of a spiritual World – I am at length a Convalescent.[43]

His joint pains did not get any better, but as he spelt out early in the next year (1804) in a letter to his wife, his grasp of his complaint at least improved: 'I am more and more convinced that it is not Gout – or at all events, that if my case be flying windy Gout, that flying windy Gout is not the same disease with regular Gout.'[44] As a result of those continuing joint pains and the indigestive problems he referred to as 'windy gout', Coleridge explained to Southey once again that for a real cure 'I must go into a hot climate.'[45]
    Like Pope's 'long *Disease*, my life', Coleridge's pains continued throughout his earthly existence. In the end, however, he convinced himself that he was not really suffering from gout – or, to be more precise, he believed that his gouty tendencies had transmogrified themselves into jaundice or erysipelas.[46] Shortly afterwards he explained to another correspondent that he was 'barely emancipated from the RED ROVER, yclept Erysipelas'.[47] These were 'a substitute for Gout which I have not strength enough to mature into a regular fit'.[48] Coleridge thus concluded along these lines that his personal medical history was one of 'failed' gout – his symptoms, unfortunately, had rarely managed actually to resolve themselves into a real gout:

I have myself been without intermission, tho' with varying degrees of intensity, ill, since we met – have every night a paroxysm of Erysipelas on my Leg, and the distress of my general Sensations, my depression of Spirits and Incapability of combining an outward act of any kind with that of Thinking, to which I have to add some nephritic symptoms, seem to hold a sort of inverse ratio to the length and severity of these local Affections. Mr Green inclines to think the latter imperfect or abortive attempts at a Gout.[49]

Even so, it is noteworthy that, to the end of his life and perhaps to keep up his spirits, Coleridge continued to refer to his condition as 'atonic Gout'.[50]

Coleridge was not the only gout-embracing nineteenth-century poet. Tennyson was, too – in his case it would seem to have been a combination of clearcut articular disorder and a multitude of other symptoms for which 'gouty' served as a flag of convenience. Tennyson grew up amid terrible family traumas, surrounded by an alcoholic clergyman father and a brood of sickly siblings. Around his twentieth year (1829), he fell into deep melancholy. 'I remember', he later recalled, 'that sometimes in the midst of the dance, a great and sudden sadness would come over me, and I would leave the dance and wander away beneath the stars, or sit on gloomily and abstractedly below stairs. I used to wonder then, what strange demon it was, that drove me forth and took all the pleasure from my blood, and made such a churlish curmudgeon.'[51] Long afterwards he claimed to have recognized the reason: 'It was gout.' The word was loosely used in Tennyson's family and it is difficult to gauge precisely what they meant. In 1885 Edmund Lushington, who married Alfred's sister Cecilia, wrote of her mental depression and disturbance: 'Many complaints that formerly had different names, are now often classed under the head of gout.'[52] Tennyson had undergone mysterious trances ever since boyhood. His father suffered from epileptic fits. Perhaps 'gout' was a respectable euphemism for what was feared to be incipient epilepsy.

With the breakdown of his physical and mental health around 1844, Tennyson went for treatment at Prestbury hydropathic centre, and then to Malvern, his son Hallam noting that 'so severe a hypochondria set in upon him that his friends despaired of his life'.[53] In 1848, on a second visit to Malvern, he was under the care of Dr James Gully, who specialized in gout. Thereafter he stopped taking hydropathic treatment and apparently never again suffered from that kind of 'hypochondria'; and he began referring for the first time to his own trances, which he ascribed either to gout or to his passing into an extra-sensory state through meditation.[54] He seems to have concluded, perhaps thanks to Gully, that the true cause of his trances was indeed an inherited disease, but that it was purely physical in nature not mental – in short, gout not epilepsy.[55] This is all the more likely in view of Gully's drastic curtailment of his heavy drinking – he had apparently been consuming a bottle of port a day. Gully allowed his patients no alcohol at Malvern, and when Tennyson left he was under orders to have no more than two glasses daily.[56]

Carlyle was another of Gully's famous patients, three years later in 1851. Gully specialized in assembling famous gouty men at Malvern, almost recruited them: the more famous they were, the more extensive his largesse. Jane Carlyle accompanied her husband during the summer of 1851, although she declined to descend into any of Gully's mud puddles and cascades of water.[57] Carlyle had been chronically ill – physically and mentally – for much of his life, never fatally, but rarely existing without one or another type of debilitating condition. His range of symptoms almost always implicated his stomach and bowels, even when in nervous combinations, so gout continued to be the suspected villain. At Malvern Carlyle was sceptical that the waters would cure him but was willing to try everything Dr Gully recommended: castor oil, cold showers, blue pills, the lot.[58] He was less enthusiastic than Tennyson about Gully's water cures, perhaps as the result of an intuition that his psyche was afflicted, not his stomach, although his family had no history of mental disorder.

Carlyle remained vigilant in his writings to gout's regal claim – the fabled monarch of disease – although he hardly violates our Smollettian paradigm about protagonists appearing in novels. Nothing, for example, in Carlyle's classic study of hero worship – *On Heroes, Hero-Worship and the Heroic in History* (1841) – suggests otherwise, and there is no mention of illness in relation to heroism. Even in his famous life of Frederick the Great, once a popular biography originally printed in seven volumes and reprinted many times, the great Enlightenment monarch's ailment, somewhat like George III's, is muted.[59] The Comte de Belleisle has gout, others too in Carlyle's narrative, as does the King. 'The King', Carlyle writes of Frederick in the early 1760s, 'fell ill of gout, saw almost nobody, never came out; and, it was whispered, the inflexible heart of him was at last breaking; that is, to say, the very axis of the Prussian world giving way.' Carlyle does not draw out the possibilities or implications, but his narrative indicates the curve of a familiar story: gout the symptom, not the cause, of a lost world mourned by all affiliated to its versions of rank and class, especially royal rank. Carlyle claims to write here as a historian, basing his work on research, narrating quite differently from the poets, Coleridge and Tennyson.[60] He assumes his research about gout is correct, and does not interrogate his authorities. However, within the lines we are tracing, Carlyle is not the most subversive of authors, but he does capitalize on the 'disease of monarchs' and strengthen its heritage.

If Carlyle's experience at Malvern persuaded him that his troubles were rooted in the mind, Tennyson's remained firmly in the body. He fell repeatedly sick, and strayed from doctor to doctor, at last settling on James Paget, who decided that he had a 'goutish affection' of the sort that he had often seen in families where gout was hereditary. It was an echo of Dr Gully's words. Some measure of how seriously Tennyson took the diagnosis is his decision to change his drinking habits: 'It will be better I think to exchange the greatest part of the port, tho' I must say I hate claret.' This resolution did not last. During the last dozen years of his life, gout constantly racked him, and he was forever giving up port on the advice of his doctors. But the numbers of times over the years that guests mentioned his most recent resolves to supplant it with whisky or brandy suggest that he was no more successful in this than at stopping smoking.[61]

As Tennyson's therapeutic endeavours make clear, water treatments were very popular.[62] Taking the waters at Buxton in 1827, Dick Dyott had noted:

> I bathed in what is called the new bath for a week, but subsequently in the old common bath, which I much preferred, as I fancied I found greater relief from it. I tried the water, but found it did not agree with me, and as my complaint certainly partook as much of gout as of rheumatism, and consequently attended with inflammation, it would have been adding fuel to the flame.[63]

Bath had gone out of fashion, but many new hydropathic establishments sprang up, with their proprietors, notably the eminent Dr Gully at Malvern, claiming that they were more scientific. Another eminent Victorian who at times at least thought he was gouty and who sampled Gully's hydropathic cures was Charles Darwin. Rather as with Coleridge, Darwin's medical history has been, and remains, one of the 'source of the Nile' mysteries of nineteenth-century scholarship. From specialists in tropical disease to psycho-analysts, all manner of medical experts have offered their divergent inter-pretations of the condition and its cause that increasingly laid Darwin flat once he had returned from the voyage of the *Beagle* and hit upon the idea of evolution by natural selection.[64]

On 13 November 1848, Charles's father, Dr Robert Darwin, died. Darwin was 'too ill' to attend the funeral. In the following months he grieved and continued to be severely sick. He consulted Dr Henry Holland, who told him that his illness was unique, and did not fit any known classification of illness; that it was not 'quite' dyspepsia, and 'nearer to suppressed gout'.[65] Then Darwin read Dr Gully's book, and may have corresponded with Gully, who impressed him as sensible.[66] 'Thank you much for your information about the water cure,' wrote Darwin in February 1849. 'I cannot make up my mind; I dislike the thoughts of it much – I know I shall be very uncomfortable there . . . Can you tell me (& I shd be much obliged sometime for an answer) whether either [of] your cases was dyspepsia, though Dr Holland does not consider my case quite that, but nearer to suppressed gout.'[67]

Gully's regime was based on the idea that chronic disorders were caused by a faulty supply of blood to the viscera and that the application of cold water to the skin would return the circulation to normal and alleviate the condition. Water was at its most effective if applied externally.[68] At Darwin's initial consultation, Gully conceded that dyspepsia was to blame. Originally only a descriptive, functional term that meant simple indigestion, 'dyspepsia' for Gully and other early-Victorian doctors included notions of physical weak-ness, depression of spirits, 'nervous indigestion' and morbid despondency. People like Darwin, used to a life of extreme mental strain, were prone to conditions in which brain activity set up and maintained nervous irritation that kept up the derangement of the stomach. The analysis was simple: the digestive organs irritated the brain and spinal cord and these in turn irritated the stomach. As Darwin put it: he 'thinks my head or top of spinal chord cause of mischief'.[69]

'You ask how I am,' Darwin responded to his friend Joseph Hooker early in January 1865: 'Dr Jenner is exhausted as to doing me any good. All Doctors seem to think that I am a case of suppressed gout: do you know of any good man hereafter to consult? I did think of trying Bence Jones; but I know it is folly & nonsense to try anyone.'[70] At this time, although the diagnosis of suppressed gout was sometimes made, it was not always accepted, as is shown by Hooker's reply: 'What the devil is this "suppressed gout" upon which doctors fasten every ill they cannot name? If it is suppressed how do they know it is gout? If it is apparent, why the devil do they call it suppressed? I hate the use of cant terms to cloak ignorance.'[71] After reading this Darwin must have had increased misgivings about doctors. He summoned Dr Chapman, and sent him a page of notes in which he unsparingly depicted the mixture of nervous and psychophysiologic symptoms which made up his invalid condition:

Age 56–57. – For 25 years extreme spasmodic daily & nightly flatulence: occasional vomiting, on two occasions prolonged during months. Vomiting preceded by shivering, ['hysterical crying' inserted] dying sensations ['or half-faint' inserted]. & copious very palid urine. Now vomiting & every passage of flatulence preceded by ringing of ears, treading on air & vision. ['focus & black dots' 'Air fatigues, specially risky, brings on the Head symptoms' 'nervousness when E. leaves me.–' inserted] (What I vomit intensely acid, slimy (sometimes bitter) consider teeth.) Doctors ['puzzled' inserted] say suppressed gout – No organic mischief, Jenner & Brinton. – Family gouty.[72]

Victorian doctors like Chapman and Gully believed that some illnesses of the nervous, circulatory and digestive systems should be diagnosed as 'suppressed gout'. Holland said that Darwin's 1848–9 illness was 'nearest to suppressed gout',[73] and wrote that there was an 'undoubted connexion between dyspeptic disorders and the irregular forms of the gouty constitution'.[74] Since gout was regarded as a 'hereditary disorder', Darwin's doctors may have postulated that he had inherited his form of gout from some of his ancestors. It seems likely that his paternal grandfather Dr Erasmus Darwin had acute attacks of gout in his joints; and his father may have had gout.[75]

The concept of 'suppressed gout' explained Darwin's illness to some of his doctors, and perhaps to himself. He came to believe that there were three causes for his illness: heredity; some of the ill effects of the *Beagle* cruise; and the pressures of scientific work. In 1838 (in the course of searching for the causes of heritable variation) he recorded in one of his evolutionary notebooks what his father had told him about the inheritance of diseases and mental and physical traits. Dr Robert Darwin had observed that when attending one patient 'he could not help thinking he was prescribing to his [the patient's] father'. In 1839 Darwin read Holland's just-published *Medical Notes and Reflections*, and made numerous annotations in the chapter 'On Hereditary Disease'. At the end of the book he wrote: 'Strong sentence on Hereditariness.' The sentence he had marked read: 'Seeking then for the most general expression of facts, we may affirm that no organ or texture of the body is exempt from the chance of being the subject of hereditary disease.'[76]

In his fourth 'Transmutation Notebook' he made a note to 'ask' Dr Holland for more details about the inheritance of certain traits. Over the years, in the course of developing his theory of evolution, he read widely about inheritance. In 1868, in *The Variation of Animals and Plants under Domestication*, he published examples of the inheritance of illness, including gout: 'With gout, fifty percent of the cases observed in hospital practice are, according to Dr. Garrod, inherited, and a greater percentage in private practice.' In that work he also published his theory of pangenesis: this held that the body cells gave off gemmules which became part of the reproductive cells, and that 'man carries in his constitution the seeds of an inherited disease'.[77] He then applied his ideas about the inheritance of illness to himself in two ways. He thought that his family was 'gouty', and that his illness was caused by his inheritance of this 'gouty' tendency. He then held that some of his children had 'inherited from me feeble health'. He may also have thought that a further cause for his children's inherited ill health was his marriage to his cousin.[78]

It is evident from the cases of Tennyson, Carlyle and Darwin that Victorian outlooks, in particular concern with the healthiness of families, were focusing attention on the hereditary aspects of disease. Gout played a complex role in such thinking. On the one hand, it was indeed seen as an inherited condition. On the other hand, as a non-lethal disease, it was a deliverance from such more threatening conditions as epilepsy. Moreover gout could still be seen as the disease of genius. As earlier noticed, Havelock Ellis was still advancing such a view early in the twentieth century.[79] A still later instance may be found in the autobiography of Osbert Sitwell. Contemplating his forebears, Sitwell wrote:

common to all four of my great-grandfathers is one other thing I have not mentioned, but have most specifically inherited: gout. Of this illness, mysterious in origin and manifestation, the late Dr Havelock Ellis wrote that it 'occurs so often, in such extreme forms, and in men of such pre-eminent intellectual ability, that it is impossible not to regard it as having a real association with such ability', and again that it would be impossible to 'match the group of gout men of genius, for varied and pre-eminent intellectual ability by any combination of non-gouty individuals on our list . . .' He adds that they have frequently been eccentric and irascible, and in the eighteenth century were termed 'choleric' by their contemporaries. Another earlier writer and most famous physician states that gout kills 'more rich men than poor, more wise than simple'. But Havelock Ellis supplies a reason for the connecting of this pathological condition with mental activity. The poison which causes it, he declares, acts as a stimulant to nerves and brain.[80]

It is interesting that Sitwell possessed such a clear historical view of the 'sick role' as enacted by famous gout sufferers:

I say to myself angrily that the decay of great men, the disappearance of consummate generals and statesmen, is in reality only due to a decline in the numbers of gouty subjects. Bound together by the tie of an agony that brings its own reward, this small but privileged community of victims to which I have the honour to belong knows no boundary of faith or creed; Kubla Khan and Talleyrand, William Pitt and the Bacons, father and son, Wesley and Darwin, Gibbon and Fielding, Milton and Newton, and many other names as famous, go to compose the roll of honour of this martyred but happy band; and of Ben Jonson, Drummond of Hawthornden tells us that the great poet 'hath consumed a whole night in lying looking to his great toe, about which he hath seen Tartars, Romans and Carthaginians, feight in his imagination.'[81]

Sitwell shows the longevity of the associations between gout and notions of talent. The late-Georgian and early-Victorian years also produced the wittiest ever martyr to the gout: Sydney Smith (1771–1845), the noted writer, *bon viveur* (he described a friend's idea of heaven as 'eating paté de foie gras to the sound of trumpets'), Whig and resident canon of St Paul's Cathedral.[82] Smith was well aware of the ubiquity of disease – 'there are above 1500 diseases to which Man is subjected'.[83] He was sceptical, cynical even, about the ministrations of medical men, implying that they grew sleek out of disease. On the death of Pelham Warren, the fashionable society physician, Smith observed in January 1836: 'Warren left behind him £100,000, with the following laconic account how he had acquired it by different diseases:– "Aurum catharticum, £20,000; aurum diureticum, £10,000; aurum podagrosum, £30,000; aurum apoplecticum, £20,000; aurum senile et nervorum, £10,000." '[84] Gout was thus apparently Warren's most lucrative disease.

Smith liked to think of himself as rather medically erudite, and skilled both at diagnosing gout in others and at prescribing for them. 'I cannot doubt (you know what a medical pretender I am)', he assured Lady Grey in September 1842, 'that Lord Grey's malady is Gout.'[85] Smith dabbled in doctoring, though – he was insistent – only within strict confines, as he protested to Lady

Grey: 'Our Evils have been want of Rain, and Scarlet fever in our Village where in ³/₄ of a Year we have buried 15 instead of one per annum. You will naturally suppose I killed all these people by doctoring them, but Scarlet fever awes me, and is above my aim. I leave it to the professional, and graduated Homicides.'[86] Smith had a rather stoical sense of the vulnerability of the human body to all manner of disorders: 'I am pretty well,' he bantered, late in life, 'except gout, asthma, and pains in all the bones, and all the flesh, of my body.'[87] In similar vein, in July 1834, he wrote to Mrs Meynell: 'Perhaps it is a perquisite of my time of life, to have the gout or some formidable illness. We enter and quit the world in pain!'[88] A chronic sufferer himself, he conveyed, almost better than anyone else, the ferocity of an attack 'When I have gout, I feel as if I am walking on my eyeballs,'[89] – though perhaps he subscribed to the traditional view that attacks of gout were salutary: 'My breathlessness and giddiness are gone, chased away by the gout. If you hear of sixteen or eighteen pounds of human flesh, they belong to me. I look as if a curate had been taken out of me.'[90] To Mrs Meynell he expressed the view that gout was in some ways beneficial: 'I find my eyesight much improved by gout, and I am not low-spirited.'[91] Certainly he was of the opinion that colchicum was little less than magical as a mode of relief. 'On Sunday I was on crutches,' he told Lady Grey, 'utterly unable to put my feet to the ground. On Tuesday I walked four miles, such is the power of colchicum.'[92]

Smith clearly subscribed to the dominant aetiological view of gout: that it was in many cases hereditary, but that it could be acquired, or triggered, through luxurious living (and it thus formed part of one's just deserts). 'I am much concerned to hear of Lord Holland's gout,' he informed Lady Holland in 1816. 'Allen deserves the gout more than Lord Holland. I have seen the latter personage resorting occasionally to plain dishes, but Allen passionately loves complexity and artifice in his food.'[93] Amusingly, Smith later wrote to John Allen himself, remarking on Lord Carlisle's appearance of good health, and asking: 'is not happiness good for the gout? I think that remedy is at work upon him.'[94]

In a further letter to Allen in November 1830, at the height of the Reform Bill agitation, Smith assumed a gloomy tone – 'I am frightened at the state of the world; I shall either be burnt, or lose my tithes, or be forced to fight, or some harm will happen to disturb the drowsy slumbers of my useless old-age' – before confessing that 'I have been visited by an old enemy, the lumbago; equally severe, as it seems, upon priests and anti-priests. I believe it comes from the stomach; at least it is to the organ that all medical men direct their curative intentions.'[95] Smith probably did accept that the stomach was the great organ of digestion, hence indigestion, hence gout. But, ever witty and inclined to scoff, he had little truck with the refinements of gout lore. In July 1836 he confided to Sir George Philips: 'What you call throwing out the gout, is all nonsense. You had the gout a little; after a certain time it would have disappeared; but you go to Buxton, it becomes worse, and then you and

Dr — say, unphilosophically, that the gout was in you before, and has been thrown out.'[96]

He told Philips later in the same year that he managed to hold gout at bay by pursuing a moderate diet.[97] Overall, Smith regarded gout neither as genuinely salutary nor as a serious, life-threatening condition, but as a kind of alarm. 'I have had a slight fit of the gout,' he explained to Lady Grey in 1837, 'a warning which will bring me back sooner than I intended; because it is a question put to me by my constitution, "What business has such an antient gentleman as you to be making tours, and to be putting yourself out of your ordinary method of living?"'[98] This was a theme upon which he could sometimes wax quite lyrical. In 1843 he wrote to Harriet Martineau: 'What an admirable provision of Providence is the gout! What prevents human beings from making the body a larder or a cellar, but the gout? When I feel a pang, I say, "I know what this is for. I know what you mean. I understand the hint!", and so I endeavour to extract a little wisdom from pain.'[99]

With gout continuing to possess such a 'personality', and often being used as a makeshift or umbrella diagnosis for all manner of aches, pains and complaints, it is no wonder that, throughout the Victorian era, a wide variety of medical systems and therapeutic innovations achieved their hour on the stage, catering to some or other aspect of the seemingly endless and inexhaustible demand for medicine.[100] Nor had the underbelly of gout – its voodoo and supernatural side – died out in the Victorian period. Stories were written as late as the 1870s about cloistered alchemists and reclusive doctors searching for the elixir of cure. The fact that such plots could sustain whole tales and novellas tells us something significant. Edward Bulwer-Lytton, the prolific novelist and story writer, published one entitled *A Strange Story*.[101]

Strange and supernatural it is, a sort of Victorian medical apologue, the story of two physicians – Fenwick and Margrave – both in love with the lovely Lillian Ashleigh: Fenwick empirical and sceptical of all things super-natural, Margrave (whose real name is not accidentally Louis Grayle) addicted to magic and mysticism. Bulwer-Lytton exploits mesmerism and gout as his main focuses, and somehow both lie within Margrave's sphere of capability. But Margrave's magical wizardry encompasses himself. As the tale unfolds we learn that for many years he has suffered from chronic gout and is in reality an old man imprisoned in a young man's body, somewhat like the painting in *Dorian Gray*. Margrave once roamed the world searching for a cure for himself and found it in the Orient, where, through magic and mystery, the sages showed him. Margrave cannot say what it is, but its restorative powers have transformed him into the ruddy young man he appears. No one, not even Lillian, can believe him to be a gouty old man. When the truth is revealed Lillian chooses Fenwick, but not *sans* Bulwer-Lytton's emphasizing the point that Margrave stood to make a fortune if he could have remem-bered what he tasted in the elixir of gout. To think, the narrator says as the curtain comes down on the tale, that 'this obstinate pauper possessed that for which the pale owners of millions, at the first touch of . . . gout, would consent to be paupers'.[102]

As the nineteenth century wore on, professors in universities had been required to search for a cure, as did Milner in Cambridge, and readers were entertained by mad-doctors, like Margrave, claiming to have found secret elixirs in the Orient. Comic novelists like George Meredith may not have been able to rival Smollett – construct a hero from gout's ridiculous ironies and inconsistencies – but gout nevertheless permeates the pages of Meredith's bulky *oeuvre* and swamps *The Adventures of Harry Richmond* one hundred years later, from whose pages we have taken the epigraph to this chapter, making the risible point about 'gout in the conscience'.

Meredith extended the podagra-pedigree conceit by reiterating what we have heard so many times: 'Gout, Mr Beltham, is a little too much a proof to *us* of a long line of ancestry.'[103] Gout's diaspora was expansive: as gothic as it was Oriental, extending over continents and countries. At home, in England, its resonances were less diverse but equally palpable, and in the fictional figure of Dr Tertius Lydgate, George Eliot's masterfully drawn fictional physician in *Middlemarch* (1872), gout becomes a symbol for an entire society. It had been so for Eliot from her early writing career. As a thinker and social critic she inherited the legacy of Sir Leicester Dedlock, evident in early passages like this one near the opening of *Silas Marner* (1861). 'The rich . . . accepting gout and apoplexy as things that ran mysteriously in respectable families.'[104]

So much has been written about *Middlemarch* that any treatment less than a full one, perhaps at book length, is destined to seem inadequate and repetitive, and we shall not belabour the obvious here. Except to say, as preamble, that it is the tragic story of a woman, Dorothea Brooke, who marries the wrong man, Isaac Casaubon, who wastes his life writing 'a key to all mythologies', and the no less tragic story of a man, Dr Tertius Lydgate, who appears to be heroic and have what everyone else wants but who ends up broken and despondent in the sense that somehow he has failed to achieve his most precious ambitions. Eliot, we believe, also suggests that Lydgate has failed because he cannot face the loss of innocence and the reality of the present. Instead Lydgate retreats into a past emblemized by gout, and, as the majestic novel ends, Lydgate withdraws pathetically into writing a treatise on gout – his surrender to the values and lifestyle of a world he despises but which has entrapped and enslaved him through a fatal marriage. We shall say much more about this surrender in relation to the topics of this chapter – gout's Indian summer after centuries of gathering cultural force – but not before we have explained how the gout also became the vehicle for explaining 'suppressed' illness, even 'suppressed' emotions and feelings, for these profoundly touch on Eliot's depiction of Lydgate's 'surrender'.

Lydgate 'surrenders' because he cannot find an exit from the prisonhouse of his marriage. Eliot's magisterial irony is not merely that Lydgate himself is a doctor who represents everything wrong with his society, but that 'surrender' into writing the treatise on gout at the end of the book becomes the ultimate judgment she can make on the world: one he has despised for long and which Eliot herself hopes can somehow be washed away. It was the 'world' all of whose values were lumped together in the symbol of gout.

Eliot develops this irony about the treatise on gout throughout the plot. The story-line builds up to it from the start when Eliot presents gout as having 'a great deal of wealth on its side'. It is the wealth and fashionability in the world Rosamond – Lydgate's ill-chosen wife – manoeuvres and the rank and class she has wanted to enter. Lydgate, on the other hand, has courageously attempted to swim socially in the opposite direction, and he has failed. Death at fifty, after having gained an excellent practice in London, is surely too harsh a judgment on a character who has typified success from the start. Death at fifty, after retreating from this 'excellent practice' into the miserable writing of a treatise on gout.

Middlemarch is divided thematically into antinomies of town and country, neither world having much commerce with the other. Dorothea, Celia and their uncle Sir James Chettam (a baronet) constitute a gentry whose natural habitat is the country, where health could reside more normatively than in the polluted city. The Vincys, on the other hand, live in town and make their money in trade. Lydgate's future wife Ros, who can discern 'very subtly the faintest aroma of rank' (Chapter 16), aspires more than anything to join this gentry world, where she thinks she ideally belongs, and she hopes to enter that world by marrying Lydgate.

Lydgate himself is the son of a baronet, Sir Godwin Lydgate, and the tainted blood about which Dickens had written so eloquently in *Bleak House* and on which Eliot had commented almost twenty years earlier in *Silas Marner* would seem to be his natural anatomical inheritance. Yet he is as healthy as can be and bears no trace of the ill health he is trained to treat. In 1830, while still a young man, he had already become impatient with the conventional activities of social rank: the army and the Church. He wants to try something new, break out into some new path, although it means going against the prejudices of his upbringing. These prejudices, including the world gout had signified, are brilliantly captured in Uncle Godwin's letter in Chapter 65. But Lydgate, unlike the biographical Dr Gully, Wells and others we have described in this chapter, is piquantly idealistic, the new-style physician hoping to combine medical research and medical provincial practice together in a new way; yet he cannot shed his origins entirely and his natural hauteur makes him countless enemies. Eliot plants his famous 'spots of commonness' about women and furniture and his good (gouty) breeding in Chapter 15, which are destined to cause his downfall and pathetically sink him into one final act before death: the final 'surrender' into writing a treatise on gout.

Marriage has often been said to be the salient theme of *Middlemarch*; indeed is a cliché of modern Eliot criticism. But rank and class are equally important, especially as they touch on all other aspects of daily life. Ros and Lydgate travel in almost diametrically opposing directions. Despite Lydgate's spots of commonness he genuinely aspires to marry intellectual endeavour in medicine and provincial life. Ros wants to escape into a world where she can hobnob with the gentry – hence her naive enthusiasm for the fatuous Captain Lydgate in Chapter 58 and her indifference to Lygdate's medical ambitions. Her conception of medical practice is the old-world view. Medicine, like the military, is in her esteem merely a *gradus ad parnassum* to a desired social end and without its steep slopes. Lydgate sees through all this myopia; hence his ironic epitome of their tragic impasse: 'I do *not* think it is a nice profession, dear.'

Medicine was never 'nice', least of all the trade in gout, but Ros wins out to the detriment of their marriage and the loss of the rural profession. The tenacity of her basic grasping nature and the force of convention prove too much for Lydgate as they sink him into the depression that causes him to recognize he ought to have married Dorothea. Hence his own despair and suppression. Here he has arrived, fifty, trapped in an impossible marriage that is as dead-ended as the no-exits of a Beckettian or Sartrean play, having surrendered his professional dream, aware that his own end cannot be far away. At this very moment he decides to abandon medical practice altogether – and compose a treatise on the gout! As we have reiterated, perhaps too often, the bitter irony of this retreat is that it is Lydgate's surrender to the values and lifestyle of a world he despised but which entrapped him through a fatal marriage. He could have fulfilled himself had his spots of commonness about women not prevented him from identifying an ideal partner in Dorothea, for she too wishes to improve this world through medical research. All this touches not merely on the Victorian medical profession, but on the vicious archetype and symbol gout had become.

Eliot's fictive vision raises genuine questions about the status of medical research and provincial practice at mid-century, matters we cannot delve into here but which should be flagged. The more pressing point is Eliot's vision and judgment of a fitting ending: the paradoxes in the treatise on gout. Lydgate's depression must be explained away in all its complexity, especially in view of the transformation of medical melancholy in the Victorian imagination; even so we never learn what specifically kills him, nor have his major critics instructed us in any depth. Can he himself literally have retreated into a 'suppressed gout' – of the very same type that gentlemen of the medical brethren were defining as the surest sources of severe male depression? Eliot mentions no organic illness, nor any possibility of hypochondria or hysteria, topics also being debated at the time. The reader's information amounts to the above facts: a pathetic sense of failure, a doomed marriage, Lydgate's retreat into a treatise on gout, followed by sudden death.

Eliot's reading in medicine remains undocumented, despite the detective work of Furst and Rothfield; in the end it may be incapable of certain documentation. We do not know which doctors, if any, she read for her protagonist's gout, or what her sense of the imaginary treatise Lydgate was writing was. But she must have imbibed from her culture *some* of these theories – perhaps several of them – about the sources of the depression of mature men. Not all the Victorians agreed about the sequitur from suppressed gout to depression. Other doctors were silent on depression but sustained the grand theme of 'suppression'.[105]

There was no end to the quack and fringe doctors touting their gout cures. A century of doubt had washed away nothing, not even magic in the service of the gout. Through all the theories and therapies and fringe cures only diversity had remained a constant – a constancy the writers, more than any other group, captured. If gout had been firmly lodged in class and rank and gender, it had also become a negative trait, something now to hide and disclaim. Sheridan LeFanu and his wife had both suffered bouts of it and his literary representations were negative. Joseph Harbottle, the judge in *In a Glass Darkly* (1872), is an old gouty man, corrupt, evil, on the road to death, not from gout but almost as poetic justice for all the evil he has committed on the bench. The story captures all the lines we have seen here: frail health, suppressed gout, loss of energy and depression, trips to Buxton for water cures, no help, visits to quacks and astrologers, and eventually death. And when he dies, 'the pomp of a great funeral attended him to the grave; and so, in the language of Scripture, "the rich man died, and was buried" '.[106] It is hard to imagine that stories like these once found their reading audience, so morose are they. But our point does not verge on discussions of literary merit, rather on the cultural ways in which gout was constructed and remained, while it was a vibrant malady, firmly within the realms of the well defined.

Sheridan LeFanu, unlike some of the other physicians we have discussed, was positively commonplace in the norms he assigned his male invalids, no less when Harbottle 'was sinking into the gout'.[107] Hard words, technical concepts, a gullible public, then and now, as our own versions of these treatments continue a century later. But we have tried to make clear that it was the Victorian era that produced the greater proliferation of new hypotheses and theories, orthodox and irregular, with the emergence of a vast public eager to share the diseases of high society and with money in their pockets to join the medical market-place. At the same time, new theories were being generated that would, in due course, help to undermine the traditions of gout. Within a few generations it would be, like hysteria, not the elusive condition but the lost disease. Only a few years earlier George Eliot had made it the unmistakable, if pathetically ironic, symbol of tragedy in her most promising hero. The idea that what may have been Victorian England's greatest novel, and greatest social anatomy, incorporated gout in this way is remarkable in itself. And it was further noteworthy that so many British writers of the nineteenth century had succumbed to its clutches, if not as 'martyr', like Coleridge, then as 'slave' like so many others. The lineage continued, through 'gothicists' like Wilkie Collins, to immigrants like Joseph Conrad. But none of these remedies helped Joseph Conrad one bit. The only difference is that he repressed it. There is not a single reference to gout anywhere in his *oeuvre*.

CHAPTER 10

Gout and Glory: Garrod and After

'A match 'twixt me, bent, wigged and lamed,
 'Famous, however, for verse and worse,
'Sure of the Fortieth spare Arm-chair
 'When gout and glory seat me there,
'So, one whose love-freaks pass unblamed . . .'

> Robert Browning, 'Dis Aliter Visum', stanza xii, in *The Complete Poetical Works of Robert Browning* (New York: Macmillan), 496.

Dozens of eminent Victorians like Wilkie Collins, the popular writer of detective fiction, and other late Victorians who now rest in less celebrated tombs, suffered from the 'monarch's disease'. Many, like Browning, were sedentary and left copiously annotated traces, only a few of which we have resurrected here, in an era when it was unmanly to discuss one's illnesses except in the most polite terms. Collins's gout was as severe as anyone's we have identified. It began when he was only in his late twenties, early in the 1850s; thirty years later, in the mid-1880s, he was still decrying 'Gout and work and age', with the G-word at the top of the list. By the end of his life, in 1889, he believed he had been burned out by the killer condition, but it had also acted as his greatest insulator over sixty-five years. 'Gout and work and age . . . try to persuade me to lay down my pen, after each new book – but, well or ill, I go on.'[1]

Before he reached his thirtieth birthday in 1854 Collins was in correspondence with Charles Dickens about his gouty condition, and his doctor, Francis Carr Beard, who was not a gout specialist,[2] persuaded him that he had inherited a virulent 'rheumatic gout' localized in his eyes. Then began the litany and life of complaints. Dr Beard prevented him from drinking all wine and suggested his condition was 'triggered by a venereal infection caught at this time'.[3] By 1855, when just thirty, Collins began his many flights to European spas: that Victorian panacea, the change of air and taking of waters – in France, Italy and throughout England, especially on the Suffolk coast – which he thought cured him but left the 'gout in the eyes' virulent. Like Coleridge before him, he grew hooked on opium (laudanum), which he claimed was the only thing keeping him alive. Later he added arsenic and nitroglycerin, staples of the gouty Victorian's druggery.[4] While still in his thirties gout prevented him from travelling abroad any further, although Dickens pleaded with him to continue.[5]

Few gouty victims took their conditions so earnestly as Collins, and his correspondence with Dickens remains one of the great archives in the annals of gout. Collins commemorated his fortieth birthday by claiming that gout had turned him grey and 'has attacked my brain'.[6] He wondered to what degree his 'Collinsian nerves' were to blame and increased the opium. In 1867–8 he claimed he was suffering his worst attack of 'rheumatic gout' ever; gout of eyes so bad that he could not read or write.[7] By fifty he was blinded in one eye by the 'rheumatic gout'. By sixty he suffered an attack of rheumatic gout, which was to last for the entire summer, 'left him so weak that his knees trembled on the stairs, though he still insisted on tottering along the sunny side of the street for exercise'. He could read or write only for a minute or two at a time.[8] His diet and habits had grown more temperate with age, while his reliance on opium and loathing of quinine and colchicum had increased. Like so many other Victorian sufferers, in his mind gout and mesmerism were inextricably linked because both were evil, and the latter was, after opium, the last resort. His wife encouraged him to try mesmerism to rid himself of the opium addiction, and Caroline Graves, an expert mesmerizer, regularly hypnotized him to remove him from its clutches. Collins also visited a local (unnamed) German doctor, and was impressed by his insistence on no medicine, only a 'full dietary rein', and all wines, but the doctor's condition was that the wines be only of the best vintages! Collins considered this doctor a 'model physician' surprisingly enough. He tried the remedy but did not improve.

What we have, of course, is the old formula in the old key: gout the insulator for the Victorian gentleman, in Collins the insulator protecting him so he could continue to write. For over all these decades he continued to be prolific, and his works incorporate illness – especially gouty illness – but never in any way that suggests anything but an Indian summer for gout – certainly no possibility of reversing the Smollettian paradigm or taking the podagra-pedigree conceit to new heights. Everywhere in Collins's detective fiction the gout represents evil, as in the prison warden in *The Legacy of Cain*.

Mr Neal, who transcribes 'old Allan Armadale's confession' in the opening passages of *Armadale* (1890), has gout in the leg. The scene takes place in Wildbad Spa, where Collins sojourned in 1863 to find relief from his own gout.[9] Neal quickly disappears from the narrative after these opening passages, figuring later only as the *evil* step-father in Ozias Midwinter's miserable past. The pages of Collins's detective fiction drip with invalids, many of them gouty, or at least suffering from the symptoms he himself had experienced, often marginally gouty shadowy figures like Fairlie in *The Woman in White* and Noel Vanstone in *No Name* (Chapter 3, scene 3), and the much more fully described Armadale. All these characters are embodied with a theme of degeneration, so hotly being debated at the time, and Armadale specifically presents the idea of the fathers' sins falling on their sons – not so far from the predicament of the Leicester Dedlocks. All are upper crust and morally corrupt, and are curiously confident in their unnamed gout-like disease. Considering that the sensation novel in which Collins was a genius was the middle class's *métier* – the form of fiction they especially liked – it is not insignificant that health and this disease so uncommon among the lower classes are presented with regularity. This is the point that needs to be made: the notion that the rising middle class would find a malady like gout so intriguing, even though in Collins's mind it was the very incarnation of evil.

Gout, however, was not such a monolithically evil beast in the mind of most Victorian doctors, certainly not for the likes of those who performed research. For this company, gout could be tamed, if only its chemistry were understood. Science advances slowly, of course, and the doctors of the 1850s, when Collins suffered his first major attacks, continued to build on the chemical advances made by Scheele, Forbes, Wollaston and their successors who stimulated new lines of scientific inquiry. Historically speaking, the expectation that chemistry held the key to pathology had been reinforced from the 1830s, as Liebig at Giessen pioneered practical techniques for furthering chemical investigation of physiological problems.[10] Yet, as suggested by the preceding analyses of the writings of Scudamore, Gairdner and others, British clinical approaches to gout were remarkably unresponsive before mid-century to the bracing winds of scientific change. Small wonder then that the likes of Collins could not be helped. The brisk transformation that occurred thereafter was overwhelmingly due to the writings of Alfred Garrod. The accuracy of his investigations and the clarity of his formulations pitched investigation on to a higher plane, giving new emphasis to the chemical experimentation, laboratory tests, animal studies and the quantifying imperative expected of mid-century investigations. It may, ironically, be significant that, unlike so many of his *confrères*, Garrod was *not* a sufferer: lacking personal interest in his inquiries, he could perhaps pursue them in a more detached spirit.

Alfred Baring Garrod (1819–1909) was a prize product of the new medical education emerging in Victorian England under the stimulus of the Parisian medicine pioneered by Bichat, Laennec, Louis, Bayle and their peers. He trained at University College Hospital, London, going on to become its physician and professor of therapeutics and clinical Medicine. And it was there that he carried out the researches into uric acid and gout that led to his *Treatise on Gout and Rheumatism* (1859). Knighted in 1887, he was appointed physician-extraordinary to Queen Victoria three years later.[11]

Combining chemical investigations with Scudamore's clinical interests, Garrod achieved a notable breakthrough: he was able definitively to identify 'the specific morbid humour which inflames all joints in which it enters': the substance was uric acid. 'The blood in gout', he announced in a paper published in 1848, 'always contains uric acid in the form of urate of soda, which salt can be obtained from it in a crystalline state.' Sodium urate crystals were found in concentrated solutions of gouty serum, in the white matter deposited on metatarsal bones, and also in gouty concretions from other body parts. What might have been called Garrod's law pronounced that gout was invariably accompanied by excessive uric acid in the blood (hyperuricaemia).[12]

It is indicative of Garrod's precise and practical temper that he spelt out in that first paper a practical method for detecting uric acid in the blood. Gouty subjects and those with Bright's disease, he found, had levels of approximately 0.05 grain in 1,000 grains of serum, whereas healthy people (and also those with rheumatism) showed notably lower values. Garrod also demonstrated that sheep and pigeon blood contained no uric acid.

These findings confirmed that hyperuricaemia was coexistent with gout – and that this was a characteristic distinguishing gout from other arthritic and rheumatic disorders. His discovery that there was no urate of soda in sheep and pigeons stimulated comparative researches and animal experiments, leading to the later conviction that there were three different types of purine (protein) metabolism, one in man and the higher apes, a second in all other mammals and a third in birds.

Noting that the concentration of uric acid in the blood dropped at the onset of acute gouty attacks, Garrod tendered the hypothesis that:

> Gout would thus appear at least partly to depend on a loss of power (temporary or permanent) of the 'uric-acid-excreting function' of the kidneys; the premonitory symptoms, and those also which constitute the paroxysm, arising from an excess of this acid in the blood, and from the effort to expel the *materies morbi* from the system. Any undue *formation* of this compound would favour the occurrence of the disease; and hence the connection between gout and uric acid, gravel and calculi; and hence, the influence of high living, wine, porter, want of exercise, &c., in inducing it.[13]

Following a further paper in 1854,[14] Garrod gave his ideas full expression in *The Nature and Treatment of Gout and Rheumatic Gout*, published in 1859, the same year as Darwin's *Origin of Species*.[15] One notable practical feature of that work lay in the instructions given for his famous 'uric acid thread test', an easy mode of establishing the presence of uric acid in the blood.[16]

Garrod aimed to render study of gout more scientific. In his book he recalled that in his 1848 paper he had experimentally demonstrated that, contrary to common belief, 'uric acid is not a product of the action of the kidneys' – the role of the kidneys was not (as once assumed) to produce uric acid but to eliminate it. The crucial point was that, for whichever reason, in gout the 'uric-acid-excreting function' was 'defective', the consequence being that 'chalk-like deposits are produced'.[17] While acknowledging that his findings were not at odds with the conventional reading of the gouty fit as a salutary act of Nature, Garrod – by temper cautious and by training localist and empirical, disposed to regard disease as specific – was sceptical towards holistic interpretations of the disorder in terms of the overall organic economy.[18]

Garrod's finding that gout essentially involved deposition of uric acid as urate of soda in the affected joints following a 'loss of power (temporary or permanent) in the uric-acid-excreting function of the kidneys' was crucial to him, since it resolved certain long-disputed questions. One surrounded 'its hereditary nature'. The evident fact, Cadogan notwithstanding, that gout ran in families could now be explained in terms of hereditary kidney disease. Another point long-puzzling but now settled was the 'frequent occurrence' of gout 'in low states of the system', for example among poor people who were patently not *bon viveurs*. This too could now be explained in terms of kidney disease, for when renal function was 'permanently injured' it would not 'require an excessive formation of this acid to cause its accumulation in the blood'.[19]

Garrod tabulated his convictions through a series of ten coherent and testable propositions of such perspicacity that they crystallized controversy for the rest of the century. Their impact was so great as to warrant reproducing them in full:

First, in true gout, uric acid, in the form of urate of soda, is invariably present in the blood in abnormal quantities, both prior to and at the period of the seizure, and is essential to its production; but this acid may occasionally exist, at least for a time, in the circulating fluid without the development of inflammatory symptoms, as in cases of lead poisoning. Its mere presence, therefore, does not explain the occurrence of the gouty paroxysm.

Secondly, the investigations detailed in the chapter on the Morbid Anatomy of Gout, prove incontestably that true gouty inflammation is *always* accompanied with a deposition of urate of soda in the inflamed part.

Thirdly, the deposit is crystalline and interstitial, and when once the cartilages and ligamentous structures become infiltrated, remains for a lengthened time, often throughout life.

Fourthly, the deposited urate of soda may be looked upon as the cause, and not the effect, of the gouty inflammation.

Fifthly, the inflammation which occurs in the gouty paroxysm tends to the destruction of the urate of soda in the blood of the inflamed part, and consequently of the system generally.

Sixthly, the kidneys are implicated in gout, probably in its early stages, and certainly in its chronic stages; and the renal affection, possibly only functional at first, subsequently becomes structural; the urinary secretion is also altered in composition.

Seventhly, the impure state of the blood, arising principally from the presence of urate of soda, is the probable cause of the disturbance which precedes the gouty seizure, and of many of the anomalous symptoms to which sufferers from gout are liable.

Eighthly, the causes which predispose to gout, independently of those connected with individual peculiarity, are either such as produce an increased formation of uric acid in the system, or lead to its retention in the blood.

Ninthly, the causes exciting a gouty fit are those which induce a less alkaline condition of the blood; or which greatly augment, for the time, the formation of uric acid; or such as temporarily check the eliminating power of the kidneys.

Tenthly, in no disease but true gout is there a deposition of urate of soda in the inflamed tissues.[20]

In support of these hypotheses, Garrod adduced evidence both experimental and clinical. His cardinal contention – that 'the blood in gout always contains an abnormal quantity of uric acid during the attacks' – was backed by case evidence from forty-seven patients. He further cited instances of lead paralysis, to corroborate his claim that abnormally high uric acid levels occurred 'prior to an attack', and thus were its cause.[21] He had for instance treated an artist, who ten years earlier had first 'felt some symptoms arising from the absorption of lead [from his paints]'. Then 'he completely lost power over both his wrists', and had a severe attack of colic. A return of the wrist-drop and a colic attack had ensued six weeks later. Through a blood test, he had shown by the 'thread experiment there was evidence of its containing abundance of uric acid'. Subsequently, this patient experienced a decided attack of gout: QED – the build-up of uric acid had been demonstrated. Such an accumulation did not invariably lead to gout, however; excessive uric acid in the blood was a necessary but not a sufficient condition.[22]

Garrod set great store by his second proposition, that gouty inflammation was always attended by deposition of urate of soda. Its presence, for instance, had been discovered in a case in which 'only one small joint had been affected' and in another where just a single attack of gout had occurred. He regarded these as points as decisive, 'because in the *constancy* of such deposition, lies the clue which has long been wanting: the occurrence of the deposit is perfectly pathognomonic': specific symptoms, specific lesions, specific disease, specific cause – therein lay Garrod's style of thinking.[23]

In establishing pathology, Garrod relied heavily on the fourth proposition: namely, that the deposited urate of soda was the *cause* not the *consequence* of the gouty inflammation. 'Several reasons' militated against the 'supposition that the deposit is the effect of the inflammation'. Patients had assured him, for instance, that they had noticed tophi on their ears previous to the first onslaught of articular gout.[24]

Further confirmation lay in the fifth proposition, 'that the inflammation of gout tends to the destruction of the urate of soda in the blood of the part'. The implication, Garrod inferred, was that 'the gout fit is, to some extent, a salutary process', ridding the system of much uric acid. Yet he was not prepared to make facile concessions to 'gout is good' lore: 'we must likewise remember', he insisted, 'that it is always attended with a certain amount of local mischief'.[25]

Addressing his sixth proposition, Garrod attempted to show how 'the kidneys were altered by the deposition of urate of soda'. Noting it had long been supposed that the kidneys are affected, he claimed to have 'fully proved' the effect of kidney action in gout. Ascertaining the fluctuating relations between uric-acid levels and the kidneys was critical to his investigation.[26]

The seventh proposition – that the cause of the gouty fit was excessive urate of soda in the blood – was, Garrod admitted, 'difficult to prove' in scientific fashion, although clinical experience was on his side:

> We have absolute proof . . . that when the urinary secretion is completely stopped, most serious and even fatal symptoms ensue; and it is therefore reasonable to suppose, that if one or more of its constituents be retained in the blood, certain morbid phenomena would result therefrom.[27]

The eighth proposition – that the predisposing causes produced increased formation of uric acid or retention in the blood – provided a key to understanding the difference between what were 'popularly known as the rich, and the poor man's gout'. Gouty attacks might involve either 'augmented formation' of uric acid or the excreting power of the kidneys being impeded; either could lead to the disease. *Excessive* production of uric acid would account for 'rich man's gout', whereas kidney *deficiency* would explain 'poor man's gout'.[28]

The ninth proposition raised the question of what precipitated infiltration of urate of soda into the tissues. It might happen in two ways, Garrod suggested: 'either by its great accumulation in the blood', or by the blood being 'less capable of holding it in solution'. Crucial was the alkalinity level. Blood serum had to be quite alkaline to hold urate of soda in solution, but there was often 'a marked alteration in the degree of its alkalinity', in some cases of chronic gout even tending towards neutrality. The critical point was that 'any diminution in the alkaline state of the blood facilitates deposition, bringing on an attack'. As was his wont, Garrod offered an experimental demonstration of that question.[29]

The final proposition was that 'in no other disease but true gout' did deposition of urate of soda occur in the inflamed tissues. Garrod had inspected numerous cases of 'genuine rheumatic fever'; none, however, had shown any indication of deposit of urate of soda. The same was true of rheumatoid arthritis. He had examined the great toe joints in at least forty cases with no known gouty history; in only two instances was uric acid discovered, and Garrod reasoned that such people would in due course have developed gout. Gout was thus specifically different from arthritis and rheumatism.[30] Garrod's Ten Propositions, in short, delivered the tables of the gouty law, and on their basis he claimed to have elucidated the requisites for a fit.[31]

His account, Garrod contended, also explained another principal phenomenon, the tendency of the gouty to suffer from oedema and the 'subsequent desquamation of the cuticle' – symptoms frequent in gout but rare in rheumatism. Much the same applied to the occurrence of chalkstones or gouty tophi, which for Garrod was easily resolved: '*every paroxysm of gout is attended with a deposit*'.[32]

What of possible objections? If the gouty fit was thus, as suggested, dependent on 'a *materies morbi*', was it a problem (pondered Garrod) that gouty attacks often supervened 'without any well marked symptoms to give warning of its approach'? Was it difficult to explain how the matter 'should have been dormant up to the time of the seizure, and why, latent thus long, it should suddenly show itself in the production of acute disease'? Such occurrences, he explained, took place because 'the mere accumulation of the urate' would not of itself automatically produce the 'inflammation'; what was essential was 'its actual deposition in tissue', which usually required a 'peculiar exciting cause'. Hence the 'poison may lie dormant for a considerable time'.[33]

There were, Garrod did not deny, other difficulties. Why did gouty inflammation 'peculiarly select the ball of the great toe'? Why did it then spread to other joints? Boerhaave and his commentator van Swieten had tackled these matters long before, maintaining that the feet were 'peculiarly liable to be hurt in walking, leaping, sudden falls, and accidents'. Garrod tended to concur. The big toe contained tissues of 'little vascularity'. Remote from the heart, it was also at the point where 'the force of the circulation' was 'at its minimum'. And once the toe was affected, the urate soda required 'more surfaces upon which to deposit itself'.[34]

Committed to localism, Garrod regarded gout first and foremost as a joint disease. Circulation played some part, and the 'great problem' of the 'migration of gout from joint to joint' was easily resolved 'if we bear in mind the fact that deposition *precedes* inflammation'. Local inflammation in one part would relieve the other, 'but only for a time'.[35]

Garrod addressed other old problems. The mystery of why women were largely exempt could be 'readily answered'. Females were less liable to excesses in wine and malt liquors. Menstrual discharges also gave them some 'immunity'. Hence Hippocrates' aphorism – that women developed gout only after menopause – was 'practically correct'. Young men also escaped gout. Why? It was because during youth, 'when the growth of the body is rapidly advancing . . . and while the secreting functions are in full activity', there was 'little tendency to engender such a state of blood as would lead to the development of gout'. And heredity? That 'tendency alone', Garrod asserted, was generally 'inadequate to cause the full development of gout' – indeed there were many men who, though 'inheriting the disorder', succeeded in passing through life 'without a single attack'. Gout nonetheless was a hereditary disease, and for that reason it was rarely radically cured. In subjects not hereditarily predisposed, on the other hand, it might be possible, through diet and lifestyle, to prevent 'a further recurrence'.[36]

The *Treatise on Gout and Rheumatism* was a landmark; quickly translated into French and German,[37] it excited Europe-wide notice. Based on sound anatomico-pathological studies, it made major contributions to the renal pathology of the disease. By distinguishing rheumatoid arthritis from gout it dealt a deathblow to 'rheumatic gout' and other hybrid and nebulous conditions. Not least, Garrod underscored the relations between alcohol and gout. In north European countries where beer-drinking was prevalent, gout was rather rare. Light wines seemed to be roughly as culpable as whisky, but port and other fortified wines were highly goutogenic. 'There is no truth better established in medicine', he avowed, 'than the fact that the use of fermented liquors is the most powerful of all the predisposing causes of the gout.'[38]

The post-Garrod decades brought extensive analysis of the metabolic role of uric acid within the rapidly expanding disciplines of organic chemistry and physiology, stimulated by Liebig in Germany and Claude Bernard in France.[39] Scientific inquiry forged ahead. Two perplexing circumstances long thwarted further elucidation of urate metabolism. One was the radical difference in urate metabolism between birds and mammals, and birds and man – differences of great practical importance, since dogs and hens were frequently selected as experimental subjects. The other problem was the idea common until around 1900 that metabolism of carbohydrates, fats and proteins involved only oxidation. The biochemical investigations involved in such problems grew more technical and had diminishing immediate relevance to medicine. Hence they will not be further examined here, except as they directly affected the clinical debate.[40]

From Garrod's day through to the close of the century, laboratory research advanced understanding of the role of uric acid within the metabolism. But science did not produce consensus. And that was not least because the relations between basic science, clinical investigation and therapeutics remained deeply contested. Divisions over gout epitomized medicine's uneasy estate in Victorian England, with its competitive individualism, professional rivalries and insecurity, its relative paucity of Liebigian laboratory facilities, and its dependence upon the patronage of rich patients. Leading figures derived the bulk of their income from private practice; most had numerous irons in the fire, having to offset scientific aspirations against the need to please their patients in a market-place in which, as George Bernard Shaw showed, the physician often had to kowtow to his fashionable patients, no trivial consideration in a disease of civilization like gout.

Indeed, most Victorian gout writings were probably produced with more than half an eye to prosperous patients, and they consequently display the physician less as the master of the microscope than as a man-of-the-world blessed with clinical acuity and a hail-fellow-well-met manner. Among such authors, unfamiliarity with or indifference to the latest in laboratory science could be represented as a positive asset.

The writings of Edward Duke Moore offer a yardstick against which to measure the more scientifically minded Garrod. Moore's *Memorandums and Recollections on Gout and Rheumatism* appeared in 1864, five years after Garrod's classic.[41] He had ascended the medical ladder thanks to aristocratic and royal connections. Becoming a member of the Royal College of Surgeons in 1826, Moore was appointed apothecary in residence first to William IV and then to Queen Victoria, and also medical attendant to the Duke of Cambridge. His main claim to attention came through his appointment as physician to the Devonshire Hospital in Buxton. 'I have had experience enough', he asserted, citing his extensive spa-town practice, to be convinced that gout and rheumatism were 'separate diseases' – though, by pointing out that 'the cause may possibly be the same', he made it clear that he had not read, or at least not accepted, Garrod's theories about the specificity of gout – his hero was a man of an older school, William Gairdner, born back in the 1790s. In the time-honoured bedside manner, Moore insisted that the finer points of aetiology might be somewhat academic: he was primarily interested in treatment, respecting which experience empowered him to speak with authority. 'I am confirmed', he wrote, 'in my favourable opinion of the efficacy of the Buxton baths, waters, and air for the cure, or, at least, for the mitigation, of the symptoms and the suffering of these two painful affections.'[42]

'The experience of thirty years', he explained, had convinced him that gout was a complicated disease. Aetiological questions often spawned footling controversies – 'the man would be presumptuous indeed who should venture to treat it on any hypothesis not well confirmed by experience'. Suspicious of systems, he would contribute the 'recollections of a long experience', because 'facts speak for themselves'. Leery of the 'theorisations of science', he presented himself as one 'content to seek for truth by a patient comparison of facts' – not laboratory data but case histories and first-hand anecdotes.[43]

Distrust of 'theorizings' went with an eagerness to tell gout in terms accessible to lay readers. One key question respected its status, since 'it has long appeared doubtful to me whether gout can strictly be called a DISEASE *per se*'. Far better to set gout 'in the same category with jaundice, asthma, dyspepsia', that is to say, to regard it as a 'symptom of derangement of the system'. The 'modern' Garrod was attentive to local lesions; Moore by contrast addressed the whole person and his constitution. In that light, gout might also be seen by way of parallel with jaundice:

> An insidious and slow disease has been for a time lurking in a patient's liver, producing the greatest distress, and a variety of alarming symptoms. At length the blood becomes tinged with bile, and jaundice is made manifest not as a disease itself, but as a most unmistakable token of a serious disease or obstruction in the liver or gall bladder.[44]

No 'simple' disease (as it might perhaps have been regarded by Paris-school localizers), gout was a complicated process. Asthma offered a further analogue. 'Derangement of various organs may produce asthma; the effect of which is to change very materially the character of the blood by overthrowing its chemical balance. We would, therefore, not say that asthma is a *disease*, but, as in the case of jaundice, a manifestation of disease.' Gout likewise. Citing Gairdner's authority, Moore suggested that gout was essentially a symptom: 'a fit of the gout is the vent-hole to the mischief which a disturbed digestion has brought about'.[45] Regular gout might thus be a salutary discharge (a 'white' disease, to revert to an earlier terminology) – though, in standard manner, Moore insisted that metastatic gout was grave ('black'). With a characteristically personal touch, he fleshed out these points by instancing, like James Parkinson, the case of his own father, 'who was what is termed a "martyr to gout"' from early life:

> A more distressing case of metastasis than his could perhaps hardly be recorded. He had at the age of seventeen lost his leg by an accident, and the stump was constantly the seat of great agony from gout. On one occasion it suddenly left the stump and the other then affected limb, and seized his nose. After intense agony it as suddenly left the nose and attacked the eye, and that so acutely as in a short time to deprive him of its sight.[46]

Because gout was so intricate, any talk of a panacea must be quite asinine, despite the fact that 'no malady to which the human frame is liable has had so many nostrums tried and advertised'. Adopting the classic clinician's pose, Moore contended that no ailment 'requires . . . more close and anxious watching by the medical attendant'. Precisely because it was so protean,

> whether it be acute gout, atonic gout, metastatic gout, every symptom must be watched, and met at its commencement. The shape that it assumes in its symptoms must be the guide to the mode of treatment; and to lay down a certain rule for the treatment of gout is quite as preposterous as the act of my fashionable friend in asking every dowager for a nostrum against hiccup.[47]

Hence Moore's clinically oriented tome was devoted to illustrating profi-
ciency in specific cases and the multifarious forms of treatment required. 'A
physician in large practice in the country was a "martyr to gout"', he recalled.

> He would leave his home in the morning under the pain of gout in the
> foot, and before arriving at his patient's house he would ride into a pool,
> and, with a small cup which he carried for the purpose, pour water into his
> top-boot, so as to make a soothing poultice for his foot; and at the same
> time he would empty his brandy-flask in another direction, for the purpose
> of putting the organs most commonly affected by metastasis, viz., the
> stomach and heart, under the influence of the stimulant, while his foot was
> under that of the bath.[48]

Apparently Moore did not feel in the least embarrassed about what today's
readers might experience as the quixotic features of such anecdotes: for
him – and his anticipated readership – here was a tale of a staunch and
sagacious physician of the bulldog breed. Four-square Englishmen were assumed to be inured to regular gout (and to wet feet and brandy): they would
grin and bear it.

So these clinical stories devoted particular attention to one specific aspect
of gout: they reassured readers – that is, potential patients – that old Moore
recognized the imperative need to keep metastatic gout, that life-threatener,
at bay:

> One of the bravest generals of the British army at the battle of Waterloo
> told me that he went into battle with a fit of the gout, but that after the
> first shot was fired all pain left him, but returned with intense agony when
> the day was over. To relieve his sufferings he made a poultice of mud,
> taking care to drink freely of brandy, as he used to say, to prevent the flight
> of the attack to his stomach or heart.[49]

Having by this rather crude device established his social connections ('this
gentleman became for many years my patient'), Moore noted that the gallant
soldier 'used to suffer considerably from shooting pains through the brain,
which I always attributed to metastatic gout'. Advice had therefore to be
formulated to keep it at bay: 'in the event of his having an attack when the
physician could not be at his bedside', he was not to be bled. Unfortunately
this was precisely what had happened on one calamitous occasion: 'a few
hours afterwards, an epileptic attack ensued, from the effects of which he
never entirely recovered'. Hence, Moore insisted, patients susceptible to
retrocedent gout should heed the great Sydenham's recommendation that
bleeding was at all costs to be avoided. He had some practical tips: 'I once
knew a man who used to go about with a collar under his neckcloth,
inscribed "Don't bleed me, it is gout".'[50]

Yet Moore was not averse to drastic treatments as such – and if this might *prima facie* seem inconsistent, it neatly illustrates the highly idiosyncratic rituals woven by clinical medicine. 'Though I shall probably encounter the prejudice against calomel and colchicum', he announced, drastic purges were to be approved: 'Both remedies have a most decided good effect in relieving the agony of acute gout, and, in a certain degree, preventing metastasis.'[51]

Moore's discussion of proper and pernicious forms of evacuation revolved around his own patients. One had recounted that 'while suffering from a fit of the gout, it shifted (as he expressed it) to his head'. An unfamiliar physician was unluckily summoned, and the next thing that the patient heard were the words: 'I must bleed him.' The stupefied sufferer protested: 'No, no, give me the calomel bottle. It is gout, and I will soon cure it.' A violent purge did the trick. And if calomel were useful, so too was colchicum, since it had a 'most powerful' impact in terminating the pains of an attack – 'although', he candidly admitted, 'it is difficult to say how it operates'. He also recommended douches and Turkish baths.[52]

The art of treatment involved the ability to compel gout to manifest itself in acute and salutary attacks, rather than lurk in the deleterious metastatic mode. To confirm his vigilance, Moore presented a tough case. An extremely gouty subject came to Buxton 'with stiff joints and thickened limbs'; 'but being *only* gout, he was allowed to live well and take his soda water and brandy; not to eat sweets and pastry, but as much animal food as he liked'. Then 'one day he was missed from his accustomed seat, and in a few hours I was summoned to his bedside, where he was laid up by an attack of gout'. The clinician discovered that his patient had taken 'four hot baths' and drunk the alkaline waters without success in converting the 'chronic symptoms of gout into acute' – the decisive blunder. Amply versed in the gout arcana, Moore rose to the occasion. The inflammatory attack 'rapidly yielded to an administration of aperient stomachic medicines, clearing out the alimentary canal, and setting all the organs of digestion in a state to perform their proper functions'. He was thus master of the situation, his forte clinical management: he knew the art of inducing acute attacks – therein lay true medical skill. What matter that he was no wizard in chemical pathology? – 'I leave that to more able chemists than myself,' he said, while coyly adding, as if to cover his bets, 'I cannot divest myself of the idea that it is uric acid.'[53]

Garrod and Moore were both active in mid-century but their methods were utterly disparate. Garrod pursued scientific pathology with the aid of organic chemistry; Moore aimed to demonstrate practical management of Quality patients. For the next half-century, contributors to the debate attempted to combine in various degrees both approaches.

A key contribution to the questions raised by Garrod came from Wilhelm Ebstein (1836–1912), Professor of Clinical Medicine in Göttingen, whose *Regimen to be Adopted in Cases of Gout* appeared in English translation in 1885.

Ebstein characterized gout as a disease of civilization – it had 'a greater number of victims in proportion as strictness and simplicity of life have been abandoned in favour of luxury and effeminacy'. But it was also hereditary, a view he supported with a host of authorities from Aretaeus onwards. Cadogan aside, 'all other observers have placed hereditariness in the front rank of predisposing causes'. The Ancients' proverb, *gaudeant bene nati*, had mutated into the modern witticism: 'we cannot be too particular in the choice of our ancestors'.[54]

Hereditariness was no simple matter, however, and Ebstein cited with approval Jonathan Hutchinson's belief that 'an individual runs a danger of contracting gout in proportion as the gouty process is developed in the parent'. Moreover, 'the disease does not show itself in all the members of a family, nor is it propagated from father to son, and thence to grandson, in a direct line'. Nor did the hereditary principle mean that the symptoms would show themselves, as in syphilis, 'soon after birth'.[55]

The aetiology of gout was thus partly Nature (inheritance) and partly nurture (luxury). As with Garrod, what was crucial was chemistry. The history of fallacious attempts to resolve the chemistry of gout was long, going back to the 'tartarus of Paracelsus', but modern chemistry had finally made the decisive breakthrough. Around 1800 the investigations of Wollaston, Tennant and Fourcroy 'had already shown that gouty concretions contain uric acid'; such advances had, however, been halted by the assurance of the traditionalist Scudamore that gouty concretions occurred 'so seldom' and 'in so few individuals' that it was 'impossible' to build a theory upon them. Hence, grumbled the scientific Ebstein, the 'sure natural basis was again abandoned', supplanted by 'vague unripe theories'. The want of 'actual data' and the 'complete stagnation of pathological investigation' helped explain how, so late as 1847, just one year before Garrod's paper, Henle could still regard the deposition of uric acid as 'accidental'.[56]

It is thus easy to see why Ebstein paid homage to Garrod: his pioneering work had finally set the pathology of gout on to a scientific basis, by demonstrating the role of urate of soda. Nevertheless even he could and should have driven his scientific investigations further, since, the German complained, 'from the facts adduced by Garrod, the conclusion could not really be drawn that the symptoms of gout were a *necessary* consequence of uric acid'.[57]

With his own particular slant, Ebstein contended that uric acid was a chemical poison producing not merely inflammatory but also necrotic pro-cesses in animal tissues. Moreover, excess uric acid was a causative factor quite independent of kidney failure. Contrary to Garrod, he thus denied that kidney damage was an essential aspect of gout: rather one should posit 'a localized retention of uric acid'. Retention of ordinary fluids produced oedema; gout was analogous but different, precipitating an inflammatory process producing 'redness, swelling, and tightness of the surrounding soft parts'.[58]

Regarding treatment, Ebstein judged it crucial to address the question of 'gouty disposition', for 'without predisposition we may say, as a rule, there is no gout'. Was there a specific hereditary tendency – or was gout essentially a product of bad diet? Was excessive production of uric acid due solely to bad diet or was there an authentic 'uric acid diathesis'? Ebstein was rather inclined towards the diathesis theory, viewing 'increased uric acid production' as deriving from a 'perhaps inherited predisposition'.[59]

To prevent uric acid building up, the aim must be to localize it in the proper tissues – the muscles and medulla of the bones. To that end Ebstein decried excessive flesh-eating and recommended vegetables. Cherries and strawberries were especially healthy, because they contained an organic acid 'less injurious to digestion than the alkaline carbonates'. Rectifying diet was crucial: there was no sense in *starving* people in the name of health, for that would only 'lower the strength'; *correct* food was more important than *less* food. Then there was the question of liquor. Water was the 'best drink'. Balance and good sense were needed, however. Experience showed that alcohol brought gout on, but it could be the lesser evil. Weak constitutions might need its stimulus, but he forbade it for 'robust patients' – they could do without it – and it was an 'absolute necessity' for those with a strong gouty tendency to forgo alcohol. 'Universal prohibition' was preferable to 'half-measures'. In line with his theory of 'local retentions', Ebstein commended exercise, from bicycling to billiards, and for this reason the gouty rich might winter in warmer climates, thereby allowing them to 'move about even during winter in the open air'. Finally he returned to questions of cure. Dismissing the hoary issue of Sydenham's nostrum, he concluded that, though 'we may obviate gout and we may assuage it', radical cure was unlikely.[60]

Honouring Garrod's view, Ebstein thus developed its implications in line with the research strategies of the Bernard era, playing down the role of specific local lesions (renal pathology) and stressing biochemical metabolic factors (acids). His doctrines (turning uric acid into the be-all and end-all of gout) were not widely accepted, though perhaps providing a stimulus for Alexander Haig; but they represented a further stage in attempts to frame a scientific theory, in the sense of identifying a single, unambiguous physico-chemical cause.

Meanwhile, patients suffered, often in vicious cycles of peaks and valleys of illness. Not all the treatments or all the water cures in Europe, for example, could remove gout from the great novelist Joseph Conrad's twisted torso, his limbs, hands and fingers. As Jeffrey Meyers has commented, 'the beginning of his writing career coincided with the onset of the extraordinarily painful gout that often crippled his hands and feet. He frequently became despondent about his literary work, but felt poor health made it dishonorable for him to accept a command.'[61] Like so many nineteenth-century writers we have looked at, and others we have omitted, Conrad used illness as a defence against a world with which he had trouble coping, and deployed the patrician disease – gout – above all.

Meyers has epitomized Conrad's type, correctly we think:

> He had a mercurial temperament and a neurasthenic personality; was a chronic hypochondriac and often maniacally depressed; and had several nervous breakdowns during his marriage . . . Moody, irritable, absent-minded, indolent and impractical, he was deeply dependent on his wife and friends, and utterly helpless when suffering from his frequent attacks of gout.[62]

A displaced Pole, he had written first in Polish and then in French, and lived in both countries, but he migrated at almost forty to England, where he made his home from 1896 onward and wrote in the impeccable English for which he has been so justly praised.

He was healthy until he settled into the routine of domestic life. Not ironically or accidentally, his first violent attack of fever and gout occurred on his honeymoon in 1896, the gout possibly having been precipitated by the malarial infection. Conrad's chronic gout may have originated in sandy urinary deposits in his bladder, which had caused him severe stomach cramps when only ten years old. His initial attacks in 1896 were sudden, causing him to wake frequently from sleep and to endure hot, red and swollen joints boiling over with shiny skin. His body grew painful and tender and the acute attacks were often accompanied by swings of mood to gave him the reputation of being neurasthenic, if not blatantly hypochondriac and melancholic.[63]

Meyers thinks 'Conrad's attacks of gout were partly psychological in origin. He did not seriously suffer from this disease, which crippled his hands, until he had to support himself and his wife as a writer.'[64] His wife Jessie witnessed his first attack on the Ile-Grande in Paris in May 1896, when he ran a high fever, and described his shivering fits:

> for most of the time Conrad was delirious. To see him lying in the white canopied bed, dark-faced, with gleaming teeth and shining eyes, was sufficiently alarming, but to hear him muttering to himself in a strange tongue (he must have been speaking Polish), to be unable to penetrate the clouded mind or catch one intelligible word, was for a young, inexperienced girl truly awful.[65]

Like Tennyson and Carlyle before him, Conrad widely consulted doctors, in England, France, Italy and Switzerland, tried all kinds of treatment and diet, eventually deciding that his condition was incurable. His letters clarify his conviction that his case was entirely physical – somatic – rather than psychological or nervous, and therefore he was willing to swallow the iodine ministered to him and wear the woollen gout gloves with the fingers cut off for extra warmth that enabled him to write. He continued to use the word 'gouty': to friends, correspondents, publishers. And he harboured a belief, as Meyers documents, that gouty people 'went out' suddenly.[66] By this dour view he seems to have believed the opposite of the podagra insulating theory, which had enjoyed such a long history. And when he told Hugh Walpole, in 1900, that he was 'a tottering, staggering, shuddering, shivering, crocky, seedy, gouty wretch', he seems to have meant he was close to the end of his life, which he was not. And he certainly did not go 'suddenly out'.[67]

Conrad suffered painful attacks of gout while writing *Nostromo* in 1902–4. He continued to have attacks of flying, acute gout for the next three years. And on 28 December 1908 he wrote to Sir Sidney Colvin, 'What with the gout (ten days) and the novel, I have been in an atrocious temper. Your letter made me feel human this morning, the first time for I don't know how long.'[68]

Next year, in 1909, he was as bad, and wrote to John Galsworthy, the novelist, on 5 June from Aldington, in North Hythe, Kent, that:

> I have been in bed all last week and am just beginning to pull myself together. The good Mac came down twice flying in his car with medicines, bandages, lotions, etc., etc., cheering me up and putting heart into Jessie, who has been quite extraordinarily worried by this bout of gout. Well it was pretty bad: the horrible depression worst of all. It is rather awful to lie helpless and think of the passing days, of the lost time. But the most cruel time is afterwards, when I crawl out of bed to sit before the table, take up the pen, – and have to fling it away in sheer despair of ever writing a line. And I've had thirteen years of it, if not more. Anyway, all my writing life. I think that in this light the fourteen vols. (up-to-date) are something of an achievement. But it's a poor consolation.[69]

Conrad never invokes the word 'suppressed' in these letters but he indicates clear lineage between gout and his interminable depressions. As he says here, 'the horrible depression [is the] worst of all'. Depression and gout were not two discrete entities in his mind but a single unity, however differently the textbooks may have explained their origins. But the patterns of depression coincide so clearly with his writing that there is no doubt it had to be added to the formula: gout, depression, composition.

Conrad wrote to Edward Garnett, in May 1917, 'I've been gouty and almost continuously laid up since February. I've just got up after the last bout.'[70] Three years later on 14 June 1920, he wrote to G. Jean-Aubry, who would become his biographer: 'I am just getting over a most severe and unexpected attack of gout, which felled me last Monday after my return from London.'[71]

And so it went for the rest of his life, to age sixty-seven, when he died in 1924. Those of a psychoanalytical cast of mind will be all too quick to interpret the psychological line: illness and writing, writing and illness, in creative counterpoints, with gout merely as the leitmotif. Even more so, they will be eager to explain psychoanalytically why there is not a single reference to gout (or, for that matter, to anything Polish) in any of his novels. But Conrad's doctors assured him he was genuinely gouty and never suggested therapists or psychiatrists, entrenched as Freud and his disciples had become by this time in England. For every Conrad, the doctors will have rejoined, there were dozens of patients who did *not* write; who were gouty without creativity. This will have been true, of course, but does not alter the plain fact that, whether he wrote or not, there was *no* cure for gout in Conrad's time. The physicians thought they had answers, and some exploited their patient's economies, but there was no cure.

In the meantime, medical debate was ploughing on. One of the most significant responses to Garrod came from Sir Dyce Duckworth's *A Treatise on Gout* (1889).[72] His description of the malady was orthodox enough: gout is a constitutional or diathetic malady, manifesting itself in very varied aspects. Beyond that, however, ticklish problems arose, for strict definitions 'belong only to sciences more exact than pathology'. Venturing yet another political metaphor, he judged that diseases were like 'nations with ill-defined frontiers, and with inhabitants intermingling, and even intermarrying'. Taxonomists had had their stab at the problem: 'gout has been placed by some of the older nosologists amongst the order of Fevers'. But he was unimpressed: any worthwhile definition must have regard to its 'constitutional nature' and to the 'essential unity' of the disorder. 'The malady is always chronic,' he remarked, 'since we must regard any one having once given evidence of unequivocal gout as goutily disposed for his lifetime.' One thing had become clear, however: like all physicians who honoured Garrod, Duckworth was insistent that gout and arthritis were not to be confused – indeed he out-Garroded Garrod, maintaining that so-called 'poor man's gout' was not gout at all but 'chronic rheumatic arthritis'.[73]

For many late Victorians, relating the history of gout doctrines became the clue to grasping its nature, and Duckworth was no exception. Gout, he insisted in a tale often to be repeated, had originally been construed within the early (and erroneous) philosophy of humoralism. At long last that paradigm had been challenged by Cullen, who had concluded that the disorder was primarily nervous: 'At the present time the humoral and neurotic theories are still in conflict' – Victorian writers loved to paint manly struggles between polar opposites: Genesis versus geology, idealism versus utilitarianism, and so forth. He noted that 'greater acceptance is perhaps found for the former' (that is, the humoral) theory, its modern embodiment being the work of Garrod and Ebstein; this rejuvenation had occurred because, at the very moment Cullen had expounded his novel 'neurotic' views, the ancient humoral theory had ironically been reinforced thanks to the triumphs of modern chemistry and the discovery of uric acid, though not till Garrod 'unequivocally demonstrated the fact' in 1848 was a key aspect of the 'gouty pathology' settled, constituting 'one of the most brilliant advances made in modern medicine'.[74]

Garrod was thus the father of modern investigation. His 'renal incapacity' theory maintained that deposition of urate of sodium was the *cause* and not the *effect* of the gouty inflammation. These views of Garrod had been resisted by Gairdner, who had regarded accumulation of uric acid not as the 'cause' but as 'a frequent symptom and consequence'. For his part, he had attributed loss of renal function to some 'great emotion or violence'. In other words, Duckworth suggested, Gairdner was of the 'nervous' school.[75]

Edmund Parkes too had dissented from Garrod's theory of renal incapacity. He believed that elimination of uric acid was impeded in gout but did not blame defective kidneys, surmising instead the 'deficient elimination' was not the cause but 'only a consequence'. Duckworth praised Parkes as 'prescient' in suggesting that Garrod's preoccupation with uric acid was myopic: excessive uric acid accompanied gout but was not its *vera causa*. Charles Murchison had also demurred, regarding articular gout as, so to speak, a 'local accident'.[76]

Another implicit supporter of the nervous theory was Thomas Laycock. Gout, for Laycock, was characterized not by uric acid in the blood but by uric acid 'in the tissues', due to 'peculiar changes in the innervation of the individual'. Jonathan Hutchinson thought along similar lines. Querying Garrod, he had denied that swollen joints and tophi were the *sine qua non* of gout. Fascinated by 'inherited gout' in the young and by 'quiet gout', Hutchinson questioned whether gout involved any proved tendency to lithate accumulation. A leading advocate of the hereditary theory of disease, Hutchinson believed there was 'a basic arthritic diathesis', which might resolve into a tendency to gout, rheumatism or any one of their various modifications and combinations: in many cases gout was 'but a superaddition to rheumatism'.[77]

In his *The Pedigree of Disease* (1894), Hutchinson argued that a doctrine of diathesis or hereditary disposition resolved certain long-standing issues in disease theory. He maintained that among the various diathetic conditions elucidated, 'by far the most important for us, as English surgeons, is gout'.[78] Not surprisingly, Duckworth placed Hutchinson in the 'neurotic' camp. By contrast, he set Ebstein, with his necrotic theory, in Garrod's army.[79]

Having thus drawn the battle-lines, Duckworth conceded that the role of uric acid had been definitively established: 'No uric acid, no gout' — it was the 'peccant matter' which worked 'much of the varied and far-reaching mischief'. But it was not the 'whole of the disorder', for constitutional factors also underlay the uric-acid metabolism. Seemingly supporting Hutchinson, Duckworth insisted, 'I would express my belief in the existence of such distinct diatheses,' and he unfolded the case for the 'neurotic theory' of gout. Duckworth was not dismissing humoral and chemical views; rather they had to be set in the context of a more basic neuropathology. In his 'neuro-humoral' theory, it was 'specially characteristic of neuroses that, being thus primarily impressed upon an individual, they tend to be transmitted by heredity'.[80]

What were the therapeutic implications? The theory explained why colchicum was effective in gout, despite having no particular effect upon uric acid: it must work, Duckworth concluded, upon the nervous system. 'The active principle or alkaloid of the drug colchicina is a member of a nitrogenized group of bodies to which veratrina, strychnia, quinia, and morphina have close chemical alliance.' All powerfully affected the nervous system.[81]

It was difficult, warned Duckworth, to distinguish *per se* diseases from mere tendencies: a man may be 'gouty without having what is commonly called gout'. Nevertheless it was possible 'clinically' to recognize such cases as gouty 'by various features in their history and progress'. Even so, modern advances 'do not place us very far in advance of that held and taught by many writers of the last two centuries'. Indeed, his theory of conjoint 'humoral and nervous causation' was not all that different, he admitted, from Sydenham's. That great pioneer had seen gout as the product of 'indigestion' – as humoral, that is – but also as resulting from a diminished 'energy of the spirits', that is, '*nervous energy*'. Sydenham thereby 'foreshadowed' the view that took account in the production of gout of the 'two pathogenic factors' of 'peccant matter' and 'misdirected or perverted nerve-force'. On the clinical side, Duckworth had little new to offer. He condemned malted or fermented liquors. Sufferers should confine themselves to diluted whisky in moderation – for 'it is useless to urge total abstinence on one who has been an immoderate drinker all his life'. A heavy drinker should 'at least be an abstainer between meals – not merely between drinks'.[82]

Another investigator who, like Duckworth, regarded Garrod's pathological bias as too narrow was John Milner Fothergill. Gout-ridden himself, he was fascinated by internal metabolic disorders, including diabetes and biliousness. Fothergill disparaged modern pathology as myopic. 'We will never understand digestion, its disturbances, and how to meet them', he insisted, in a manner characteristic of the broad, English clinical approach,

> by poring over the morbid changes found in the post-mortem room; even when aided by the microscope. We might as well attempt to study the construction of a building from the examination of it in ruin, and by minute inspection of the material of which it consisted.[83]

The science necessary was physiology not pathology. For instance, he insisted, it had finally been discovered that 'biliousness' was 'connected with disturbance of the digestive process in the liver'. For long almost nothing had been known about the liver, but thanks to the late Claude Bernard 'our knowledge has of late made giant strides', and, at last, 'enlarged physiological knowledge' had 'broken a path for a rational comprehension and treatment of the disturbances of the liver'.[84]

Fothergill was vexed at the protean connotations of the term gout. Not only did it come in many varieties – 'Regular', 'Recurrent', 'Retrocedent', 'Irregular', and 'Suppressed' – but its usage was actually broadening: 'a term once applied to an affection of the joints, is now used to cover a very wide field of ailments, viz., all the outcomes of a condition of blood laden with gout-poison'. Medicine was in a cleft stick over nomenclature. Lithiasis or lithaemia were more precise terms for a condition when the blood was laden with uric or lithic acid, but such neologisms were unevocative. 'Gout', on the other hand, was useful, clinically speaking, since it suggested the good living and indulgence which were the 'well-spring' of gout: 'the fathers have eaten sour grapes and the children's teeth are set on edge'.[85]

The role of uric acid had been definitively established by Garrod and others. But this was not the whole scientific story and clinically it did not help much, for in the individual case gout had a complicated history. Exposure to cold, for instance, was one common cause, and strain on joints another, as in the butler's celebrated great toe. Alongside these external triggers there were internal causes. It was vital to grasp the effects of gout-poison upon the vascular system. Many troubles could follow, including apoplexy, aneurysm, angina pectoris and fatty degeneration of the heart with angina.[86]

Taking the wider clinical perspective, Fothergill agreed that gout was good for you. 'There is a widespread opinion', he wrote, 'that a fit of gout clears the system,' noting Mead's dictum that 'gout is the cure of gout'. Garrod had been wary of such readings but Fothergill demurred, protesting that many sufferers 'abort' attacks by resort to colchicum, and so 'bottle up' the gout in the system.[87]

What were its causes? Fothergill conventionally divided them into predisposing and exciting. Of the former, he argued that there was 'none so potent as heredity' – 'breed is stronger than pasture'. Yet once admit that good living in the past caused gout in the present and 'we are compelled to admit that good living in the present will give rise, in all probability to gout in the future'. Hence lifestyle was no negligible factor in creating predisposing causes. It also provided 'exciting' causes. These were, broadly speaking, 'excess of animal food, leading to much nitrogenized waste; imperfect oxygenation, leading to the formation of uric acid, instead of urea; mental causes affecting the liver; and lead-poisoning'.[88]

And not all attacks were acute and external. 'When the great toe is suddenly affected', Fothergill observed, a 'tyro' would avoid the error of mistaking gouty for ordinary inflammation. But with acute articular attacks elsewhere, the 'ready diagnosis' dwindled away into 'uncertainty', except by the man who 'has got his eye in for it' – like the writing on the wall of Belshazzar's hall, which Daniel read with ease. True Daniels among doctors needed the capacity to differentiate gout from 'what was commonly called rheumatic gout'.[89]

Among the key questions raised by Garrod was the role of the internal organs in the excretion of uric acid. This was taken up by Robson Roose (1848–1905), a fashionable Brighton practitioner and a noted society host. His *Gout and its Relations to Diseases of the Liver and Kidneys* (1885) presented it in time-honoured manner as a protean malady. 'The disease may be almost entirely latent,' marked by 'obscure symptoms, slight in degree, and evanescent in character', grasped only when a 'decided family proclivity', or the 'subsequent progress of the case', guided the diagnosis aright. Roose thus endorsed Hutchinson's idea of gouty diathesis. This explained why gout was capable of assuming widely different forms involving 'a vast number of symptoms, disturbances, and complications', many 'inexplicable' until an acute attack furnished the 'key to the diagnosis'.[90]

To support his position, Roose returned to Cullen. Not least Cullen had clarified the different types, a classification, Roose noted, which was 'really based on clinical observation'. Yet the uric-acid theory was also a sheet anchor, one unambiguous advance. In view of Garrod's work, Roose was dissatisfied with Duckworth's claim that 'primary gout' was a '*diathetic* neurosis' – such readings were problematic as a 'difficulty arises in accounting for cases of gout occurring in the absence of any neurotic taint'. He preferred the 'neuro-humoral theory': uric acid must exist in the blood before the disease could be produced, even if its presence was not the *sole* or *sufficient* cause for an attack.[91]

Roose also roped in Edward Liveing's 'neurotic' theory. In his classical work on megrim, Liveing had stressed the connection between gout and such disorders as migraine, asthma, angina pectoris and certain forms of 'transient mental derangement'. Hence Liveing had believed gout was the manifestation of a disorder seated in the nervous system. And Sir James Paget too had drawn attention to the part played by the nervous system. All these were complex issues, Roose confessed, and he feared much theorizing was flimflam. But one need not despair: medical rigour was bearing fruit. For example, among Cullen's varieties of gout, 'the terms *atonic* and *wandering* are at the present day almost obsolete'. Modern classifications were superior, yet gout was not easy to resolve, and it was still impossible to suggest any 'really satisfactory explanation of the so-called "metastasis"'.[92]

Despite these enigmas, Roose was adamant that, *pace* Garrod, gout was not merely a joint disease. It certainly attacked the stomach, indeed in two different forms, *spasmodic* and *inflammatory*. Diagnosis was difficult, and he noted Buzzard's suggestion 'that many cases of so-called "gout in the stomach" would be found, if examined by the light of our present knowledge, to be examples of tabes dorsalis' – that is, a form of neuro-syphilis. All said and done, there were ample reasons for believing that 'many slight affections of the nervous system' were referable to the 'gouty diathesis'.[93]

Thus Liveing, Duckworth and Roose all gave some credence to the 'neurosis' theory of gout; another vocal late-nineteenth-century advocate was Willoughby Francis Wade. In *On Gout as a Peripheral Neurosis* (1893), Wade argued that 'the nerve was the anatomical seat' of gout. For Wade, two main questions arose. First, what was the nature of the gout 'neuropathy'? Second, what was its relation to the gouty joint? Like many authors, he suffered from gout and wrote in part autobiographically. Like Roose, Wade returned to Cullen for support. 'It is in the peripheral nerves', he argued, that the 'real and chief bond of union' would be found.[94]

At the close of the century the great synthesizer of Victorian medicine, Sir William Osler, summed up developments by reiterating in *The Principles and Practice of Medicine* (1898) that 'the nature of gout is unknown'.[95] Thanks largely to Garrod, certain things had been elucidated, for instance the role of lead. But most of the rest remained 'theory'. At best, 'gouty diathesis' was a useful shorthand. It is time to examine the two leading theoreticians of the turn of the century. The pillar of orthodoxy was William Ewart (1848–1929). In *Gout and Goutiness: and Their Treatment* (1896), he pondered recent developments. He too was worried about the relation of words and things, disease and classification. Was the concept of 'gouty diathesis', so popular with Hutchinson, Duckworth and others, one of those 'mere names' ever threatening to 'take the place of facts'? 'Gouty diathesis' involved semantic hazards: its 'lack of definition' led him to avoid its employment in favour of 'straightforward expressions', such as 'disposition' and 'special liability'.[96]

The diathesis concept was slippery, even circular, especially when one began to speak of a 'diathesis which is acquired' alongside one 'inherited'. Was the supposed 'gouty diathesis' to be applied equally to such 'opposites' as the gluttonous, full-blooded individual and the starving?[97]

Progress was inherently enigmatic, and the way to untangle confusion, Ewart thought, lay in surveying the evolution of ideas about gout. Names and things had been unambiguous among the Ancients. The expressions 'podagra', 'gonagra', 'omagra', 'chiragra' 'indicated merely the seat of the painful affection', irrespective of any theory. Substitution of the umbrella term 'gout' did not clarify matters, intimating the existence independently of 'articular troubles' of a '*constitutional* disease' which, Ewart confessed, had always 'been impossible strictly to identify'. Use of the term gout 'suggested a theory as to its nature', and by consequence much of the gout literature had largely been devoted to discussion not of an articular but of a supposed constitutional disease.[98]

Modern trends were towards specificity, resulting notably in Garrod's localizing work, which had the strength but also the shortcomings of excluding 'all unknown and all theoretical matter'. For Ewart the 'extreme development' of that localizing tendency was Haig's view (examined below) that identified the condition with 'uric acid in the wrong place' – one which, on the principle 'no uric acid, no gout', excluded latent constitutional factors. The big issue was how uric acid related to gout. Gout, Ewart believed, was really made up of the 'uric acid trouble' plus 'something else'. The triumph of bacteriology meant that other diseases were being 'cracked' while gout remained a mystery.[99]

In view of this aetiological ignorance, it could be profitable to describe gout as a 'functional disorder' for 'we know gout only through its manifestations'. These, in any case, were quite complicated enough! There was '*Gout itself . . .* apart from its manifestations' – in other words, the still unknown prime mover of all gouty phenomena; there was '*Declared gout*', gout associated with definite structural change. Then there was '*Goutiness*, or the condition of imperfectly declared gout', usually consisting of varied functional disturbances with merely clinical symptoms. Such variety seemed to demand the concept of diathesis, but that was highly problematic, for was a 'diathesis which is acquired' the same as one which is 'inherited'? Overall, diathesis was a highly nebulous concept: should one talk of a gouty diathesis? Or a 'uric acid diathesis'? Not least there loomed the question of aetiology. At least half the cases of gout are *inherited*, Ewart maintained. The notion of inheritance had but limited explanatory power, for gout was '*modified in transmission*'. Nor could the possibility of a racial diathesis be left out:

> The Anglo-Saxon and the Dutch stand, in respect of gout, in a marked contrast to the Scotch and to the German or Scandinavian. Both England and Holland are remarkable for the humidity of their climate and for their liberal dietary. On the other hand, Scotland and Ireland, the recognised homes of frugality, are no less humid than England, whilst Germany enjoys a relatively dry climate.[100]

Such cases tended to show that dietary factors predominated over the climatic and the racial, for 'races so far removed from the regions of prevalence of gout as even the African tribes' have provided gouty specimens 'acquired in the individual after emigration, owing to rich living'. Faced with all these puzzles, Ewart surveyed alternative theories, and concluded that the history of pathology showed 'oscillations' between 'two great theories' – the 'humoral' and the 'solidist'. In most diseases that dichotomy had been resolved, but the gout controversy has lasted 'almost to the present day'.[101]

'Humoralism' ('of which Sydenham had been the last great representative') had been challenged by Cullen, who 'adopting his teaching, carried it to its ultimate conclusions'. But though 'they had done service in effectually breaking through the old tradition, their views were too uncompromising to obtain a lasting hold on medical thought', not least because Cullen's nervous theories had been straightaway challenged by the new chemistry.[102]

Uric acid had latterly moved stage-centre. The conception of a 'uric acid dyscrasia' was, Ewart noted, 'almost exclusively humoral'. But it was a queer sort of fluidism, since 'the mischievous property is in this case identified with a solid, the sodium biurate crystal'. So long as uric acid remained fluid, no trouble ensued; 'but with its precipitation in or about the joints, and in other situations as biurate, it becomes harmful'. Such theories had spawned the 'pure humoralism' of Alexander Haig.[103]

Tricky questions remained. Why did the crystallization 'occur in the wrong place and in abnormal quantities'? Was it excessive *production* of uric acid or undue *accumulation*? Haig's theory of faulty diet suggested over-production; Garrod's view suggested retention (renal defect). But the 'renal block' theory had the problem that 'commonly no morbid change can be detected in the kidney'.[104]

Ewart admired Garrod for his *hypotheses-non-fingo* scientific rigour, his 'philosophical reticence' respecting any 'more remote element in the disease'. The responses to Garrod from Gairdner, by contrast, 'were merely inferences from clinical observation', lacking the support of any such 'physical method of demonstration' as Garrod had put forward. Yet Garrod hadn't solved all the problems. Difficulties still attending the understanding of the workings of uric acid had led to the revival of the 'nervous theory' by Duckworth and Wade.

Ewart also addressed the vexed question of gouty cachexia. Duckworth had traced this either to original frailty of constitution or to 'unbridled indulgence' in the 'predisposed'. Truly robust constitutions did not suffer in this way, or only in due course. Gouty heart was another unresolved question – was that a separate clinical entity? Trickiest of all was metastatic gout. A patient might become prone to pulmonary, gastric or other troubles; such 'visceral trouble' was still a 'gouty trouble', though it might not be a true 'retrocedence'.[105]

Ewart believed his historical analysis had established various points. The concept of the 'unknown factor "diathesis"', so dear to Duckworth, was 'superfluous'. Yet the theory of 'goutiness' was useful as a companion to gout itself. Goutiness 'inclines almost fatally towards declared gout'; and those once attacked with 'declared gout' lapsed sooner or later into 'goutiness'. If 'diathesis' was redundant, the constitutional notion of gout was helpful. 'Goutiness' was applicable to all conditions in which the constitutional change was manifest. Gout was commonly structural, 'but in all cases it is also *functional*, and is made up of the gouty visceral manifestations'. Garrod's early elucidation of the local accumulation of sodium biurate had, ironically, 'largely contributed' to a perhaps premature acceptance of the uric-acid theory.[106]

Goutiness was to be distinguished from gout: its main feature was '*increased irritability* and *lowered resistance*'. Was this 'degeneracy' merely the work of a long continuance of the 'acid dyscrasia'? That was difficult to resolve.[107] Discarding idle talk of 'gouty diathesis' and viewing the gouty disposition as lying in some 'deviation from healthy metabolism induced by a prolonged course of toxic alimentation' afforded practical benefits. Conceiving of a 'healthy habit' would encourage belief in the 'curability of goutiness, though not of the late results of articular gout'. To understand gout, Ewart insisted, it was essential to understand the metabolism, notably the stomach, the pancreas and spleen, and, above all, the liver. Modern models of metabolism constituted a major advance. 'Whereas plethora was once believed to be crucial' (Scudamore and Gairdner), there was no evidence that 'undue vascular fulness' was principally to blame. By contrast, 'gout is largely a *renal question*'. Even so, gout was not reducible to kidney disease for then all sufferers from granular kidney ought to present evidence of accumulation of uric acid. Hence Ewart concluded that some other factor besides renal inadequacy must be involved. In short, writing around the turn of the century, Ewart was able to make an informed historical assessment of the gout dispute, but was completely unable to resolve it.[108]

The radical figure around the turn of the century was Alexander Haig, whose *magnum opus, Uric Acid as a Factor in the Causation of Disease* first appeared in 1892 and proved so popular that it had gone through seven editions by 1908. Haig was the Cadogan of his day. While, in the opinion of many, creating a lot of new nonsense of his own, he dismissed all the archaic gout palaver. Gout was not constitutional, it was not hereditary, it was entirely due to bad diet. All now hinged upon the modern demon, uric acid. Haig thus took Garrod and made him into a god. He also had scientific pretensions: and for him modern science had demonstrated that the very concept of gout was *passé* because of the discovery of the role of uric acid. Gout had become a pre-scientific label. And times had changed. It was an age of democracy; scientists and physicians had to address a far wider audience than the old gout doctors. This was a point upon which Haig was emphatic. 'Fresh food', he argued, at the very opening of his great work,

> has as yet been possible only for a small portion of the race, and till quite recent times its use in large quantity was still only possible for the richer fraction of that portion. It brought with it its own diseases, formerly confined to the rich, now spreading far and wide through all classes, hand in hand with the cheapening of flesh and tea. This volume suggests that these diseases can be prevented or cured by leaving out the poisons and reverting to the foods most in accord with the anatomy and physiology of man, which were more common here a century ago, and are still common

in other countries. There can be no doubt, however, that here, as else-where, prevention is better than cure.[109]

Here was a new language of gout. In one respect, however, Haig resem-bled the traditional gout doctor. He spelt out his views on gout and on health by way of autobiography. 'Having been a life-long sufferer from migraine,' he explained, 'in the autumn of 1882, in despair of obtaining complete relief from drugs, and not without some fear that I was suffering from organic disease, I gave up butcher's meat and replaced it by milk and fish.' Change of diet completely changed his body sensations. By 'altering uric acid' levels he found he could 'alter the related symptoms'. This perception had led him to understand not just headache and neuralgic pains but gout as well, for he had discovered that 'in curing a headache by giving an acid to diminish excretion of uric acid', the result had been 'pricking and shooting pain in my joints'; he had naturally concluded that 'the uric acid was retained in these joints and produced the pains'. Library research led him to discover that Garrod had described 'similar joint pains as occurring in gouty subjects after the ingestion of beer or wine'. All beers and wines were strongly acid. Hence 'a simple explanation' existed for gout.

> I have since ascertained that this was a single instance of a general law, and that all substances increasing the solubility of uric acid increase its excretion in the urine and do good in the joint troubles due to its irritating presence; while conversely all substances diminishing the solubility of uric acid, diminish its excretion in the urine and increase these irritations in joints and other fibrous structures.[110]

Thus he had unearthed metabolic relations: 'the explanation of the arthritis or gout has never seemed to me to be a very difficult matter'. Indeed, Haig was willing to lay a wager: 'I am quite prepared to undertake to produce a uric acid arthritis in anyone, provided my instructions are carried out, but the clinical result will often resemble what is described as the arthritis of rheumatism rather than that of gout.'[111] From this he concluded that 'the arthritis in both diseases is due to uric acid'. Rheumatism was the disease in which uric acid was driven into 'a large number of joints', whereas 'in gout a great part of the uric acid in the blood is . . . concentrated on one particular joint'.[112]

Overall, gout had been misunderstood. Despite all the blather, it was not a unique and specific disease but merely one of a multitude of pathological consequences of surplus uric acid. Thus Garrod had been both very right and very wrong – right to incriminate uric acid in gout, wrong in thinking that that connection between uric acid and gout was unique and specially pathognomic. The truth was the reverse: practically all diseases were caused by excess uric acid!

This enabled Haig to spell out some broad propositions, aimed to set understanding of gout and all joint diseases on a new footing:

> GOUT is the old name of that form of arthritis caused by uric acid which commonly affects people in middle life, and is more often, at least at first, to be found in a single joint. Rheumatism is the old name of the arthritis produced by uric acid which commonly affects young people and many joints at a time . . . This we can now see is not, strictly speaking, a disease at all, but a reaction of the physiology of the body to food-poisons.[113]

This food-poisoning theory had drastic implications for traditional concepts, for it meant – and here the echo of Cadogan is almost audible – that 'gout is not a constitutional disease due to any defect in the formation or functioning of the body. It is a form of "diet" disease due to food poisoning.' Hence it could be cured by 'leaving off the poisonous foods'. Haig argued that uric acid was exceedingly poisonous. 'To-day we can produce all forms of arthritis and other so-called diseases simply by swallowing uric acid.'[114]

The implications of these positions have been well elucidated by James Whorton, who has emphasized the significance of Haig's auto-experimentation on what he called 'the human test-tube'. It was clear to Haig that deposits of the poison uric acid in the tissues would produce irritation. He believed that elevated blood pressure was the immediate cause of his headaches and migraine; hence there was a direct relation between acid in the blood and blood pressure. He had already observed that test-tube solutions of urates could be chemically manipulated to form gelatinous colloids; a similar phenomenon must be occurring in the blood – 'collaemia' ('the presence of uric acid as a colloid in the blood stream and its action as an obstructor of the tiny capillaries').[115] By impeding blood flow, colloidal uric acid raised blood pressure throughout the body, and, he contended, depressed the metabolic rate (acting like 'a wet blanket on a fire'). Various disorders would follow, including melancholy and gout. The uric-acid deposits would grow in the tissues as constitutional vigour dwindled, until at last 'the long pent up store of urates breaks its dams and rushes into the circulation with an overwhelming flood'. Apoplexy might follow, heart failure or Bright's disease, which Haig supposed was caused by long-term irritation by uric-acid deposits. From 1911, he tried to cure several cases of inoperable cancer with a diet of nuts, fruits and biscuits, free of uric acid and its metabolic precursors. None of the patients recovered.[116]

Haig campaigned to educate all classes respecting the dangers of uric acid and the need for diet reform: all foods containing uric acid or its purine precursors were highly toxic. Conversion of the human race to the 'uric-acid-free diet' was his goal. A uric-acid-free diet would cure the craving for alcohol, tobacco and other stimulants. He occasionally envisioned a future 'which will be ... truer, nobler and better, as man slowly realizes how much of his sordid past has had its origin in unnatural food'.[117]

For all his eccentricities and zealotry, Haig is an important figure. While derided by the medical profession, he attained a wide public following, not least because of his crusade for dietary reform. Almost unconsciously, his significance lay in dissolving the very concept of gout. Gout had always been elitist; Haig's uric-acid disease was a malady for everyman in the new age of the masses.[118]

Gout also began to dissolve in the writings of one of its most intriguing twentieth-century students, who may be seen as rounding off the movement begun by Garrod: Richard Llewellyn Jones Llewellyn. Welsh-born, he began in practice at Aberystwyth but, becoming interested in arthritis and rheumatoid conditions, he moved to Bath, starting a specialist practice there, and being appointed physician to the Royal Mineral Water Hospital.

In 1920 Llewellyn published *Gout*, which concluded that gout was a disease of civilization. Unknown among 'native' peoples, it was 'the Nemesis that overtakes those addicted to luxurious habits and dietetic excesses'. Experiencing the need, in the wake of the Great War, for a comprehensive explanation of human health, sickness, biology and destiny, Llewellyn unfolded a grand historical theory, relating disease, race and civilization: nations too, like individuals, when fallen on hard times, 'lose their gout'.[119]

Llewellyn had little respect for early theories of pathogenesis. The 'fanciful views of the humoralists' exercised almost undisputed sway till Cullen repudiated a doctrine 'unjustifiable in conception'. But Cullen's theory secured few adherents, being overtaken by the new chemistry, since when opinion inclined to the view that the 'life history of gout was bound up with that of *uric acid*'. Scientific proof was lacking till in 1848 Garrod's 'epoch-making discovery' allayed all doubts.[120]

Garrod made uric acid the 'alpha and omega' of the disease. But this was unsatisfactory, for investigators remained unsure as to the 'why and wherefore of that accumulation of uric acid in the blood' which Garrod held to be a necessary antecedent. Garrod attributed this to a 'functional renal defect', but to many 'renal inadequacy' was not wholly satisfying, hence subsequent hypotheses as to pathogenesis.[121]

Llewellyn summed up the main alternative positions. The primary alteration in gout was variously assumed to be:

1. In the blood or tissues (histogenous theories).
2. In the bodily structures, either inborn or induced.
3. In hepatic inadequacy.
4. In hyperpyraemia.
5. In the nervous system.

Of these the first to be considered were the 'histogenous theories', those stressing the role of the cells. Llewellyn identified these theories with Parkes and Laycock. In 1872 Ord argued for an inborn tendency in the fibroid tissues of gouty subjects to undergo a type of degeneration, and most important among these theories was Ebstein's, who concluded that the primary factor in gout causation was necrosis of the damaged textures.[122]

Others, especially Murchison and Latham, stressed the role of the liver and hepatic inadequacy. Some, like Liveing, emphasized the nervous theory. Doubts, however, accumulated as to the propriety of the terms 'uric acid diathesis', so long credited for nearly all the minor ailments flesh is heir to.[123]

Having sifted this heap of alternatives, Llewellyn offered his own definition:

> Gout is an hereditary disorder, the *intrinsic* element of which is an inborn instability of nuclein metabolism which may remain latent, but under the influence of *extrinsic* factors, *infections*, becomes manifest, as betokened by local inflammatory tissue reactions in joints or elsewhere the specific character of which is attested by the associated *uratic deposition*.[124]

Gout was hereditary, indeed the most hereditary of all arthritic disorders. For confirmation he cited Scudamore and Garrod; Roberts had found that three-quarters of the cases of gout occurring among the easy classes could be distinctly traced back to a gouty ancestry, and Luff had disclosed a 'definite family history' of gout.[125]

Llewellyn queried whether gout was ever truly acquired *de novo*. It was (almost) necessarily the surfacing of a latent tendency. 'The *innate predisposition* thereto is *always inherited*,' he wrote, 'and the predisposing factors, that we presume may originate gout, are in reality mere *excitants or determining* agents.' With this proclivity gout might, however, skip a generation.[126]

The gouty, in other words, had an inborn error of metabolism, as stated by Alfred Garrod's son Archibald. The vague phrases 'constitutional' or 'nutritional', applied by older writers, were thus rather obsolete. Llewellyn offered some preliminary conclusions.

1. Gout is always an hereditary disease.

2. The factors currently regarded as predisposing agencies are in reality merely *determining* agents, not the cause of gout, but the *occasion of its appearance*.

3. In the absence of an hereditary taint, these same are powerless to evoke the *specific* manifestations of true *'gouty' inflammation* as estimated by associated *uratic deposition*.[127]

Environmental factors played a part. Lead-workers were specially prone to develop gout – Llewellyn noted with pride that two of his predecessors at the

Royal Mineral Water Hospital, Bath – William Falconer and Caleb Hillier Parry – had drawn attention to the frequent occurrence of gout in those exposed to lead. Gout also had its exciting causes, including addiction to the 'fleshpots'. Local trauma – and local foci of infection – were extremely common. Thus he judged that:

    1. Heredity is the sole *predisposing* factor in gout.

    2. That the differentiation between the usually cited predisposing and exciting causes is unwarrantable.

    3. That both alike are merely *determinants*.

    4. That their influence as such in exciting outbreaks is exerted through the medium of *infection*, this achieved either directly or indirectly.[128]

Overall, however, the role of inborn errors of metabolism was crucial. Gouty individuals, Llewellyn insisted, were the victims of some inborn defect or eccentricity of metabolism, rather like sufferers from alkaptonuria, cystinuria and pentosuria. Here Llewellyn drew on Sir Archibald Garrod's theory of inborn errors in metabolism. It was a similarity Llewellyn believed crucial, for 'all members of the group, including gout, display hereditary tendencies. All occur much more often in males than in females. They all alike tend to persist through life.' And the analogy applied despite the fact that 'the clinical features of alkaptonuria, etc.' were 'colourless' as contrasted with the 'vivid arresting phenomena of gout'![129]

Llewellyn nevertheless had reservations. Before 'gout could with justice be relegated to the same category of disorders' it would be necessary to prove that uric acid was an 'intermediary' and 'not a terminal product of metabolism'. But research indicated that uric acid was an end-product. Hence, though gout might have kinship with alkaptonuria, there were differences too.[130]

Gout's profile was changing in medical theory and popular parlance alike; the 'nervy side' of gout was diminishing. 'Gouty' headaches had almost disappeared, and certain medical euphemisms were in retreat. Acute 'gouty' delirium had been in many cases but an euphemism for alcoholism. 'It would be held rash to-day to speak, like our forefathers, of "gouty" *cystitis, urethritis,* or *orchitis,*' for there was no evidence of any pathological connection between them. Llewellyn was therefore deeply suspicious of irregular gout, for 'experience' suggested that it was an 'abstraction'. All this led him to the 'melancholy' conclusion that the gouty had 'suffered much of many physicians'.[131]

Diet was one of the doctors' fads and frailties. Once 'uric acid' had been regarded as an infallible index of gout, the inference seemed obvious: the ideal diet for the gouty was a diet free from any uric-acid-forming material. But was this so? 'For who has not met with gouty veterans who, having run the gamut of endless dietetic experiments, still remain "gouty", though, *mirabile dictu*, still avid for fresh ventures?'[132]

Ancient gout folklore was on its last legs, including the 'Honour of the Gout':

> The absurd delusion, not wholly dissipated even to-day, that to have gout, 'Morbus Dominorum', was highly creditable, a mark of good breeding, was firmly ingrained in our forefathers. We all recall the story of the old Scottish gentlewoman who would never allow that any but people of family could have *bonâ fide* gout. Let but the *roturier* aspire to this privilege, and she scouted the very idea − 'Na, na, it is only my father and Lord Gallowa' that have the regular gout.' As to the origin of this mistaken ambition, it most probably was the outcome of the fact that it was peculiarly an appanage of the great, the wealthy, and alas! those of intellectual distinction![133]

Not only gout lore, but gout itself was on the wane. This was the outcome of many factors, not least the rise in national sobriety.

These were issues to which Llewellyn returned in a later work, *Aspects of Rheumatism and Gout* (1927). The question of diatheses, inborn errors and the role of medicine still preoccupied him. Earlier theorists 'argued, if the husbandman could eradicate weeds by changing the character of the soil, then why could not the physician do the same in respect of disease? . . . the control of the diathesis was their objective.'[134] The doctrine of diatheses had declined. Why? Not, Llewellyn judged, 'due to any inherent fallacies in the conception itself, but to the growing conviction that there were *exogenous*, as well as endogenous, factors concerned in the production of diseases'. Physicians had turned with relief from the recondite mysteries of diatheses to more accessible fields of exploration thanks to the epoch-making discoveries of Pasteur. Specificity and bacteriology had swept the board and the doctrine of diatheses suffered temporary eclipse. The riddle appeared solved. The causes of disease were no longer 'without form and void', but living organisms; all that was needed was the mere bringing together of pathogenic germ and susceptible host to suffice for the production of this or that specific malady. But bacteriology did not solve all the questions. Attention therefore shifted from *le grain* to *le terrain*, from the microbe to the individual. The result was the recent revival of the term 'diathesis', in an effort to look at disease by tracing 'the record of its long descent'. Despite Mendel, however, seeking the source of inborn morbid potentialities still savoured too much of the 'incomprehensible'.[135]

For Llewellyn the resurgence of the term 'diathesis' was inevitable. The word 'soil' had come back in − but with a new twist, 'for to-day we no longer look upon "soil" as dead, inert material, but rather as a chemico-physical aggregate teeming with bacterial life'.[136]

Llewellyn therefore offered an ecological vision of disease, bearing affinities to the ideas of social medicine, while stressing heredity.[137] The evidences that man and his environment were one and indissociable 'rapidly accumulate', bringing out the fundamental *unity* of human, animal and plant life. Grander organic rhythms were at work:

> The tendency to rhythm is deep ingrained in protoplasm – writ as plain in the systole and diastole of the heart, the inspiratory and expiratory phases of respiration as in the recurrence of the menstrual cycle. Do not our body cells, too, like the 'laughing soil', respond to the call of the seasons, the biologic action of light, heat, and electrical stakes or disturbances?[138]

Llewellyn thus announced the need for an 'Enlarged Etiologic Outlook', built on the idea that man and his environment were one organic whole: ceaseless adaptions to cosmic forces, and no less infinite scope for *maladaptions*, with resulting *metabolic* obliquities making or not for disease or infection.[139]

He also drew practical conclusions. Was it not a 'tradition' that persons of 'rheumatic' or 'gouty' diathesis were notoriously deficient in their power of adaptation to cosmic or climatic vicissitudes? Under such circumstances, 'we must envisage the human organism not simply as a *nidus* for microbes', but rather as an 'organic unity' upon whom 'multiple *cosmic* forces of most varied type are constantly impinging and to which it must as constantly adapt'. This being so, was it not equally certain that '*maladaptions*' would bring 'Nemesis' in the shape of '*altered metabolism* of divers kinds and therewith lowered resistance?' Hence the idea of diathesis should be revived. The relationship between inheritance and clinical manifestations was 'complex'. A new way of thinking about medical causation was needed, superseding the 'traditional habit' of dividing 'causes into *predisposing* and *exciting*'.[140]

It was standard to say that, given the absence of the specific organism, the affiliated disorder would not have occurred. But this was shallow because its presence within the body did not necessarily entail infection. Witness the 'carrier' phenomenon. In that light, Llewellyn proposed that notions of rheumatic and gouty diathesis be re-established, and he reasserted the hereditary nature of gout.[141]

Llewellyn represents a critical juncture and suitable outpost for the conclusion of these convergences of medical theory and 'felt life' in the Jamesian sense. But not before comparing Llewellyn briefly with two of his contemporaries: the famous brothers Henry and William James.

To sum up, Llewellyn felt himself at a threshold. Traditional doctrines of gout were obsolete; traditional gout was itself in rapid decline. Unexplained disorders remained – of course – and these Llewellyn was still inclined to deem 'gouty'. But, for all its advances, disease theory itself still hadn't cracked the problem of the understanding of constitutional or chronic conditions and the James brothers were living proof. William had been healthy enough while alive, but he died in 1909, leaving his brother Henry, in England, to fall into renewed illness at Rye. Henry consulted Sir James Mackenzie, the London heart specialist, for fear of angina pectoris and was reassured that the problem lay in his mind – there was nothing to fear. But Mackenzie's reassurance counted for little and Henry sank into depression and fever, claiming he was suffering attacks of acute gout, becoming anorexic through aversion to food, and having difficulty getting in and out of bed in the morning. Gout and depression he yoked in opposition to angina, a most curious symmetry. He wrote to a confidant that ultimately the doctors had failed him; that he was pathetically suffering from 'the black devils of nervousness, direst damnest demons'.[142]

Llewellyn would no more have been able to help Henry than Mackenzie did. Over the decades of the nineteenth century doctors had generated mounds of disease theory, none of which could explain to Henry James, let alone cure him of, the chronic malady from which he claimed to be suffering.[143]

Perhaps this lacuna between theory and credibility is what had eluded the doctors. As the condition *par excellence* signalling excess and guaranteeing insulation, gout was too precious, if too comic, to surrender, even to the doctors' superior wisdom. For writers like the James brothers – or Hemingway for that matter – it provided a virtual guarantee of long life and sustained creativity. Few men within the social history of excess cultivated it more assiduously than Ernest Hemingway, a man of excess in every sense of the word, whose medical problems rival those of Samuel Johnson, though Hemingway's were primarily self-inflicted.[144] Oddly, there was no sign of gout in his life, but he suffered sore throats from childhood, anthrax infection in the foot, dysentery, liver ailments, eyesight problems, erysipelas, keretitis sicca, wounds to head and knees, jaundice and malaria, dozens of head injuries and multiple concussions throughout his life, shot himself in both legs, was told to give up drinking or die, endured throat pneumonia, cirrhosis, oedema – and final collapse into death. Hemingway even used 'uncertain health' as his alibi not to attend the Nobel ceremony (though generally he tended to downplay his ailments).

Gout seems the only condition he did *not* endure. Still, it crops up in his works, as in *Farewell to Arms* in the section where Frederic Henry, the hero, and Catherine, his lover, compare notes on their respective fathers:

'Wine is a grand thing,' I said. 'It makes you forget all the bad.'
　'It's lovely,' said Catherine. 'But it's given my father gout very badly.'
　'Have you a father?'
　'Yes,' said Catherine. 'He has gout. You won't ever have to meet him. Haven't you a father?'
　'No,' I said. 'A stepfather.'
　'Will I like him?'
　'You won't have to meet him.'
　'We have such a fine time,' Catherine said.[145]

Perhaps Catherine's pronouncement *is* the last word. 'We have such a fine time' – the epigraph for all gouties. The insulating condition and guardian of excess had also brought an almost comic relief to its victims. After the theories and therapies of generations, beyond the spas and newfangled water cures, what had all the doctors in the world been able to do for a Collins, Conrad, James or Hemingway except ensure that their patrician disease kept them going?

GOUTOMETRIES

CHAPTER 11

Podagra Ludens: *Disease and Discourse*

I. *Podagra ludens: ludic representations*

... homo ludens, podagra ludens[1]
(man the playful, gout the playful)

We have surveyed a condition now reduced to such chemical simplicity that a blood test reveals its presence and drugs rectify the chemical imbalance it brings. But gout also had a representational and visual evolution whose contexts from the start have been ludic – playful – as if to suggest the wide chasm between its chronic afflictions and basic insulations from calamity. Johann Huizinga, the Dutch historian, has commented on *homo ludens* in relation to the 'anatomic foot' that 'nobody will expect that every language has one definite word for "hand" or "foot"'.[2] And Georges Bataille cautioned scholars in *Literature and Evil* (1991) against equating the lexical history of such words as 'play element' with their representations. If Bataille's or Huizinga's agenda inclined them to explore realms medical, they may have gleaned how germane these concerns were to the 'monarch's disease'. Gout's 'play' included the sport embedded in its discursive metaphors of rise and fall, push and pull, even the battle of the sexes. In time these representations of play – verbal and visual – were amalgamated to other forms as unseen processes and pathologies.

But what kind of 'presence' was gout? Who can be said to have had it? When did it commence? Given the obsession with onset, when did its presence count as news? What could be publicly reported?

These questions can be raised for all disease, but for gout the metaphors implied another 'body politic'.[3] Gout's rise and fall, swelling and reduction, rendered it a prime metaphor for the political state. The analogy was noted in printed medical treatises and diplomatic discourses. 'Political gout', as in an anonymous *Podagra politica seu tractatus podagricus*, elevated gout to stratospherical metaphoric levels.[4] It appeared the natural liaison between private self-diagnosis and public self-fashioning, in the senses we described in Chapter 3. Gout, as the general human potential for 'swelling', also elicited questions about the *imaginary*: the imaginary rise and fall, the imaginary report and intelligence, the imaginary enemy and ally. Given the consequences, gout exceeded mere malady and designated a moral and metaphorical limbo whose signposts emblazoned the monarchs of Great Britain, of whom George III's crippling condition was but the best example.[5]

These conditions already applied to the medieval world. If the sufferer's aches were chronicled, they were enumerated in the language of extension and increase. Dante and Chaucer understood this monolith despite the absence then of a coherent theory of podagra.[6] Linguistically speaking, the world of Petrarch and Boccaccio retained this similitude about physical extension: all 'gouty discourse' referred to physical rise and fall, as if gravity existed before the phenomenon was conceptualized.[7]

This monolith of extension conveyed jocund energy by virtue of predictability: always the *same* comic rise and fall. Even in the grotesque Rabelaisian underworld, where random events are commensurate with linguistic deviation, gout's predictable rise and fall elicited similar comic expectations. On this constancy the Renaissance world superimposed two further linguistic traditions: an unending play on words, and the linking of gout's metaphors to the affairs of state.

The former had been especially linked to the foibles of doctors, a *topos* Rabelais embroidered;[8] the latter – the body politic – formed one of Western civilization's most tentacular configurations. Old wives' tales in Rabelais' era denigrated the healer by claiming his gout was the sign of his taste, a silly homology of 'gout' and 'goutte'. 'Aux tierres à le goutte, les médecins ne voient goutte' – in matters of taste, doctors have none. Variants existed in the dictionaries and encyclopaedias of general knowledge of the time.[9] According to Mikhail Bakhtin the doctor presided over natural and supernatural realms in Rabelais' milieu, the arbiter of plagues as well as newer menaces, syphilitic and bubonic.[10] Rabelais' satires, influential for the development of the early novel, privilege podagra and syphilis as emblems of the human condition, building on their heritage of 'rise and fall'. About this lost continent Bakhtin wrote eloquently in his book about Rabelais and medicine.[11] But Rabelais' conceptual framework was also Aristotelian, especially as it underpinned his notions of tragic and comic sensibility; the 'Ancient' who penetrated the core of reality's binary modes – comic and tragic – as if the two spheres of man's mind.[12] Gout was woven into the comic vision as rise and fall: the verbal wheel on which linguistic gymnasts could practice their rhetorical wit. By the sixteenth century a *topos* about podagra had developed built on analogies of physical matter's rise and fall and captured in gout's comic potential to exceed ordinary linguistic boundaries. It blossomed into a subgenre incorporating levity into the older Lucianic and more recent Menippean, neo-Latin traditions.[13]

II. The Lucianic and Menippean heritage

this tedious unconnected epistle is an infallible symptom [of the gout] . . .

Smollett, Humphry Clinker, letter of 26 June

So Smollett's prickly Bramble to his 'doctor' in one of his characteristically *disjointed* – as if the epistle itself were arthritic – letters. Bramble believes that malady and representation are reciprocal, even causal: the disjointed fragment reveals his symptom, not vice versa. Fragments fuse with swellings and reductions in the stomach, legs and limbs. This disjointed fragment – gout's linguistic sign – also enjoyed another heritage derived from Lucian, the second-century dramatist who wrote at least two mock tragedies about 'Podagra'.[14]

Lucian's plays were revived in the Renaissance when his 'gout tragedy' was widely read.[15] The palaeography is corrupt: it is unclear whether Rabelais' contemporaries judged them as one or two plays; even our classicists are uncertain of their authenticity. But this lapse did not impede their rediscovery: they influenced *Gargantua* and *Pantagruel*, as Rabelais' modern commentators note. Sydenham himself was steeped in Lucian's Latin gout-play and composed a commentary on it that appeared in his famous treatise.[16] Medical authors after *c.* 1600 were keen to cite Lucian's bombast when touting 'the gout'; others of non-medical bent turned his 'gouty wit' into their own Menippean satire in the Erasmian tradition of the *Praise of Folly*. Set the dials to approximately 1620 or 1630 and these ludic strains are combining into an undergrowth of subgenres: verse exploiting gout's risibilities through praise, folly, attack and overthrow. To these were superadded the themes of progressive folk societies in utopian and dystopian versions, life as spectacle, realism as theatre, as in Jacob Biedermann's *Ludi theatrales* (1666): a pastiche of witticisms extolling game and play, celebrating spectacle, bombastically trumpeting utopias where mankind would be salvaged.[17]

This heritage energized Burton's *Anatomy of Melancholy* (1621) and Philander Misaurus' *Honour of the Gout* (1720) as well as European 'praises' that blended genres into anatomies or dissections, 'graveyards' of ancient knowledge and gnostic wisdom, in the paradoxical–encomiastic tradition, flaunting rhetorical bravura in pedagogical exercises.[18] Such Menippean 'praises' dramatized the uncertainties of medical diagnosis by exploiting metaphor, especially gout's notorious rise and fall, and cultivating the gymnomastery of punning on the 'feet of verse' and 'feet of the gouty'.

Christopher Ballista's *Overthrow of the Gout*, published in Latin in 1528, is such a blended work.[19] The French Ballista wrote with Lucian's dialogic fragment at his side, imitating, plagiarizing, parodying the ludic elements Huizinga described. We resurrect it and its poetic genealogy here to

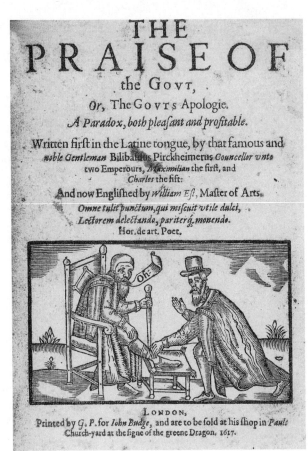

1. Title page of Pirckheimer, *The Praise of the Gout, Or, The Gouts Apologie*. London, 1617.

adumbrate gout's generic resonances and rich metaphoric heritage rather than its medicinal therapies or the *male* pessimism it continued to evoke. The late-medieval and Tudor rhetorical tradition was diverse: even texts in grammar were viewed as 'ludic' sport, as in the sprawling *Ludus grammaticus* (1612). Ballista and his best Elizabethan translator, Barnabe Googe, amalgamated these exercises with Lucian's 'podagra' fragment, while building on the paradoxical–encomiastic tradition driving Pirckheimer's *Praise of the Gout* (1617).[20]

But why *gout*? Other old maladies, fever and mania, had not been similarly rhetoricized because they lacked the base of folly inherent in medical gout. That is, the 'praise of gout' was central to this popular form (always 'low' among literary 'kinds') because folly was proclaimed to lie at the base of the gouty condition: its veritable foot; and folly, like knavery, was paramount in canonical satire from Horatian and Juvenalian times.[21] Bakhtin has captured its essence within the contexts of 'gout comic-tragedies' when noting that:

Some forms of parodic-travestying literature issue directly from the form of the genres being parodied – parodic poems, tragedies (Lucian's *Tragopodagra* ['Gout-Tragedy'], for example), parodic judicial speeches and so forth. This is a parody and travesty in the narrow sense of the word.[22]

One specimen was Michael Maier's (1568–1622) *Lusus Serius: Or, Serious Passe-time. A Philosophical Discourse Concerning the Superiority of Creatures under Man*, a disputatious dialogue debating which animal, vegetable and mineral is most useful to mankind.[23] Maier was a prolific Dutch polymath, doctor of medicine, alchemist, a Rosicrucian steeped in this Menippean tradition – he could have been gouty himself. Phylogenetic warfare in heaven constitutes Maier's centre-stage within a ludic aim to distract the reader from everyday cares. Mercury vanquishes all contenders throughout realms animal, vegetable and mineral – proof that he is the most precious substance. Touting himself, Mercury claims he can banish gout – proof of superiority – when powdered and mixed 'with Gold or any other body'.[24]

His vaunts extend to taxonomy: 'In the Gout, it is the surest remedy which may well suffice, since under that name there are almost an hundred diseases compriz'd, though frequently lurking under more common or different shapes . . .'[25] The bombast, as well as the insulating status of gout, is predictable: a full 'hundred diseases'. If gout had become a catch-all for myriad maladies, one wonders what the 'Menippean Mercury' would have claimed had he returned to his *lusus serius* a century later. By then satire demonstrated that it adjoined these disconnected, if swollen, 'limbs' into verbal organisms propelled by rising and falling, inflating and deflating techniques of composition. The connection between medical theory and rhetorical polish was cemented.[26]

The context of Maier's dialogism is warfare, the point of his paradoxical prose, antithetical wit. Only learned readers, trained in schools, could understand his flights of fancy. Sharpest are his metaphors of rising and falling motions, permeating even the smallest units of the dialogue's wit. This theme of warfare extended to other ludic works in this subgenre, as in the *topos* of *the overthrow of the gout*. Here topsy-turvy mock-exchange constitutes the main action. Battle bursts out between patient and malady: who will triumph, victim or illness? A fight ensues emplotting the trope of warfare routinely assumed today when we stave off our own post-Sontagian maladies. Works then were called 'overthrows' and typified by jocularity and stock elements of play.[27]

By the mid-seventeenth century this form amalgamated to other praise-of-folly varieties. 'Gouty inactive limbs' wax comic, as dangling joints and swollen feet coalesce into the armchairs and stools clamping them into rhetorical inflations. The proverbial author compares his metre to his 'swollen feet'. He derides his gouty limbs, amazed they can write down these ditties and speculates on the 'rise and fall' of this mock warfare. His rapport with

readers is familiar and he wonders about the audience 'consuming his literature'. Diversion from podagra was a primary function, and this deflection may
have been exactly what Laurence Sterne, the comic author of *Tristram Shandy*
(1760–68), alluded to later when noting that his Rabelaisian dissertation was
written in a post-Lucianic mode. 'What is it?' Tristram asks about his
autobiographical memoir: "'tis a Dissertation writ against the spleen'.[28]

III. The rhetoric of swelling

> There dies not above one of a thousand of the gout,
> although I believe that many die gouty.
>
> John Graunt, *Bills of Mortality*, 1662

For centuries disease had been conceptualized within war's metaphoric
matrix.[29] As far back as the Old Testament commentary, the hubristic and
deformed sick 'swelled' just as war proliferates. War was also applied to
written 'forms' militaristically swollen out of size. Spenser, the concise poet,
noted in *The Present State of Ireland* (1633) how 'this [warlike] humour in
historians hath made the body of ancieentt [sic] history in some parts so *goutty*
and monstrous' – hence Herodotus and Thucydides.[30] Samuel Johnson
remembered these resonances and reproduced them in his entry on 'gout' in
the dictionary of 1755. But swelling also had a more recent profile in the
'swollen size' of newspapers from a single sheet into globs of print.[31] The
emergence of newspapers in the seventeenth century is too complex to be
told within a single book, but it is sufficient here to notice that news depends
on acts of verbal bloating, puffing this or that intelligence: the 'body of the
news' as the 'body of the person'.

Readers, like news, were also worthy of puffery, especially when patients.
Milord so-and-so is in the progress of a gout: this was noteworthy, hence
newsworthy, when 'swollen' by rhetorical realism. Language determined the
patient's public status. The ailing reader was, moreover, a certifiably diagnos-
able patient, as well as consumer of these intelligences. During the outbreak
of civil war in the 1640s the trope of the 'gouty army' swelled to a derisive
commonplace to attack the political opposition. The denigration of the Other
was made in ludicrously bloated prose, so mischievously inflated that it verged
on the absurd. No such thing as a 'gouty army' existed: gout was neither
contagious nor prone to striking hordes of soldiers or sailors. Nor was it in
gout's inherent nature to produce *any* type of epidemic. Yet its chief metaphors were transported from human bodies to written bodies and are found
in newspapers and ephemera, as in this passage on the outbreak of the second-
phase Civil War from *The Parliamentary-kite*, an organ of Royalist propaganda,
for 29 June–13 July 1648:

If any manner of Man or Woman in Town, City or Country, tell any Tale or Tydings of a loather [sic] Trayterous and Rebellious *Parliament*, and a *Gouty Army* of Cut-throats (called by some Saints;) consisting onely of Murderers, Robbers, Blasphemers, Atheists and Schismatics, (whose Trade is to Murder, Massacre, Ruine and Tyranize) they were both begotten in an ill hour, brought forth in division, bred up in gouty Faction and Oppression.[32]

It is hard to gauge how these passages were interpreted by their original readers, but this early periodical prose is permeated with 'swollen metaphors', even if less directly referential than these military versions. Swelling as a topic in physics had interested naturalists poised between Harvey and Boyle, one of whose goals was to reduce its mysteries to mathematical laws of fluids and solids.[33] Metaphysical poetry, saturated with conceits and artifices despite its gravitation to human love, was also prone to 'swelling' as a metaphor for the erotic, as in Donne's famous 'extasie poems' about his mistress lying swollen as a 'Pregnant banke':[34]

> Where, like a pillow on a bed,
>   A Pregnant banke swel'd up, to rest
> The violets reclining head,
>   Sat we two, one anothers bed.

Donne – master rhetorician and invalid – suffered 'flying attacks' of a malady he diagnosed variously as fever, consumption and gout.[35] From early maturity he had been ill and read up on his symptoms.[36] Later, when he thought he was dying, he chronicled his 'crisis' in *Devotions upon Emergent Occasions, together with Death's Duel* (1624), a symptom-by-symptom dissection. Donne's imagination was suffused with the idea of the human body as the natural site for metaphoric and analogical extrapolation. He invokes 'gout' as a metonymy for old age and chronic cramp. But Donne also assimilated the rhetorical traditions of the body politic and in his satires generates coinages about the 'swollen bladder of the court' and the joy arising when 'the state doth swell'. Still, this pre-Restoration Civil War puffery paraded tropes aimed at breaking the back of rhetorical aggrandizement, in whose domain things 'gouty' could still be configured as centrally important.

A representative moment from *Perfect Passages of Each Dayes Proceedings in Parliament* adumbrates the point. This was a Royalist newspaper of the 1640s intent on decrying 'mad Malignants', a common designation for anti-Royalists. The more significant context is its language of swelling: a heap of grotesque images built on entrails grown out of proportion: 'See how mad Malignants are! O how they *swell* with gout, to hear that we prosper; and now they are resolved to spin out their owne bowells to make a web to catch us for their prey . . .'[37] The malady is male specific and viscerally aggressive. But it was not merely rebellious armies and religious sects who 'swelled' but crowds: the mob, who under any regime, could become swollen – at least 'swelling'. To enlarge itself was the most apparent, if logical, of its tendencies, like the female body in pregnancy and childbirth. Hysteria, then known as 'the mother', was another state of 'swollen' female bodies where enlargement occurred as 'the wandering womb' rampaged through interior female spaces, but hysteria was rarely a metaphorized malady in this new Grubbean ephemera of the English Interregnum and Civil War;[38] nor was consumption or plague. Gout assumed centre-stage, as gouty swellings became riots of news, revolt, war and the mob in bloody revolution.

We dwell on a seventeenth-century moment to illustrate this metaphoricity because it affords such concrete textual and historical evidence: England in bloodshed, a transformative leap in the dissemination of information, medicine and language.[39] No doubt other 'moments' exist, especially in later centuries. The discourse of luxury in Georgian Britain and the language of insulation in Regency England would have equally made the point. Yet another reason exists for selecting this convergence: theory about gout *c.* 1650 – although Sydenham had not yet made it *the modern condition* – and an almost epistemic break then occurring in information practices.[40]

Newspapers were bred in the cradle of revolt; a vocabulary of enlargement – 'swelling' – their metaphoric *sine qua non* for reporting news. Their sudden emergence occurs amid national turmoil and chaos. Concurrent with this birth is a metaphoric infrastructure of rising and falling derived from medical theory. However, what differentiates the mid-seventeenth century as a moment of 'gouty' bands and 'rising' sects is its restraint compared to later 'puffery'. In the eighteenth century, this new topology increases as threatened upper classes seek to differentiate themselves from lower ranks. Before social stratification adopted a vocabulary of 'nerves and fibres' as anatomic guides to distinguishing persons of rank, war news ransacked medical terminology.

Throughout the Royalist crisis 'gouty prose' grew from the popular press, while the 'news' formed a novel protean cultural 'swelling'. After the Restoration, pride and gout were linked by those decrying 'the disease of insulation' as protecting its victims from the heinous sin of pride.[41] No less astute an observer than Sydenham doubted any necessary connection, claiming that he himself was hardly 'proud' to have contracted gout. The codes of the 'bloated body' – normal and pathological – were thus emplotted in narrative practices, as in Sydenham's celebrated tract. By the Restoration such 'swellings' routinely became a trope for rebellion and the swollen anarchic mob. This language framed the lexical context in which Sydenham – transformer of gout theory – generated his treatise: a forest of analogies, subgrowth as metaphor, as in things 'goutily military'.[42]

IV. Homo ludens and the neo-Lucianic heritage

Gout continued to be encoded in these Lucianic and Menippean genres after the English Civil Wars. One of its mordant representations was astrological, as in the 'Lucubrationes Podagricae': 'gout diversions',[43] predictions of 'gout attacks' – war again – based on astrological charts. Another Restoration specimen is Robert Witty's *Gout Raptures*, composed for students at Cambridge University.[44] The playful scribbler claims to be 'helpful to those who study astronomy', as gout 'afflicts' sedentary students of the heavens. He dubs his ahistorical rhapsodies 'Historical Fiction', ponders the meaning of gout and sublunar things 'romantic', cautioning against over-study. These gouty fabrications extended to broadsides and illustrated versions, especially in ditty and panegyric. When Edmund Calamy (1600–66) and Thomas Manton (1620–77), popular divines, were arrested and incarcerated, gout kicked in as a dominant image and produced a flood of poems. Robert Wilde's first rendition (1662) versified:

> Old Bishop Gout, that lordly proud disease,
> Took my fat body for his diocese,
> Where he keeps court, there visits every limb,
> And makes them (Levite-like) conform to him.[45]

A 'gouty fantasy' follows, personifying the sufferer as well as the culpable bishops who have 'burned the toes' of their victims. A later swipe surfaced in 'Wipe for Iter-Boreale Wilde: Or, An Infallible Cure for the Gout',[46] an iambic-pentameter satire by 'I.B.' of dissenting preachers engraved on a broadside as 'a cure for gout'. 'I.B.' refers to a troika of mythical misters 'Monk, Browne, Wilde' – Jonsonian humoral stereotypes – and the historical Manton, allegedly demented by gout, who was in jail during composition.[47] Political satire abounds, punning on 'wild' root and the runaway villain, 'Mr Wilde'. Feet, gouty and poetic, strut, just as sottish divines like Manton hit at the 'foot' of the matter in juxtaposing 'Gout' and 'Elegie':

> Gout! I conjure thee by the pow'rful names
> Of Monk and Brown, and their victorious fames,
> To tell me (speak no doubt thou canst): speak, come,
> Why didst thou shackle the Poetick feet
> Of thy lov'd Master, when it was most meet
> They should be jogging. Can Monk and Brown die,
> And Wild be tame? not write an Elegie?
> Gout! thou't ingrateful: Hast so soon forgot
> Who made thee Bishop, did he make thee sot?

Lucubrationes Podagricæ.

1. **S**Aturnus *Capricorno* postremus Planetarum Oftentat fe Regem noĉte fpreto ordine Stellarum.	♑ Capricornus. ♄ Saturnus, Infortunium majus, Planetarum altiffimus.
2. Is *Lunæ* invidendo fe mente cruciari Dixit, Sexum fœmineum tam latè dominari.	♑ Domus diurna. ♄. ♄ ☽ ♂. Luna eft minus Cœli lumen in natis dominium conditum.
3. Hanc infimam Stellarum & Tropicum tenere ! Quis toleret ? mox decidet, quod jam vult promovere.	Tropici duo ♋ & ♑ ♋ domus ☽.
4. Invidit *Caffiopeiæ* in Cathedrâ locatæ ; *Andromedæ* Celicolæ, *Ariadnæ* Coronatæ.	Caffiopeiæ Cathedra, Syd. Andromeda, Syd. Ariadnes Corona, Syd.
5. Nec *Geminis* pepercit, infantes non amabat ; Cincinnum & divelleret, his diĉtis intonabat.	♊ Gemini. Coma Berenices, Syd.
6. Mulieres regnare ! id univerfi vetant, Morigeræ fint fœminæ ac à me Jura petant.	

7. *Aqua-*

2. Title page of 'Lucubrationes Podagricae', *c.* 1600.

Gout Raptures.

ΑΣΤΡΟΜΑΧΙΑ;

OR AN

Hiſtorical Fiction

OF A

War among the Stars :

Wherein are mentioned the 7 Planets, the 12 Signs of the Zodiack, and the 50 Conftellations of Heaven mentioned by the Ancients. Alfo feveral eminent Stars, and the moft principal parts and lines of the Celeftial Globe with their Natures and Ufes are pointed at.

Ufeful for fuch as apply themfelves to the Study of Aftronomy, and the Celeftial Globe.

By *Robert Witty*, Dr. in Phyfick.

CAMBRIDGE,

Printed by *John Hayes*, Printer to the Univerfity : and are to be fold by *John Creed*, Bookfeller. 1677.

3. Title page of Robert Witty, *Gout Raptures*. Cambridge, 1677.

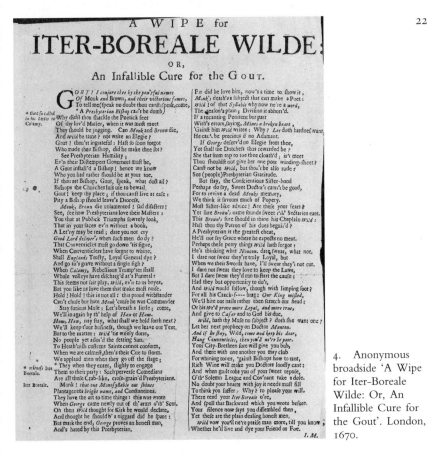

4. Anonymous broadside 'A Wipe for Iter-Boreale Wilde: Or, An Infallible Cure for the Gout'. London, 1670.

To some, gout-writing was a new province waiting to be tapped. Others later demanded the 'muse of gout', occasionally invoking Sydenham, as did Newton in these sardonic ditties about 'infallible cures':

> The *Gout* I think, remains as yet unsung,
> In antient Language or the modern Tongue,
> Then tho' unskill'd in learned SYDENHAM's Rules,
> Without a Science of the *Physick-Schools*,
> Nay, without Prospect of a golden Bribe,
> A *Gouty Prisoner's* Cure I dare prescribe,
> And Oh! what fitter Subject can I choose?
> To suit the *Lameness* of an *hobling Muse*,
> Short curtaile'd Lines in HUDIBRASTICK Verse,
> Will best the *limping Malady* rehearse.[48]

The 'hobling Muse' could also evoke conventional images in vulgar rhymes:

> O Gout thou puzzling *knotty Point*,
> You nick Man's *Bones* in every *Joynt*,
> Like Surgeons Hall, you Richness gain,
> By screwing mortal Limbs to pain,
> First MINER like you work below,
> To sap Mans Fabrick by the Toe.
> So footing take, where footing ends,
> As HEBREW reading backward tends
> If Med'cine can the Smart dislodge,
> From *Bone* to *Bone* you play the Dodge.

Gout's personifications also mirrored villains in the drama, wreaking havoc and racing up, militia-like, the body's scale:

> But in Revenge, like flying Foe,
> You barn and cripple as you go,
> For if compell'd to quit the Feet,
> You wound like PARTHIANS by Retreat
> The restless Humour upward flies,
> As Dregs disturb'd fermenting rise,
> From *Ancle* forc'd you climb the *Knees*,
> And run the rounds by fore Degrees.
> You sour Sap from Crab-tree Roots,
> Begins below and upward shootes,
> And where malignant Juices flow,
> Close *knotty Knobs* in Sharpness grow . . .

The scribbler recounted that the 'monarchical malady' was as ancient as the Greeks, afflicting kings, not queens:

> Old OEDIPUS the *Theban* King,
> Felt *swelling Joint* and *Gouty Sting*,
> And tho' the Sage could SPHINX explain,
> The Sage cou'd nere unriddle *Pain*,
> Tho' Stoicks crack of *Indolence*,
> Man's Flesh retains a feeling Sense,
> And what is worse the affected Part,
> Finds small Relief from *Doctor*'s Art,
> Great RADCLIFF's Skill confounded stands,
> When Patient roars my *Toe* my *Hands*.
> The *Gout* supplies the Jail with Chains
> And fills the Tenement with *Pains*,
> Corrosive Pains that cramp the Bone,
> And stop all Morion but it's own,

> But as *Apollo* God of Wit,
> Besides his Physick keeps a KIT,
> No doubt to sooth the Patient's Heart,
> When Doses can't remove the Smart . . .

Poetry as therapy, as in the old copula – an 'elbow world' where 'certain lenitives' (palliating drugs) equate to 'verse':

> A certain Lenitive admit,
> Perhaps a Verse may lull the Fit,
> When cutting Teeth or ill plac'd Pin,
> Molest the tender *Babie*'s Skin,
> Shrill-Lullabys in Cradle strain,
> Aswage the sroppish *Bantling*'s Pain,
> Then as the Humours throb and ake,
> This easie fake Prescription take,
> In *Elbow-Chair* Majestick fit,
> In full high Twinge yet scorn to sret,
> Suppose your self in *Papal See*,
> Extending *Toe* to *Devotee*,
> Consider too how Princes bear,
> The royal *Gout* with royal Care,
> From these Examples cease to sume,
> But in the soothing Flannels Roam,
> Wrap round the Joynt this healing Verse,
> 'Tis PATIENCE proves the *kindest Nurse*.

Such repertoire was exploited in too-facile analogies redrawn by dunciads and aspirants alike. The hungry poet in his Grubbean cell felt vulnerable to both states: poverty and impoverished verse. But gout was a disease of *rank* and *class*: poor poet, why the consternation?

> 'Ah! what's that gastly Form I view,
> With shrivell'd front of livid hue,
> and dim his hollow eye;
> His crippled Feet Support refuse,
> His knotted Joints deny their Use,
> It's all Infirmity.
>
> Is there a Doctor, whose Degrees
> Serve only to enhance his Fees,
> Bred regular to slay;
> Or lawyer, who first makes a Flaw,
> Then robs by Letter of the Law,
> And deems you rightful prey?

> On these, and such a thousand more,
> O Gout, exert thy keenest Pow'r,
> Thy sharpest Pangs prepare;
> With honest Indignation maul
> The Vulgar great, the Vulgar small,
> But the poor Poet spare.[49]

Sparring versifiers hardly conceived of their belly's woe as ludic, yet their burlesques remained playful despite hunger's panic. Canonical poetic satire – Dryden and Pope – held ambitions too lofty for such pursuits but even Swift in his most ludic verse abuses words by 'playing' on their hidden meanings. Works both retained and omitted their 'Lucianic' designations, as when William Brownsword commingled these traditions in *Laugh and Lye Down . . . a Poem Serio-Comic*.[50] Brownsword was a country vicar in Sussex, bored by dreary English winters. His forty-six pages aim to elicit play to fill vacant hours, his 'gout remedy' a metaphor for man's ludic capability: *podagra ludens* (playful podagra) could be the poem's epigraph. The 'Serio-Comic poem' is cast as a dialogue between Sir Hans Sloane, then President of the Royal Society, and an aspiring 'gout doctor' of the lucrative type we have surveyed throughout this book. The eight-page prose preface is self-deprecatory, followed by an inserted poem consisting of 496 lines of bouncy Hudibrastic tetrameters punctuated with Butlerian notes and burlesque asides:

> If any Critic dares attack,
> I'll lay him flat upon his Back:
> Or else I'll give him such a Squeeze,
> Shall make him – Down upon his Knees . . .

'Laugh and Lye Down' is glossed as the supreme prescription for gout because its releases soothe and divert the reader from aches and pains. In an era converging on the muse of laughter and championing ridicule as the test for human enterprise, the medicine of laughter was salubrious advice.

Such authors as Brownsword assumed their largest audiences to consist of other gouty valetudinarians. Brownsword therefore concluded with a digression on the 'perennial foot', saluting the reader as 'an old *Roman* Comedian . . . a jocularity (Merry and Wise) . . . Fare you all well'. The 'foot' remains the essential site: supine as well as doubled up in the dilogism (two or more meanings, one word) of one word. Foot of furniture, foot of verse; swollen and normal feet; aesthetically ambiguous; curative metaphoric incarnations if we will just 'laugh and lye down'.

Such bagatelles often teased out the 'swollen limb' as well as 'arthritic arm' composing them. The ode, a more ponderous if emotive form than couplet verse, also captured these gestures. In 'Satirical Trifles: Consisting of An Ode, written on the first Attack of the Gout',[51] the anonymous scribbler narrates as

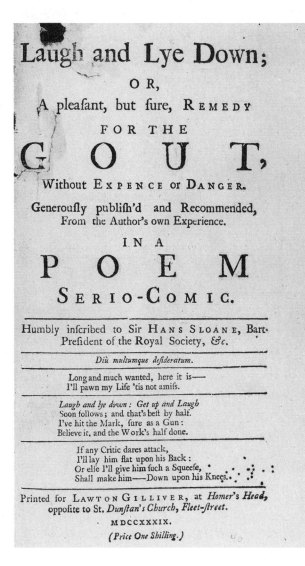

Laugh and Lye Down;

OR,

A pleafant, but fure, REMEDY

FOR THE

GOUT,

Without EXPENCE or DANGER.

Generoufly publifh'd and Recommended,
From the Author's own Experience.

IN A

POEM

SERIO-COMIC.

Humbly infcribed to Sir HANS SLOANE, Bart.
Prefident of the Royal Society, &c.

Diù multumque defideratum.

Long and much wanted, here it is——
I'll pawn my Life 'tis not amifs.

Laugh and lye down: Get up and Laugh
Soon follows; and that's beft by half.
I've hit the Mark, fure as a Gun:
Believe it, and the Work's half done.

If any Critic dares attack,
I'll lay him flat upon his Back:
Or elfe I'll give him fuch a Squeefe,
Shall make him——Down upon his Knees.

Printed for LAWTON GILLIVER, at *Homer's Head,*
oppofite to St. *Dunftan's Church, Fleet-ftreet.*

MDCCXXXIX.

(Price One Shilling.)

5. Title page of William Brownsword *Laugh and Lye Down; or, A pleasant, but sure, Remedy for the Gout, Without Expence or Danger.* London, 1739.

if penning a case history, and suggests that the attack itself amounts to trivia, so 'soft' you can 'stroke' it (to echo the poet Thomas Gray in his poignant letters about gout's attacks). By the mid-eighteenth century, weeklies and monthlies 'swelled' their pages with these ephemeral insertions, as in David d'Escherny's grandly titled *Essay on the Causes and Effects of the Gout,*[52] palpably a satire on the pharmaceutically mysterious *regulus folis*, but actually an attack on the disease endemic in Grub Street called *cacoaethes scribendi*: rampant scribosis or the illness of shitty writing.

Some portion of this exuberance was autobiographical, especially the psychomachia of gout's 'first attack'.[53] But leisure was needed if one was 'to

SATIRICAL TRIFLES:

CONSISTING OF

An ODE, written on the firſt Attack of the GOUT.

To MANKIND, an Ode.

The FAREWELL, written at *Woodcote*, near *Epſom*.

EPIGRAMS.

By B. A.

— — — — — Quittons la Satire,
C'eſt un mechant metier que celui de medire.
Motto to Dr. TOTTIE's *Sermon.*

LONDON,

Printed for FLETCHER, in St. *Paul's Church-Yard*; FLEXNEY, near
Gray's Inn Gate; and ſold by FLETCHER and BROUGHTON in *Oxford*;
and MERRIL in *Cambridge*. M. DCC. LXIV.

(Price One Shilling.)

6. Title page of the anonymous 'Satirical Trifles: Consisting of An Ode, written on the first Attack of the Gout'. London, 1764.

disclose' the menace of gout's 'fits' and 'attacks', however comically insulating, and this fact raises questions about gout's economics in a world of dunciads. By the early eighteenth century all sorts of writers – paid and unpaid – hacked away, as in the *Spectator*, where grubstreet 'Abraham Thrifty' confesses to writing while lying in a 'fit of the gout'.[54]

Gout-economics makes for an intriguing chapter in the history of commercialism. Publishing in Bath alone raked in thousands in its self-do manuals and *vade mecums*, encouraging printers to harvest its profits before 'Moneyraker Anstey', Christopher Anstey, incorporated gout as the centrepiece of his lucrative 'Bath guides', reducing the malady to the babble of five-year-olds:[55]

> Lord Ringbone, who lay in the parlour below,
> On account of the gout he had got in his toe,
> Began on a sudden to curse and to swear;

I protest, my dear mother, 'twas shocking to hear
The oaths of that reprobate gouty old peer:
'All the devils in hell sure at once have concurr'd
'To make such a noise here as never was heard;
'Some blundering blockhead, while I am in bed,
'Treads as hard as a coach-horse just over my head;
'I cannot conceive what a plague he's about!
'Are the fidlers come hither to make all this rout
'With their d—'d squeaking catgut, that's worse
    'than the gout?'

Such drivel and couplet confusion emphasizes the 'sport' within this deflating scribble:

Ods bobs! how delighted I was unawares
With the fiddles I heard in the room above stairs,
For music is wholesome, the doctors all think,
For ladies that bathe, and for ladies that drink;
And that's the opinion of Robin our driver,
Who whistles his nags while they stand at the river:
They say it is right that for every glass
A tune you should take, that the water may pass;
So while little Tabby was washing her rump,
The ladies kept drinking it out of a pump.

But *comic* malady and literary limpness could not long be separated:

I saw, t'other day, in a *thing call'd an ode*,
As it lay in a snug little house on the road,
How Saul was restor'd, tho' his sorrow was sharp,
When David, the *Bethlemite*, play'd on the harp:
'Poor thing! tho' she hobbled last night to the ball,
To-day she's so lame that she hardly can crawl;
Major Lignum has trod on the first joint of her toe . . .'

About these domains of pains and print the social historians have been virtually silent.[56] Yet between the belletristic Georgians and commemorative Victorians – the period of gout's steepest rise and fall – gout affiliated itself with print culture in manifold ways. Apart from its growth as a new species of medical literature it grew enough to be classified and annotated *in itself*. In this sense gout became a region of the mind now lost. Consult the indices of works printed in seventeenth-century France or during the English Restoration before Sydenham's paradigmatic leap: gout rarely appears *outside* medical literature. By the Regency and Victorian era it fills columns in correspondences and swells (again!) their pages, so much that readers consuming them must have thought *every* gentleman enjoyed 'the honour of the gout' and that these bouts required chronicling for posterity. It is worth citing just one, the *Greville Memoirs*, to show what representative entries on gout amounted to:

> C.C.G. [Greville] suffers from, II 167, 184–5, 233, 289, 324, 364, 412, III 21, 90, 103, 176, 199, 201, 210, IV 15, 135, 173, 323, V 83, 85, 89, 123, 125, 127, 146, 152, 205, 314, 328–9, VI 122, 146, 187, 268, 324, 335, 418, 437, VII 42, 58, 105, 107, 131, 139, 216, 254, 307, 379, 391, 417, 445; Lord Eldon suffers from, III 205; Sir John Tyrell waves a crutch in the H. of C. when suffering from, IV 33n; Lord Chatham went to Bath for his, IV 186; Lord Stanley suffers from, IV 354; C.C.G. attends a Council on crutches when suffering from, V 135–6; Lord Stanley suffers from, at Goodwood, VI 336; Sir James Graham laid up with, VI 339; Lord Beauvale dies after an attack of, VI 396; Clarendon suffers from, VII 440, 472.[57]

But where patronage, puffery and profit resided plagiarism was not far away. Since the post-Sydenham decades theft in the gout trade – medicinal as well as printed – had been rampant, nowhere more callously than in 'Sir' John Hill's claim, almost taken to the courts, that Dr Cadogan (as we saw in Chapter 7) had lifted his theory. It continued as reviewer upon reviewer detected echoes of previously published tracts; James Kirkpatrick, a perpetual reviewer for the *Monthly Review,* discovered that 'J. N. M. D. Stevens' had plagiarized his ideas from Sydenham himself virtually without acknowledgment.[58]

The public was endlessly duped, but insufficiently so to halt gout's diversions. For gout continued to be as much a diversion as a deflection: whether in the frolic or jolt of travel, it remained the jolly disease. Even writers of the most diverse sort who adumbrated gout – John Gay, Benjamin Franklin, musicologist Charles Burney, our scribblers – had conceded this playful deflection. The huge annals of printed matter, amounting to literally millions of words, are permeated with formulations to the effect that Milord this or that has lingered in the gout and therefore been *diverted* from political cares and mundane chores.

Gout was thus a *diverting* disease, sufficiently luxurious to afford its proprietors the leisure to bend the language of everyday use, not merely by punning playfully, in the ludic sense, and parading their command of vocabulary, but also by coining new words. Popular periodicals such as the *Critical Review* complained that 'gouty men' were corrupting and thereby changing the language (can this campaign have been Smollett's?). Grub Street hacks like Charles Martin, today rightly forgotten, reiterated the formidable accusation that those who consumed excessive meat and wine lacked linguistic clarity.[59] Yet gout mandated the new language: neologism and other coinage became forms of puffery perceived as renewed power, this though the 'puffed' potion was ineffective or poisonous. Its metaphors intensified.

V. The metaphoric heritage

Gout also appealed to the rhetorical frame of mind, tapped into its already acculturated versions of analogy and personification by creating a new discourse of the fallen. Another book à la Susan Sontag's *Illness as Metaphor* would be required to demonstrate the forms this metaphoric habit took.[60] Gout also continued to be resurrected metaphorically as the 'condition of the fallen'. Luxurious creatures whose excesses were legion constituted 'the fallen', normatively as if already dead. Hence the widespread emblem of 'the gouty old man' about which we have descanted above and will see more in the next chapter. Disease itself has been personified throughout history – think no further than the visualizations of cancer and AIDS in our time – but the early modern representations of gout show how inherent to language these processes of personification are: as family member, brother, cousin, enemy; as 'monster', 'imperious mistress', 'transient visitor', in Gibbon's invocations.[61] Gibbon was chilled by the protean diversity of his fierce 'enemy', soothed that his flying attacks were benign. In this tension he summoned his 'mistress gout' – notably feminine – as his 'sweet visitor'.[62]

A grey zone exists between the medical condition gout and the play on words its sufferers generated. This *double entendre* elicited a tension between 'being in a humour' – sick and diseased, as in a 'fit of the gout' – and 'being humorous' – funny and witty. Gout, as we have argued throughout this book, entailed a ludic and comic state of affairs for the whole 'body', perhaps owing to the need to trivialize its ponderous moral links to sex and debauchery. 'Wit' in debauchery was said to be the secure knowledge that marriage amounted to a shield, and that libertinism should be cultivated as an end in itself. Gouty old men were proverbially lecherous, their walking canes physical emblems of their three-legged disabilities. The sequitur was that *all* males 'in the gout' – old and young – were debauched. Excess led to gout; to be '*in* the gout' was animate proof that one already had 'been' debauched. The nuance of difference was only a standard of verbal articulation. One line suggests that the 'wits' verbalized debauchery rather than actually engaged in it; another, that gout was idealized precisely *because* it was stronger than verbal articulation. But it is impossible to know whether our received notion is the idealized or historically empirical one or some blend.

These links with debauchery served to underscore the fragility of male sexual ties. Ambivalent valences in male bonding had already come under terrific stress in the early-modern period.[63] Dryden's earliest poetry, for example, sneers at 'old three-legg'd gray-beards with their Gout'.[64] Dryden himself had allegedly been a fellow traveller, and the ageing Dryden of the

Oldham poem, walking with a cane after his injuries in the Rose Alley incident of 1679, developed a complex view of youth and senescence and the homoerotic attachments in both states.

Gout was thus the ambiguous emblem of those no longer able to 'perform'. Age and decrepitude formed one symmetry, potency and virility another. However, asymmetries of age and vigour also flourished in incongruent forms. William Constable, a Georgian Yorkshire landowner and collector, Fellow of the Royal Society, had been a corpulent man whose chronic illnesses afflicted him more than they might have if he had been a diminutive ectomorph. At sixty he collected, travelled, his mind sharp, and gave up London to return to his country seat. Though 'gouty' he continued to garden, collect, and manage his money. The tropes of impotency were as ambiguous as their opposites.

Gout's symbols also included the 'bridge' between life and death: the last passage. Tennyson, the great apostle of death, understood its metaphoric resonance as well as any English poet. He invokes it in just this sense in the climax of his moving poem on 'Columbus', when the explorer is racked with age and 'gout' – at the end – and, alone in his Spanish cell, hallucinating about 'one last crusade':

> Who wept with me when I returned in chains,
> Who sits beside the blessed Virgin now,
> To whom I send my prayer by night and day –
> She is gone – but you will tell the King, that I,
> Racked as I am with gout, and wrenched with pains
> Gained in the service of His Highness, yet
> Am ready to sail forth on one last voyage,
> And readier, if the King would hear, to lead
> One last crusade against the Saracen,
> And save the Holy Sepulchre from thrall.[65]

But it is hard *not* to like the chap with swollen and ulcerated legs, even if his ruddy lady recoils. Non-contagious, he poses no threat of infection. William Rowley, a scribbling, quasi-pornographic eighteenth-century doctor who had been an army surgeon, believed contagion the secret of morbid pathology. He wrote tracts on many medical topics: female breasts, male testicles, venereal diseases. His theory of gout lies far from the 'divinity-of-gout' tradition persistent among the pious doctors and was based on excess: '*Bacchus pater, Venus mater, ira obstetrix arthriditis.*' His funniest writing is a description of 'swollen legs' in a 1770 treatise rife with regular, irregular, misplaced, flying, atonic and other sub-varieties.[66] Rowley believed gout to be inherently – almost risibly – contagious; entire military units could be afflicted. But he never sucked the verbal humour of its 'swellings'.

'Atonic' gout – gout *contra* health – amounted to the weirdest of these subspecies: afflicting one organ, the stomach, its poison said to produce instant shaking, chills, hallucinations, wild phantasms, death. Fanny Burney's males in *Camilla*, especially Jacob's master, are afflicted with it, as are the coachmen of her correspondence. Its metaphors are of loss: in appetite, digestion, equilibrium, sanity; its stasis that of virulent nausea, flatulency, eructations, abdominal swelling. The authors of 'atonic gout' in the *Encyclopaedia Britannica* (1797) claimed its deliriums the fiercest of any variety, causing 'palpitations, faintings, and asthma'.[67] This species was everything deadly at once, and could rip through the stomach wall as viscerally as Blake's worm eating through the sick rose.

Other varieties offered an insulation so predictable it required a new vocabulary to describe them. Besides, since the Renaissance, gout's predilection had been for the robust, in the pink of health, who could tolerate excess.[68] One ate and drank well, slept and slept around, kept late hours, spent fortunes, collected objects, travelled distances, all of which were proofs of heritage and masculinity. But the 'strong' could also be 'chronically' ill, and gout's declensions encompassed 'chronicity' as if synchronous with 'chronic insulation'.[69] The protection was against infection, especially 'infection of alien social class'. No wonder gout's crown continued unchallenged through the Victorian era as the 'monarch's disease'. Jonathan Hutchinson epitomized this delicate balance to his friend William Cowper, the poet of *The Task*:

> I shall be happy to hear that my friend Joseph has recovered entirely from his late indisposition, which I am informed was gout; a distemper which, however painful in itself, brings at least some comfort with it, both for the patient and those who love him, the hope of length of days, and an exemption from numerous other evils. I wish him just so much of it as may serve for a confirmation of this hope, and not one twinge more.[70]

Medical debates about 'insulation' reified cultural anxiety about luxury. 'Insulation' from corruption became the secular *cri de coeur* rather than any localized medical malady like gout – except that gout was then also a region of the mind, not merely a localized medical malady. Still, the insulation debates raised questions: *insulation from what*? The antistrophe in these dialogues was that gout had never really 'insulated', just reproduced itself into other maladies, protean, as Sydenham had claimed.

Robert Drake, another of the dozens of now obscure Georgian 'gout doctors', deemed it 'false to believe [gout] extends life'. Invalids in North America often referred to deaths specifically caused by gout as 'in coffin': to show 'Death's Cruelty' in taking them to the grave.[71] Drake groped for a simile to challenge the insulation thesis: '. . . this salutary disease . . . kills us with a lingering death, and like Prometheus's vulture, gnaws us into fresh torment.'[72] Sweat was the culprit: '*Morbidly swollen sweat*', as if perspiration itself could swell and kill. 'Gout-Drake' derided the great 'arthritic tyrant' lording over the realms of luxury in further personifications, claiming that gout-the-monarch should be confined to 'his proper seat: the extremities' rather than penetrate into the head, lungs, stomach, intestines.

These 'acquisitions' were as vexed a metaphoric domain as gout's tissues of insulation. First and foremost, gout was an 'inheritance'. One 'acquired' it similarly to rank or political sway: by right, *de jure*, not by labour or merit. Whether as pedigree, lineage or (more self-righteously) heritage, its language amounted to imbrications of the father–son filigree: this was its superlative conceit. It could not be copied, imitated or feigned. Thus a 'pretentious' or 'pretending' gouty old man could only be conjured in a contrived fiction or play, and, as such, rarely is to be found.

These metaphors of pedigree and acquisition implied patience as its funda-mental prerequisite: 'sit tight and acquire gout like political influence' could have been its epigraph. Its rightful acquisition was thus a positive force despite any compensating inconvenience. Once acquired it was 'consumed', in the way one 'consumed' wealth or inheritance. Routine 'consumptions of gout' scattered the metaphors recklessly to fly *en masse*: illness, money, class, rank, in any jumbled order. F. M. Cornford's jesting advice to academic novices unpacks these juxtapositions: 'Political influence may be acquired in exactly the same way as the *gout* [italics ours]; indeed, the two ends ought to be pursued concurrently. The method is to sit tight and drink port wine. You will then gain the reputation of being a good fellow; and not a few wild oats will be condoned in one who is sound at heart, if not at the lower extremities.'[73]

Such tropes are typified in Anne Finch's 'The Goute and Spider: A Fable – Imitated from Mon de la Fontaine And Inscribed to Mr Finch After his first Fitt of the Distemper'.[74] Heneage Finch, the fourth Earl of Winchilsea, embodies an accident waiting to happen. During the revolution of 1688 he was arrested for sedition, persecuted and jailed. Afterwards he was barred from court, prevented from taking any post, grew depressed, retired to the Kent countryside, and buried himself in antiquarian pursuits.[75] He joined antiquarian societies and corresponded with 'gouty [William] Stukeley' of Stonehenge fame, who, like Anne, wrote poetry about 'spleen' and about whom we have heard in Chapter 7. After milord and his lady secluded themselves in the countryside, Heneage became sedentary and unable to accompany Anne on her rambles. Her inspired poem is part consolation to her husband for his affliction, part therapeutic for her own loss of the literary life she had in London, and part poeticization of the myth of the patient spider.[76]

Finch's rhymed pentameters begin with the common *topos* of the patient spider:

> When From th' Infernal pitt two Furies rose
> One foe to Flies and one to Mans repose

> Seeking aboue to find a place secure
> Since Hell the Goute nor spider cou'd indure
> On a rich Pallace at the first they light
> Where pleas'd Arachne dazzl'd with the sight
> In a conspiccuous corner of a Room
> The hanging Frett work makes her active Loom.
> From leaf to leaf with every line does trace,
> Admires the strange convenience of the place
> Nor can belieue those Cealings e're were made
> To other end than to promote her Trade . . .[77]

But patience is soon invaded by 'the hungry Fiend' as the enemy, an image that will be extended, amplified and sentimentalized as the century wore on:

> Where prou'd and prosper'd in her finish'd work
> The hungry Fiend does in close Ambush lurk
> Until some silly Insect shall repay
> What from her Bowells she has spun that day.
> The wiser gout (for that's a thinking ill)
> Observing how the splended chambers fill
> With visitors such as abound below
> Who from Hypocrates and Gallen grow
> To some unwealthy shed resolues to fly
> And there obscure and unmolested lye
> But see how eithers project quickly fails
> The Clown his new tormentor with him trayles
> Through miry ways rought Woods and furrow'd Lands
> Ne're cutts the Shooe nor propp'd on Crutches stands
> With Phoebus rising stays with Cynthia out
> Allows no respitt to the harrass'd Gout.

Mock battle soon ensues as the 'maid' clears out the spider's web, only to reveal she has uncovered the 'battering ram' of that stinging pest, the 'gout':

> Whilst with extended Broom th' unpittying Maid
> Does the transparent Laberynth invade
> Back stroke and fore the battering Engin went
> Broke euery Cord and quite unhing'd the Tent
> No truece the tall virago e're admitts
> Contracted and abash'd Arachne sitts
> Then in conuenient Time the Work renews
> The battering Ram again the work persues.

Finch has captured the energy of these personifications (gout as wilful insect) so deftly combined in classical allusion ('Colwort' and 'Cataplasus') as a type of dramatic insectomachia:

> What's to be done? The gout and Spider meet,
> Exchange, the cottage this; That takes the feet
> Of the rich Abbott who that Pallace kept
> And 'till that time in Velvet curtains slept
> Now Colwort leaues and Cataplasus (tho vain)[78]
> Are hourly order'd by that griping traine.
> Who blush not to Prescribe t'exhaust our Gold
> For aches which incurable they hold
> Whil'st stroak'd and fixt the pamper'd Gout remains
> And in an easy Chair euer the Preist detains.

Finch commends the patient spider – an endearing message to her husband – while damning the verminous Rowlandsonian gout:

> In a thatched Roof secure the Spider thrives,
> Both mending by due place their hated liues.
> From whose succeeding may this moral grow
> That each his propper Station learn to know.

Fable yields to consolation, as the narrator addresses 'my Dear' who is not sufficiently rich to assuage the gout with excess, nor poor enough to scare it through penury.[79] Transforming herself into a loving 'Ardelia', Finch closes her poem on a hopeful note of Edenic conjugality that not even the state of gouty ill health can dissolve:

> For You my Dear whom late that pain did seize,
> Not rich enough to sooth the bad disease
> By large expences to engage his stay
> Nor yett so poor to fright the Gout away
> May you but some unfrequent Visit find
> To prove you patient, your Ardelia kind
> Who by a tender and officious care
> Will ease that Grief or her proportion bear
> Since Heaven does in the Nuptial state admitt
> And to allay the hard fatigues of life
> Gaue the first Maid a Husband, Him a Wife.

Thus Ardelian wife abides doting husband, as nurse to patient. But gout's acquisitions were not always countered with such conjugal patience; it could also elicit, commemorate or initiate enduring friendship in an age when male bonds were metonymies for other attachments than romantic intimacy.

Hence if gout was the hidden conceit of pedigree, it was also the guarantor that friendship would endure, in part through insulation. Thus, the juvenilian Eros, especially among friends in Italy and on the Grand Tour, was transformed in old age into a nostalgic Erotics of Gout. Even more: these huge double and triple all-male Georgian correspondences read like mountains of print couched in coded language, with interludes of comic relief sandwiched between outpourings of sadomasochistic pain: 'Madame de Bouzols, Marshal Berwick's daughter, assured me there was nothing so good for the gout, as to preserve the parings of my nails in a bottle close stopped,' Horace Walpole in Paris wrote to Thomas Gray at home.[80] Years later, Gray lamented to intimate buddy William Mason exclusion from the triumvirate of health:

> You are wise as a serpent, but the devil of a dove, in timing both your satire, & your compliment. When a Man [Gray] stands on the very verge of Legislation with all his *unblushing* honours thick upon him; when the Gout has nip'd him in the bud, & blasted all his hopes at least for one winter: then come you buzzing about his nose, & strike your sting deep into the reddest angriest part of his toe, wch will surely mortify.[81]

Gray and his homosocial circle ultimately integrated gout's grand metaphors: pedigree, politics, friendship, misogyny, insulation, long life. As Gray wrote to his youthful 'schoolboy lover', Horace Walpole, after they repaired the wounds of their Grand Tour: 'I plead no merit in my sympathy, because I have the same enemy [gout], & am daily expecting *her* [italics ours] attacks, the more violent perhaps for having been now for some years suspended; talk not of round windows, nor of dying in them: our distemper (remember) is the means of health & *long life*.'[82] So Gray adjudged gout's assurances but not so William Cole to Walpole a few weeks after Gray's death: 'He went off pretty easily, considering the nature of his disorder, the gout in his stomach, which occasioned a sickness and loss of appetite; neither would anything stay in his stomach.'[83]

If gout was construed as an essentialist politics camouflaging pedigree and misogyny, its excesses were as legion as its versions of acquisition and insulation. Lexically excess had enjoyed a venerable history as a metonymy for 'greatness': the 'excessive man' always larger than life. This had been the classical 'Vanity of Human Wishes' tradition: progression from the discovery of talent to meteoric rise to fame, conquest and challenge, followed by overreaching and collapse based on the reckless and excessive. Dryden rendered it lapidary in the preface to his translations of Juvenal's satires:

> This very rev'rend lecher, quite worn out
> With rheumatisms, and crippled with his *gout*,
> Forgets what he in youthful times has done,
> And swinges his own vices in his son.

But the famous and mighty were not to be envied, a literalist poetaster claimed in the mid-eighteenth century, when their 'distorted limbs' were bared.[84] The incongruities were appalling to the naked eye, even if they memorialized excess and pedigree. Benjamin Franklin had been the most talented man of the Enlightenment, in Philadelphia, at home, as well as in Paris: the 'man of the future'.[85] It was inconceivable he would not be '*in* the gout', the proverbial 'in' capturing the brick-and-mortar of his insulatory assurance. So it was – his case history extraordinary. In his now little-read *Dialogue between Franklin and the Gout* he probes whether his excesses were *sufficient*: 'Many things you have ate and drank too freely, and too much indulged those legs of yours in their indolence.' Still, 'you eat an inordinate breakfast, four dishes of tea, with cream, and one or two buttered toasts, with slices of hung beef, which I fancy are not things the most easily digested'.[86] Excess as proof remains the quince of the matter.

On these benighted constellations confirming natural inheritance and rightful ownership was bestowed *honour*: hence the commonplace 'honour of the gout'. Synonyms existed – 'freedom of the gout' – each implying elevation to something grander than what existed before; but 'honour of the gout' – as proof of decoration – remained the favoured phrase, suggesting privilege and pre-eminence. To 'honour' was attached the solitary privilege of polite declension, for which nothing except death outstripped the 'honour of the gout'. When, in the mid-eighteenth century, Earl Nugent failed to appear before his patron, the Duke of Newcastle, his reason was predictable: 'Mr Nugent sends his most respectful Compliments to the Duke of Newcastle. He received the Honor of his Grace's Card here, where He has been detained by the Honor of the Gout.'[87]

Eventually it became widespread that gout arrived in groupings or pairs; in doubles, as in the neoplastic cupola of 'the gout *and* the stone'. For Gibbon it was 'waves *and* tides'.[88] The mature idiom at the crest of the gout-wave at the end of the eighteenth century was that 'gout and stone' arrived together, like brothers; and that those under 'visitation' were disturbed more if one 'brother' had arrived without the other: gout without stone, stone without gout. Visitation and its antithesis, quiet, were imagined in relation to convenience; as the poet Andrew Marvell had written in 'The Church Militant':

> It did not fit his gravitie to stirre,
> Nor his long journey, nor his goutt and furre.[89]

Those afflicted prayed for non-concurrent arrivals, were grateful for seriatim episodes.[90] The visitations indicated the 'honour' of physical motion, as well as the dignity of gout's 'arrival', especially the patient's migration to a higher plane – which was construed, in turn, as a process of bodily flux. This metaphor of 'migration' was spatial and captured gout's crucial 'travelling pains'. Nicholas Hawksmoor, the noted builder, wrote to Lord Carlisle on 29

March 1729 that he would travel if the journey were free of 'racking gouty pain'. Pain was to be endured, through breeding, but the affliction amounted to a 'penetration' resulting in crisis.

'Crisis', like its cousin 'excess', was proof of gout's verisimilitude. Without 'crisis' one could never be sure the *real thing* had established itself, as Dr Samuel Pye cautioned.[91] These 'crises' produced constellations of 'fits' in the form of sudden seizures, stupefactions, deliriums. The 'fits' could not be forced: a 'fit' of the gout arrived solitary and unpredictably, its appearance like crashing waves and bolts of thunder. 'The lightning of the gout', William Stevenson wrote in his tract championing the virtues of blistering, 'flashes downwards to the foot.'[92] The action gravitates to the anatomical foot; if the 'attack' can be withstood through blistering, afterwards 'all is sunshine and calm after the volcano has burst and spent itself'. The 'fits', in turn, brought on spurts of creativity, sudden explosive energy, anything but the steady calm of workmanlike productivity.

These were pictures in words. In real life sufferers personalized these social fables according to individual need. Gout was thus less a communal 'essence' than the private tales people told themselves. Alexander Pope, the poet of pith, could capture these antitheses in a single elliptical line: 'See the same man, in vigour, in the gout.'[93] In other Popean versions, inertia and vitality alternate, 'As sober *Lanesb'row*, dancing in the Gout'.[94] For Smollett's gouty Matthew Bramble, as we saw in Chapter 7, a 'fit of the gout' required balance: the control of explosive energy by balancing the sudden 'crisis' with the 'arrival' of passion itself, as when Bramble's heart-strings are plucked to the limit when viewing his native Scotland. These 'crises' were spatially rather than temporally visualized, nowhere more dramatically than in the dreaded 'flying gout', about which so much medical theory was generated throughout the long eighteenth century.

Mrs Piozzi, Samuel Johnson's constant companion, thought she saw gout 'fly' to her husband's neck, breast, sides, back and head all at once on 23 January 1794. She 'saved him' with sudorifics, only because he was 'strong in the extremities', but not before the damage to his 'head' was perceptible.[95] As with the preying 'Promethean vultures' Robert Drake had described, the sharpest seizures always 'flew' to the head. Horace Walpole thought he knew why. The 'flying gout' is drawn, it seems, from the skies: 'The first [gout] goes, when it has had its swing, and does not return, till, like a comet, it has made its revolution. The other may never leave one, or come back the day after it has disappeared.'[96]

'Flying gout' had its correlative in 'wandering gout': no coevals for the expert doctors who finely discriminated these taxonomies. 'Wandering gout' was unpredictable, fickle, fussy, not to be trusted from one day to the next. The difference lay in degrees of morbific variance and in the interior spaces of the afflicted body. These 'attacks' arrived in a dozen declensions, proof of gout's terrific consumer-edge. In a 'flying gout' anatomic matter suddenly

grew unsettled, topsy-turvy chaos; in 'wandering' regional matter was implicated. A 'flying gout' was experienced as a sudden 'eating up' of the 'self'
accompanied by a sense of impending doom, instant retreat its only solace.
The antidote to these 'wandering crises' was calm, quiet, patience; 'sure gout',
which was even milder than 'flying gout', was analogized to these halcyon
states. Walter Scott wrote in his journal on 8 April 1826:

> We expect a *raid* of folks to visit us this morning whom we must have *dined*
> before our misfortunes. Save time, wine, and money, these misfortunes so
> far are convenient things. Besides there is a dignity about them when they
> come only like the Gout in its mildest shape to authorize the dignity of diet
> and retirement, the night gown and the velvet shoe. When the one comes
> to chalkstones and the other to prison though, there would be the devil.
> Or compare the effects of Surre Gout and absolute poverty upon the
> stomack – the necessity of a bottle of laudanum in the one case, the want
> of a morsel of meat in the other.[97]

Manored dignity, mild visitation, 'Surre Gout' – the picture of the well-
bred guest. If 'Surre Gout' tiptoed in, it arrived as a civil visitor whose class
identity was indelible. Another sign embedded in this notion of chronicity
was the gout relieved by exercise. Relief was as crucial as the exercise itself,
but the oddest activities elicited relief, nothing predictable by the 'doctors'. A
list compiled over 200 years would raise hackles, as when Eustace Budgell,
one of the early 'Wits', claimed to have experienced these delights and
anthologized them in Addison's and Steele's *Spectator*. The list contradicts
popular notions of 'disturbance', claiming that attack to some was panacea to
others. Reviewing complaints about being awakened by noisy workmen,
Budgell documents the advantages of being stirred at an early hour. A 'gouty
valetudinarian' chronicles how he was 'relieved from a Fit of the gout by the
sound of old shoes'.[98] Such instances were printed and regularly chronicled as
'gout news'.

Chronicity was the flip side of *crisis*, gout the proof of both. 'Constancy',
with its embedded notions of fidelity and reliability, cemented itself linguistically to gout by an ingrained personification: a husband or wife who could
be relied upon. The least suggestion of 'crudity' disturbed these delicate
balances. Perhaps this is why 'vexation' represented such ambiguous claims on
the body's economy: always less than a root cause of gout but forever a
greater 'enemy' than 'crudity'. The midriff was the chief interior battleground
of these disturbances, the warzone susceptible to 'interruptions' precipitated
by a lapse of 'constancy'. Metaphorically speaking, gout was 'manifestly a
disease of crudity and indigestion', a reviewer wrote in Smollett's popular
monthly, his gaze focused on 'the stomach and bowels'.[99] Little wonder that
for all these hacks interpreting and vulgarizing medical theory, yet also
shaping it, gout was 'the chief representative of all chronic diseases'.[100]

Inevitably it was also construed as 'monstrous': monstrous attacks, monstrous joints, monstrous limbs, monstrous interruptions, a phantasm of contorted shapes and dangling limbs – except that nothing dire ever occurred in that little elbow world. Elbows, like mock-epics, routinely engaged afflic-tion, the 'elbows' that described pains 'nightmares' more accurately than 'peccant eruptions'. The mythology about gout was that it was monstrous for reasons extending *beyond* violence to the body, but these were rarely verbal-ized. Monstrosity also expressed itself spatially, as in Queen Anne's gout, a source of public befuddlement: widely remarked on, the sphere of endless speculation, given her comic corpulence, its chief miracle the fact that it could have 'swelled' her *already* vast internal organs. Infiltration and penetra-tion were described as 'corrupted substance', her condition owing to the 'degree' of putrefaction. 'The gouty body castive, putrid, and fetid' attracted synonyms equally morbid, if comically inscribed: the body 'concoctive', 'peccant', 'morbifick'. The image was of elements 'cooking' and putrefaction 'forming', as in architectural moulds. All this monstrosity reduced the body to a 'ruin', a rubble, as in surrounding neo-gothic piles.

But once 'formed', gout's poison commenced its journey to the interior. 'Immiscible matter' corrupted healthy tissue on an unseen interior road and invaded the healthy processes of digestion. The peccant matter could be located anywhere on the body's map, even in the moist and nether genitals. Hence the body's 'boggy' parts originally signifying 'gouty land' and the terrain sexually charged. Wine and women, drink and sex, remained the *fons et origo* of these 'putrid fomentations' in the land of bogs. From the start the theory had been associated with the erotic, in tropes about Bacchus and Venus. The Enlightenment encyclopaedists continued this tradition, as in Johann Heinrich Zedler's declensions on gout, listed under 'arthritis', where Venus surfaces for the umpteenth time.[101]

As 'Stonehenge Stukeley' warned, gout was the most 'violent' of the diseases of passion;[102] little wonder it attracted the language of recklessness. Hester Thrale narrates her husband's seizure of 'flying gout' as if some hedonistic, almost Dionysian, act of 'exquisite torment'. His passion and pain combined, 'gout flying to his neck, breast, sides, and back . . . on the Lungs once'. Despite the 'flight', insulation in the 'extremities saved him, with sudorificks in aid', but 'thoughts of his breeding Gout so fast shocks me'.[103] Such usage (breeding, flying) continued well beyond Robert Browning's jottings about gout in the nineteenth century. Oliver Sacks might ask what attendant migraine lingered here; Foucault what torture or bondage. The drama lay in violence shared between victim and observer, despite Mrs Thrale being no Sunday stroller when she caught sight of this 'breeding'.

Violence to the 'heads' – even the 'brains' – of the gouty was caught in the language of pain. Charles Burney, already mentioned, noted that 'the pain is now more general: – & renews its attacks in [cur]ious quarters. I do not like it, – yet I drink no wine – & eat little or no meat . . . All will not do to keep this Noddle of mine painless and Steady.'[104] The 'pate' was attacked more than other organs, but what seizure was this? Addison recognized it as delectable that his 'visitation of the gout' had occurred *sans* pain. When he commenced his informal study of 'Physick' he 'found in my self all the Symptoms of the Gout, except Pain, but was cured of it by a Treatise upon the Gravel, written by a very Ingenious Author, who (as it is usual for Physicians to convert one Distemper into another) eased me of the Gout by giving me the Stone'.[105] The protean cupola (gout and stone) would not have surprised Sydenham or gout's lexical students.

Pain in this elbow world was legitimated by the assurance of comic relief, as when 'Mr Spectator' (this time Steele) laments having to attend a party wearing 'high-heeled shoes with a glassed wax – leather instep'. Though an afflicted 'Coxcomb' he wants to impress the ladies. A guest replaces his shoes with regular heels, which both embarrasses and relieves the 'Spectator'.[106] Modern theories of pain rarely include comic relief, except as mock-epic attempts to flay dead horses, but goutometries are explicit on this comic relief, lexically and biographically. When the hypochondriacal Immanuel Kant suffered nocturnal gouty attacks he defended himself with 'concentration' against these leeches of the night. Concentration? Only the pompous and earnest could fail to grasp the joke in the curative power of 'concentration' in a philosopher's obsessing on a single object. Kant's choice for 'concentration' was Cicero and he records that the next morning he would be uncertain whether or not he had suffered the 'attack'. The 'sight of the glowing red toes of the left foot, however, removed his every doubt'.[107]

Few phrases survived so long in the malady's natural history as 'martyr to the gout', one who slavishly surrendered. The slavish component was fundamental, as Dr John Arbuthnot had written in his 'John Bull' tract on diet: 'Most commonly a *gouty* constitution is attended with *great* acuteness of parts, the nervous fibres, both in the brain and the other extremities, being delicate.'[108] No wonder these slavish 'martyrs' were imaged heroically, their minds bright mirrors to absorb and reflect abstract ideas. Queen Anne's last days summoned images of a lucid mind fit to lead the nation. A team of recent expert medical historians epitomized her:

> She died in coma at the age of forty-nine . . . her constitutional gout flew to the brain, and she sank into a state of stupefaction, broken by occasional fits of delirium. The great Dr John Radcliffe was called to her last illness but refused to attend. He commented: 'Here we are all in the dark, as well as her doctors. At first they said it was an ague, and then gave her Jesuit's bark [quinine]. She took but three doses, and that was left off; so that I suppose they found it no ague, or she would have taken more or none at all. Then it was conjectured to be the gout in her stomach; and now it is

thought to be the gout all over,' and he [Radcliffe] added sarcastically, 'excepting the joints.'[109]

For Dr John Adair, the high-fee Scottish celebrity physician, 'surrender' paradoxically amounted to 'satanic leprosy'.[110] He claimed to be able to derail the old enemy (masculine in his and Benjamin Franklin's version, but feminine in Gray's and Walpole's)[111] by 'strengthening the nerves'. 'Strong nerves' were thus a doubly inverted anti-Christ of gout implying freedom over opposition. The military–political thrust is patent in this warfare between submission and nervous antidote, the latent paradox being that the patient had never conquered the enemy, merely himself.

Gibbon, prose stylist though he was, indulged all these metaphors: enemies of gout, tyrants, villains, militias, attacks, allies, prisoners, escapes, retreats, warriors knocked down.[112] Historically he descanted on 'the first martyrs of gout', ranking them by nation and announcing that Switzerland had the fewest number owing to clean air and Calvinist recoil from excess.[113] Richard Cumberland, the neurasthenic dramatist who became the lifelong butt of Mrs Thrale's homophobia, decoded the signs at once when recounting how Horace Walpole had evolved into a 'martyr to the gout':

> Walpole had by nature a propensity, and by constitution a plea, for being captious and querulential, for he was a martyr to the gout. He wrote prose and published it; he composed verses and circulated them, and was an author, who seemed to play at hide-and-seek with the public.[114]

Gout was equally a spiritual guide as a consequence of these lessons of relief. 'Relief' was its great message, especially for the *patient* (the double meaning intended) who could learn from its ancient wisdom. Its lessons in 'patience–impatience' were varied: not merely fatigue through exercise but the warnings it proffered against the sedentary life. The monastic and scholarly were especially susceptible – that is why they should 'move the limbs' and work in the fields. Some wished the gout more 'regular' in its 'visitations' so it could keep them *more* monastic. But the doctors insisted that motion, not wisdom, would be the salvation of the learned; motions of such jabs and jolts that a social history of motion is needed to probe their varieties. In these lessons gout assumed the dignified garb of the learned 'physician' himself.

Why then had he arrived disguised in rags, a niggardly pauper? The miser always was gouty, twisted, deformed in the visual imagination, even when an old hag. Miserliness was a symptom, not root cause, of gout, as in the miser's ritual progression from generosity to meanness, mirroring in small the decay into twisted organs and limbs. Sherlock Holmes' 'Adventure of the Missing Three-Quarter' exposes the gouty old boys and their internal contradictions. Lord Mount-James is one of the richest men in England but racked with gout and proverbially miserly:

'And your friend was closely related?'

'Yes, he was his heir, and the old boy is nearly eighty – cram full of gout, too. They say he could chalk his billiard-cue with his knuckles. He never allowed Godfrey a shilling in his life, for he is an absolute miser . . .'[115]

Such 'holding in' amounted to a type of anal retentivity but, again para-doxically, was said to render the victim sharper in mental acumen. The metaphor of 'progression' here was old. Even in Robert Herrick's sixteenth-century 'progress' poems in *Hesperides* – 'Upon Guesse' and 'Upon Urles' – gout 'progresses' from feet to arms.[116] These metaphors were widespread throughout the realms of prose and poetry: not merely in medical texts or panegyric verse. 'Progression' was also more abstract, as in the sequence gout–self–identity. Robinson Crusoe's ancient father is 'gouty', a feature Defoe makes clear at the opening of the book.[117] He is a strong patriarchal figure whose authoritarianism drives his children to sea: one son has perished, another is about to. He is a flat character representing the emblem of paternity: guiding his sons through life by influencing their movements; the possessor of gout – the 'fathering disease' *par excellence*. But one wonders whether Defoe's intelligence about gout (Defoe himself was apparently not a sufferer) derived from the travel literature in which he was so heavily im-mersed rather than medical lore.

Thomas Phelps, a travel writer Defoe could have read, was one of many who recounted the peril of gout among his crew while collecting slaves on the Barbary Coast:

The night following, we intended to proceed, but it pleased God, to strike me lame with the Gout, so that I was not able to stand . . . The readiest expedient to remedy my distemper, which I could think upon was this, we make a fire in a hole in the ground, and I put my Foot into the hole to draw away the pain, having also a Lancet with us, I endeavour'd to breath a Vein in my Foot, but I could not affect it, for the Lancet would not enter, however, I found some ease by the force of the fire: My company being sensible of the delay which my distemper occasion'd, began to be mov'd . . .[118]

A harrowing account follows of his attempted escape with his 'foot on fire'. Such flight was extreme but that Defoean mind-set also inherited a 'gout of the middle' whose motto – as Defoe's father cautioned – was 'stay home and acquire gout' as a *positive* force. Such domestication formed part of the downward filtering process, as fathers, like Robinson's, attempted to prevent their sons from oceanic peril, their own gout a necessary condition for the plea. Domestic gout was also the arbiter of the parlour, as the Shandy males learned: a malady keeping them at their hearth, defining their 'Shandyism'.

A gout of extremities – if we continue in this line of classification based on social perception and expectation – amounted to pornography: the radical lewdness of the old man, the ageing, well-heeled husband, forever usurped by the younger, more virile man. This is the very stuff – as we shall see – of some of gout's most visual representations. Less iconographic accounts swarmed in memoirs – in those of invalids and in other secret diaries of the geriatric, fearful for their wives, as in an anonymous *Secret Patient's Diary: Also the Gout and Weakness – Diaries Being each a Practical Journal or Scheme* (1725):

> The happieſt man that ever breath'd on earth,
> With all the glories of estate and birth,
> Has yet some care or pain to make him know,
> No grandeur is above the reach of woe,
> Your lordship feels it in your gouty toe,
> But in the keenest agonies of grief,
> Content's a cordial that gives some relief.[119]

Numerous traditions converged to render gout the jungle of metaphor it became by the Victorian era. Gouty self-fashioning gentlemen in the late Renaissance had 'risen' to self-puffers in the eighteenth century only to 'self-reflect' about their social standing in the nineteenth. A single dominant strain – for example, that to be 'in' the gout was to 'stand apart' from the crowd – diminishes the verbal undergrowth gout became. However, such forests of metaphor must not reduce the biographical fact of self-professed sufferers. Three generations were chronicled in Edmund Marshall's published narrative:[120] Edmund's father and son alike received case histories. All the Marshalls, similar to the nearly castrated dynasty of Sterne's Shandy males, were gouty and scoured southern Europe for cure. Marshall himself developed gout in the summer of 1769, thereafter travelling to Spa where he ingratiated himself with the Belgians and encountered the 'arch-hero' who has cured him: a French doctor named similarly to, but spelt differently from, Sterne's character, Le Fevre, possessing a hermetic secret cure.

Although Marshall's *Specific for the Gout* is permeated with asides – the reportage that has enabled the composition of case histories of such obscure figures as the Count Rougrave, the Grand Vicar of Liège, and a Mr Blavier – his prose sprawl amounts to the gout pathography flourishing at mid-century. He is particularly informative on female gout, especially a Mrs Myers who suffered as acutely as any man, and Belgian Mother Angélique who diagnosed the malady among her nuns in Liège.[121] Marshall also explains how his gouty father (à la Robinson Crusoe) entreats him (Edmund) not to lead the dissipated life. To his Crusoean father is attributed the warning not to 'live too freely in juvenilian years'.[122]

A CANDID AND IMPARTIAL
STATE of the EVIDENCE
OF A VERY GREAT PROBABILITY,
That there is discovered
BY MONSIEUR LE FEVRE,
A REGULAR PHYSICIAN, Residing and Practising
at LIEGE in GERMANY,

A SPECIFIC for the GOUT.

CONTAINING
The Motives which induced the AUTHOR to listen to the
Pretensions of the LIEGE MEDICINE; with an Account
of its Operations and Effects in his own Case.

TO WHICH IS ADDED,
A NARRATIVE
Of the CASES of several other PATIENTS, Persons of Rank
and Reputation, who have been cured, or are now in a Course of
Cure of the GOUT, by the EFFICACY of Dr. LE FEVRE'S
POWDERS, communicated by themselves to the AUTHOR,
during his Residence at LIEGE.

IN AN APPENDIX IS GIVEN
An ACCOUNT of a HOUSE fitted up at LIEGE, for the
Reception of the ENGLISH only; with a TABLE of the
EXPENCE of the different Accommodations.

Also a DETAIL of the best and most approved INNS upon the
ROAD to LIEGE, either by the ROUT of CALAIS or OSTEND.

By EDMUND MARSHALL, M.A.
Vicar of CHARING in KENT.

Nec quia desperes invicti membra Glyconis
Nodosa corpus nolis prohibere chiragrâ? HOR.

The SECOND EDITION.

CANTERBURY:
Printed for the AUTHOR, by SIMMONS and KIRKBY.
Sold at the King's Arms Printing-office, Canterbury; and by
W. GRIFFIN, Bookseller, in Catharine-street in the Strand,
MDCCLXX.

7. Title page of *A Candid and Impartial State of the Evidence of a Very Great Probability*. By Edmund Marshall. Canterbury, 1770.

POSTSCRIPT.

SINCE the above was written, the author has, at the request of ten Gentlemen of fortune and condition in this Country, dispatched an invitation to Dr. Le Fevre to come over to England—it has been already intimated, that this Gentleman had given me authority to declare his readiness to visit these kingdoms, whenever he should be respectably called hither—The invitation made him by these Gentlemen, appears to me so clearly to come within this idea, that I have warmly recommended it to the Doctor's acceptance—Should nothing have happened to make it necessary to him to have chang'd his resolution—the public may be assur'd, that due notice shall be given of the time he may appoint for his journey to England——

As Dr. Le Fevre against his own sentiments, has been, in a manner, constrained to name some certain sum for the administration of his medicine—

8. Postscript of *A Candid and Impartial State*.

The Senecan advice went unheeded, as in Robinson's case; but rarely cropped up between *mothers* and sons. Old Mrs Purefoy's constant lament to her London agent is an exception: 'I thank God his [my son's] gout does not return.'[123] Fathers mentored their sons through this *rite de passage* which sympathetically bonded them in that Chesterfieldian world, even though some were unable to write such letters to their sons.

Marshall's first-person narrative, influenced by the novel form, chronicles him from birth to the moment when the 'crippled' protagonist first presents himself to Le Fevre. Within weeks Marshall returns to London, cured by Le Fevre's 'long-acting white, tasteless powder'; however, it is not Le Fevre's pharmaceutical powder but Marshall's assumptions and language that command our attention in goutometries. His self-reflective narrative addresses an 'English gouty reader' who is regularly invoked, flirted with, and – Shandylike – taken leave of. Where is Marshall's son in all this? Did he take his father's second-generation advice? Did he contract gout? The reader is not told: instead every 'lithe gouty throbbing' is vividly recorded, suggesting an audience ready to consume this 'gout romance' of three generations.

Marshall's book was widely reviewed; within months taunts appeared among which one long review stands out.[124] The belligerent reviewer doubts Marshall's veracity, suggests he is a 'young man paid off' by Le Fevre to puff his panacea and intimates that Marshall has been taken seriously because English physician James Johnston, a student of the famous Edinburgh Dr Robert Whytt – the 'philosophical doctor' – also claimed to be in Liège at the same time.[125] The conclusion is that readers of the memoir, as well as users of the powder, have been swindled. 'Mr Le Fevre's theory of the disorder [of gout], and of the medicine, is so *romantic* and *wild*, that we cannot avoid suspecting he had something *else in view* than to explain the nature of the one or the other, when he *formed* it.'[126] Puffer and puffed – Marshall and Le Fevre – mattered to the attacker. However, similar works make plain that readers often had other more sentimental motives: release from despair, comfort from pain, the solace of discovering others similarly suffering.

Hence gout, through a slow process of social transformation and metaphoric evolution, came to symbolize in the popular imagination essentially two bodily zones: the afflatus of old age and the indignity of cramp loosely construed. Both were resistant to earnest interpretations and proof of Horace Walpole's *aperçu*, divulged to his constant 'gout correspondent' – milady Ossory – that 'gout and pain and confinement have made me hate everything *serious*'.[127]

Gout was also comic cramp, no matter how socially disdained and culturally reconstructed. Cramp – as Walpole and his gossipy ladies were aware – represented the body in essentially grotesque postures and 'windy' contortions. Here the metaphors went wild. The doctors had written reams about cramp between the eras of Sydenham and Garrod, always suppressing its anatomo-pathology into polite elisions and, later on, forgetting that the caricaturists had penetrated its basic indignities through comic deflation. Cramp, although the possessor of a colourful discourse more readily captured by the Rowlandsons and Gillrays than medical doctors, lacked a language except for the declensions of 'corruption' it could muster. Even Walpole danced around cramp when proudly celebrating to Cole – his constant male confessor in the gout – that he had suffered from all three types:

> How there can be a doubt what the gout is, amazes me!. . . It may be objected that the sometimes instantaneous removal of pain from one limb to another is too rapid for a current of chalk – true, but not for the humour before coagulated. As there is evidently too a degree of hollow wind mixed with the gout, may not that wind be impregnated with the noxious effluvia, especially as the latter are pent up in the body and may be corrupted![128]

Such morbid effluvial 'corruption' voided in bodily 'wind' was the state of affairs to be talked *around*, not through or into. 'Cramp' was thus the poor cousin of the internal organs: one could more politely discuss the vagaries of spleen or the vomitorium of pancreatic overspills than cramp's noisy concatenations. The cramp produced by 'gout in the stomach' – as in Queen Anne's acute case – was euphemistically called 'hysterical affections', but decreased to 'vapours' when migrating to the head.

'Cramp' suggests inherently comic configuration detracting from any 'honour' gout bestowed. When Walter Scott disentangled them – 'cramp' and 'honour' – in a humorous letter to Joanna Baillie, sister of the anatomist Matthew and niece of the Hunter brothers of anatomy fame, one wonders how she construed his yoking. 'The *cramp* I believe [is] in my stomach for I have no pretensions to the honour of the *gout* – with which I have been assaild three or four times this season with the greatest possible violence.'[129]

The violence of cramp was more abrupt, 'honour' suggesting expected arrival despite accompanying pretension and ulterior motive, neither of which were commensurate with the groans and grunts of 'cramp'. Perhaps this is why Lewis Carroll's miniature allegory of gout, in the story of the pig, has such enduring, almost childlike truth:

> There was a Pig that sat alone
>   Beside a ruined Pump:
> By day and night he made his moan –
> It would have stirred a heart of stone
> To see him wring his hoofs and groan,
>   Because he could not jump.
> A certain Camel heard him shout –
>   A Camel with a hump.
> 'Oh, is it Grief, or is it Gout?

What is this bellowing about?'
That Pig replied, with quivering snout,
  'Because I cannot jump!'[130]

Gout, however humorous, incorporated a sunny optimism capturing the essence of the comic spirit through which its regimens had peaked among the fun-loving Georgians and transcended its tragic-comic origins. The Duke of Portland's 'remedy for the gout' gave proof of the doctors' guarantees if the patient diligently took his medicine in a graduated course, with no hope of improvement during the first three weeks. In the second three months, the amount decreases, as it continues to do over the next twenty-four. The recipe warns: 'you must not be discouraged tho'; the *rite de passage* is insulating the patient against graver calamity. If the above fails, the patient must take ever decreasing amounts with nothing but a strong brandy. So the patient returns to his favorite remedy, and all ends well. As one of the perpetual scribblers of gout in a ditty merely titled 'Doctor' declaimed:

> Doctor once dubbed – what ignorance shall baulk
> Thy march triumphant? Diagnose the gout
> As cholic, and prescribe it cheese for chalk –
> No matter! All's one: cure shall come about
> And win thee wealth – fees paid with such a roar
> Of thanks and praise alike from lord and lout
> As never stunned man's ears on earth before.[131]

Stunning it was, this essential profile of the metaphoric and discursive heritage. Gout's visual legacy was more constricted, for reasons we now explore.

CHAPTER 12

Gout: The Visual Heritage

Two threads run through gout's visual heritage: its male, almost phallic, grotesque objects — swollen, inflated, protruding feet, arms, bellies — and the hint that the gouty male is forever ready for erotic play that is less than direct; if not physically capable himself, at least an observer of, and ancillary participant in, the action. This is true of *all* the epochs surveyed in this book: especially Georgian and Victorian satire — the vast tradition of caricature extending from Hogarth and Rowlandson to Cruikshank — flourishing in the heyday of gout during the eighteenth and nineteenth centuries. Another strain derives from silence: the scarcity of female representatives. Perhaps this absence should be expected in view of gout's gender base: until the eighteenth century few cases of gouty women are described. We searched without success on several continents for visual representations of women, only to be repeatedly thwarted. We do not claim none exist — merely that they are so scarce they have eluded us. A decade's search produced not even the occasional caricature or ephemeral cartoon of women.[1]

Rather than represent women, the pictorial tradition devoted itself to podagra and the gout diagnosis, however construed, and captured the ludic elements of title pages and emblems. Little is known about the 'H. S. Beham' who put his name on a 1607 black and white print that survives in the Warburg Institute in London catalogued as 'Podagrae Ludus'. But by *c.* 1600 the conjunction of gout and play has been cemented.[2] A godlike male figure, dressed in Roman garb, waves his wand as if commanding heaven and earth to obey the edict inscribed above his crown: *podagrae ludus*. The other words — *solvere nodosam nescit medicina podagram* — embellish the notion by summoning doubts about the gazer's construal of these two essential words (*podagrae ludus*) and the concepts underlying them.

Does the god mean man is inherently *gouty* or, vice versa, that podagra is inherently *male*? Or that gout itself is mysteriously playful (compared to other maladies)? What exactly *is* a playful illness — assuming gout was a sufficiently stable signifier *c.* 1600 to consider it an illness? Or does it mean that gout should *lead to play* during affliction or after recovery? There are other ways of interpreting this conjunction of seemingly disparate signifiers: the one of a diagnosis (*podagra* or gout) that was old by the time of this engraving; the

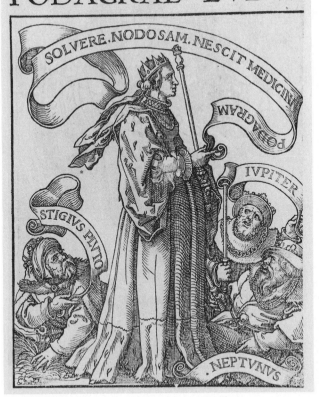

PODAGRAE LVDVS

9. H. S. Beham. *'Podagrae Ludus'*. Black and white print. 1607.

other (*ludens* or play) of a cultural potential and anthropological propensity antedating the Greeks.

The remarkable feature of this convergence of gout and play, however interpreted, is that the visual tradition documents it in parallel with, or in accompaniment to, the verbal legacy already discussed. Engravings yoking the two must have drawn on the commonplace understanding, as in so much other Renaissance emblemology, for Beham's version of the *podagra ludens* tradition was one among many.[3] The flowering of the theme in visual representation occurred during its maturity in the Classical period, especially in the works of the great caricaturists, from Hogarth and Rowlandson to Cruikshank. Hogarth's presentation of 'the marriage contract', the first plate in 'Marriage à la Mode' (1731), set the stage for later copies. Here, among the six figures, the gouty father occupies the position of power and rank. None of the others – daughter, groom, their representatives – is as prominent. His fine suit, powdered wig, surroundings (lavish paintings on the walls and a canopied bed), the contract for the impending dowry flowing down his right side, the huge town house across the square, the magnificent chambers

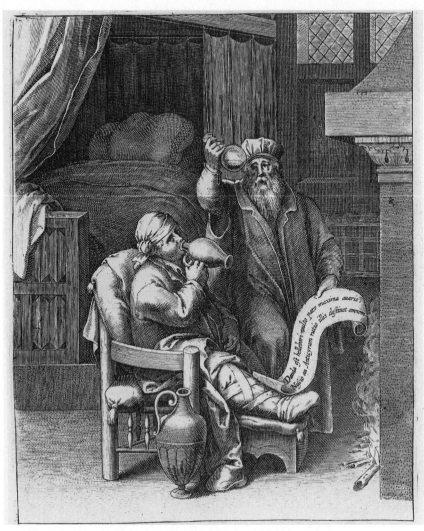

10.   Vaenius. Gout in *Emblemata Horatiana*. Black and white print. 1607.

surrounding him: all these set the stage for a story that will unfold in
subsequent plates. The geriatric's swollen right leg, high on a gout stool,
occupies the centre of this moralistic print in Hogarth's marriage series. And
this gouty leg and stool reveal the podagra conceit in fullest visuality.

Through the 1740s and 1750s derivatives of this almost archetypal father-
figure appeared, imitating Hogarth, retaining his conceit about pedigree.
Some prints situated *señor podagra* surrounded by his family, others solitary.
There was sufficient interest in the 'gouty father' as an archetype – or at least
he was comic enough to be scrutinized visually – to stand on his own two
feet, as if he could. For example, one of a number of cheap copies of

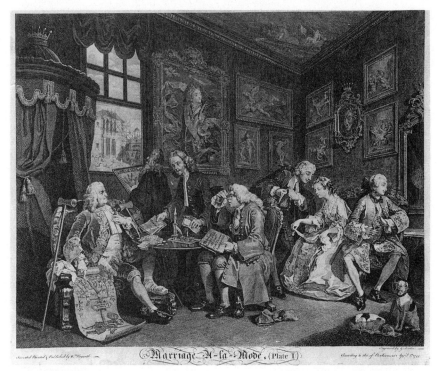

11. 'The Marriage Settlement'. One of a series of copies of Hogarth plates by Davison of Alnwick. 1745.

Hogarth's marriage series – there were many – is called 'the gout'.[4] The black and white detail is limited but shows a larger-than-life gouty patient alone in his room, his left leg lifted on a gout stool. The imitation is similar to the 'gouty Frenchman', a plate we do not reproduce, in the Countway Library of Medicine, in Boston, vividly capturing male renascence and decay through the gouty metaphor: Jeaurat's 'La Vieillesse'.[5] Here his left hand nervously clutches the servant's bell, his expression suggesting he has chided his valet for lax attendance upon him. The young man departs bewildered: why are these gouty patients so demanding? The gaze of puzzlement captures the satire's moral sentiment: the gouty valetudinarian's reliance on his overburdened servants. Viewed from the patient's perspective, however – upper-class gentry – the moral is in reverse: servants underperforming and failing to comply. Point of view counts for much in interpreting these prints.

Thomas Rowlandson continued in this line, perfecting the gouty-old-man cartoons and fixing him within the *podagra ludens* tradition. More remarkably than Hogarth, Rowlandson understood how the gouty caricature should combine into an organic whole – each part relating to all the others.

Rowlandson's 'Old Husband' may be his most masterful case in point: a story within a story aiming to capture the convergence of gout as Eros and gout as Play within the revelries of the day.[6] We dwell on this narrative in view of its significance to our subject.

The action is familiar (the ménage), the place Bath (where the couple may have come for the season). The gouty old husband has swollen to the limits of his frame, his huge foot resting on a pillow larger than, but in tandem with, the lines of his protruding belly; his eyes glance upwards, almost oblivious to the venereal scene occurring behind him. His only residual joy is his wine (the decanter suggesting wine rather than spirits) and glowing fire. A mean-looking cat sits near by facing the fire. His wife and her military lover have been *en embraces* in their closet. She sits on their canopied bed with the door wide open, just about to be penetrated in sexual intercourse by her erect partner. A horrified female servant discovers them and flings up her hands at the sight.

The satire reveals the typology of the old, worn-out and sexually incompetent husband in contrast to the young, vigorous, lusty and always beautiful wife: a pair of contrasts running all through the visual heritage. So much for story and action; other details render Rowlandson's morality more explicit of his intentions. Two paintings on the walls – a portrait of a scion or male relic; a baby, perhaps the old man's son – frame and guarantee the gouty husband's lineage: three generations of pedigree, the essential 'podagra conceit' before the viewer. Five phallic objects stand erect in contrast to the old man's horizontal mass (a rotund shape all across), punctuated by a bright candle celebrating the lovers' bacchanalia. A remarkably phallic picture pole, whose tip simulates an erect penis glans, is also apparent. On the mantel is a plaster of another rotund old gentleman with erect penis; a vertical fire stoker is ambiguously placed to make the observer wonder whose fire is to be put out. An equally phallic end of the fire's grate is evident, containing a round head that can also be understood as one of the phallic objects ready to perform.

These are in parallel to the military lover's penetrating shaft. Nothing else in the old man's room can console him. Rowlandson's lines are vertical and straight, in contrast to the invalid's flaccid protrusions, suggesting anything *but* phallic capability. The details tell an unequivocal story: husband and wife were once lovers who produced progeny, but he cared more for his port wine and family pedigree than for his wife. The predilection landed him in gout and prompted her to take a lover. *His* medical condition is irrevocable, rendering his past irrelevant; *her* future ensures strings of lovers, especially the prospect of money and gout-free longevity after his death. Her worries are few; she can expect to inherit his fortune once he is dead.

'The Old Husband' was imitated and applied to other ailments. There is no space to reprint others here, but we do wish to mention Joseph Seymour's series illustrating William Hayley's *The Triumphs of Temper*, often reprinted in the 1780s and 1790s.[7] Seymour's plate ('gouty Recoil') shows a young woman recoiling from an old man with his swollen foot held up on a gout stool. In others, the gouty husband is victimized by theft and burglary rather than his wife's or paramour's infidelity. In all these caricatures the threshold of morality is checked by playful comic action and framed by the *podagra ludens* theme. Playfulness abounds inside the dominant action, especially in lust for sport and motion rather than erotic adventure.

Our second point about gout's visual heritage pertains to the grotesque: the almost phallic imagery of this accumulation. After 1700, prints endlessly circulated showing an upper-class male possessed by a very large foot usually raised to a stool or 'gout table', as in Jeaurat's 'Old Age'.[8] This is the stereotype: upper class, well dressed, decked out in good accommodations, yet despondent for reasons extending beyond arthritic complaints. The engraving, after a painting by Jeaurat, shows 'Old Age' explicitly represented by huge gouty legs. A middle-aged man occupies the centre of attention, holding forth somewhere in an elegant room with large swing windows and foliage and clouds outside (a country house?). His expression suggests the sudden awareness of decrepitude, especially the loss of desire and capacity for erotic arousal – as the lines from Jean-Jacques Rousseau's poem make plain, punning on the old banality between 'gout' and 'goute', despairing over the confluence of infirmity and old age:

> Vieux, on le méprise, on l'évite,
> Toux, gravelle, goute, pituite,
> Mauvaise humeur infirmité,
> Assiègent sa caducité.

The pitcher has been thrown over or accidentally tipped, its contents spilled, as the gaga patient rings for his servant in exasperation. The morality is conveyed in the French text but the print bears another meaning: the swollen leg becomes the visible emblem of male loss through exorbitant size, inertia and immobility. This incongruity of size and immobilization – matter and space – creates the other level explored in this chapter. Matter is clear enough but immobilization in relation to the canvas's space, and to the gazer's eye in the act of observing these enlarged limbs, is something to be probed.

Both points – ludic and erotic – incorporate gender. If the early critical heritage of Smollett's *Humphry Clinker*, for instance, had included female responses another profile would exist of this most risible of gouty inventions.[9] Likewise gout's phallic visual representations. If no early female commentators on paintings like Jeaurat's survive, there is still no doubt that the 'masculine interpretation' gleaned disappointment and loss above all else. For these satires

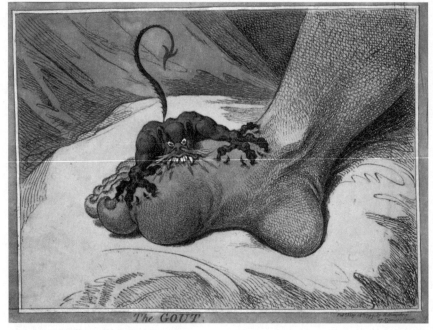

12.   James Gillray, *The Gout*, 1799.

were 'read' as parables of loss: men, sow your seeds now before you become gouty as in the picture before you. Rowlandson's famous depiction of the enlarged foot with the devils of gout hovering round the toe is an exception rather than the norm.[10] The message here extended loss into the realms of anatomic realism and Goyaesque torture. A foot is blown up: neuter, ageless, sexless, deformed, gnawed at by the devils of podagra. Its viewers can only have surmised what pain the foot's owner endured. Rowlandson chose not to show more for good reason, leaving the consequences of pain to the viewer's imagination. The afflicted anatomical organ is the site of focus – the only known illustration in the long eighteenth century to blow up the foot in this way. Fat old men are imitated and parodied but not this inimitable, besieged, genderless toe.

In Joseph H. Seymour's 'Young woman recoiling from an old man seated with foot on gout stool',[11] the storyline is a commonplace. The old man's lower torso is swollen, curbing the lady's erotic desire, his phallic apparatus merging with other swollen and inert blobs, prompting her to recoil. In other versions not produced here the female protagonist is younger or older, depending on the artist's intention and the further meaning he wished to imbue the canvas with, but always sustaining the two points about erotic play: (1) if only the male had not been so immobile, and (2) lingering potential.

In earlier chapters we glimpsed the gouty patient's insulating energy. The visual heritage from Hogarth to Gillray and Cruikshank incorporated it as well, but not always as grotesque; and when grotesque through deformity or enlargement, the male body was distantiated from its own symmetrical centre. The gouty male body endured, of course, as a depressing site on which to situate erotic loss and lamented desire. Insulation continued within this small margin for idealization. Elderly gouty male subjects resisted sitting and posing: who wants to be remembered as a septuagenarian freak of Falstaffian glob? – a state of affairs explaining the paucity of portraits, even when the artistic mood lent itself to portraiture in the eighteenth century.[12]

Before then, the visual record is empty: indeed, we have found no representations of gouty patients – of any gender – before the early eighteenth century. After this approximate period, gouty patients appear in prints, caricature, portraits and – once china and porcelain begin to be manufactured – as mass-produced objects. From J. J. Kaendler's work (plate 14) in Meissenware to the porcelain produced in Delft and Stafford, sufferers of gout were routinely found.[13] Here realism commemorates patients and reminds spectators of bygone eras; nostalgia and memory also reminded male viewers of gout's clutches. The insulating malady was never far from the rest of domestic life in these decorative pieces adorning bourgeois European houses.

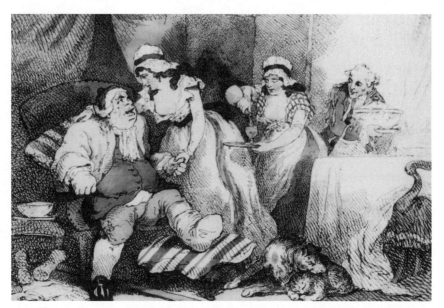

13. Plate attributed to Joseph H. Seymour, 'Young woman recoiling from an old man seated with foot on gout stool'. This is found as plate 3 in William Hayley's *The Triumphs of Temper* (Newburyport, Mass., 1794).

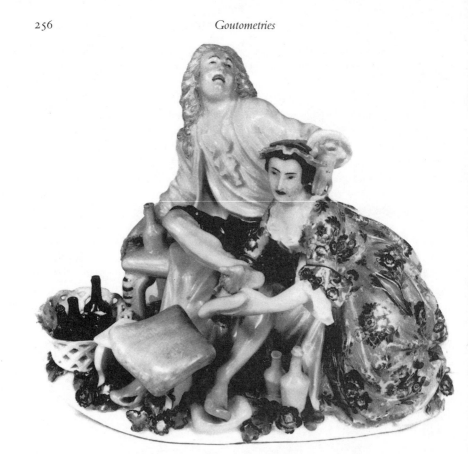

14. J. J. Kaendler. 'Meissen group gathered around the gout sufferer'.

Before the eighteenth century, gout's visual heritage was limited to portraying the 'gout doctors' and their remedies. Thus it would be surprising not to find portraits of Willibald Pirckheimer (1470–1530), the author of *The Praise of the Gout* discussed in Chapter 5. Several are extant and the one by Dürer appeared on the title page of the first English translation of his Menippean encomium of 1617: *A Paradox, Both Pleasant and Profitable. Written First in the Latine Tongue, by that Famous and Noble Gentleman Bilibaldus Pirckheimerus Councellor unto two Emperours, Maximilian the First, and Charles the First. And now Englished by William Est, Master of Arts.*[14] The Horatian epigraph about the nature of paradox is relevant by virtue of insulating the sufferer while keeping him gouty. As Pirckheimer's subtitle reads, 'both pleasant and profitable': pleasant because never indicating fatality, profitable for guaranteed insularity. Pirckheimer himself is captured as masculine, hairy, almost bearded, symmetrical, erudite – the image of gravitas.

Pirckheimer's significance surpassed his links to Albrecht Dürer, who painted his portrait in 1524. The Dürer connection segued into gout *and* melancholia as a single unit, both predicated on the belief that the sedentary life produced chronic lowness of spirits.[15] Pirckheimer himself suffered from chronic podagra and wrote about it in his *Apologie sue podagra* (1522). A recent *Festschrift* celebrating his contributions to Renaissance medicine demonstrates how keen interest is today in his overlaps with Erasmus, Thomas More and Dürer himself.[16] Pirckheimer's own chronic gout renders him central. It arose from an insatiable lust for knowledge and overly zealous application in study: hence his condition as embodying the radical Faustian paradox posing fundamental dilemmas for his life. Dürer's portrait captures these ambiguities: a broad face, thick, almost goitre-like neck and nape; manically tossed hair blending in with his lace shirt, literally insulated; a stylized male aggressiveness. Pirckheimer's 'look' celebrates gout as the malady of insulation: insulatory but not yet comic (the comic gaze was a late arrival), the guarantor of longevity, the condition affording time to devote to contemplative study.[17]

Less than a century later, William Atkins was not so raffishly fashioned in his only extant portrait: 'the effigies of W. Atkins the Gout Dr. who for Gouts, Rumatisms, Palseys, and Convultions, and all Pains in any parts he exceedeth all men, both for safest and speediest Cures'.[18] Atkins amassed a fortune and fame as a 'specialist doctor' in a Restoration milieu when these were rare. His grim face exceeds the predictable: dour, labelled 'gout doctor', it was copied in an identical version in the Georgian period and reprinted with the portrait of 1694. The anonymous portraitist has imaged him in earnest: a harbinger of bad news, Hermes of Death, not merely the author of *A Discourse Shewing the Nature of the Gout* (London, 1694).[19] Crowning the solemnity is his appellation: 'gout doctor'. His solemnity bore no relation to his speciality: the image of the gout doctor had not yet been transformed into the mercenary but gleeful countenance of his medical counterparts. That came later at the end of the eighteenth century.

'The learned doctors of gout' – as Walter Shandy might have invoked them – retained an identity of pomp and circumstance lost in the British Isles by approximately 1700. Before then, their portraits and works were virtual insignia: artefacts of technology as well as self-advertisements. Such imaging lingered on the Continent, an indication of different styles of presentation and professionalization across the Channel. It is unthinkable, however, that a title page such as the one illustrated here could have appeared in England as late as 1751. In England gouty erudition gave way to bibliographic merriment and comic joy. An anonymous German print entitled 'Gichtkranker und Tod'

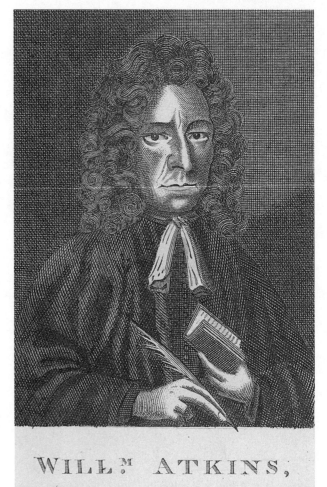

WILL.ᴹ ATKINS,

(Gout Doctor.)

15. Anonymous portrait. 'Willm. Atkins, Gout Doctor'. *c.* 1700.

shows the gout patient confronting Death itself (plate 17).[20] The print is hardly British in its sombreness; it remains the solitary example of 'confrontation' we have found, although the iconographic genre abounds for other maladies: bubonic plague, ague, consumption.

Death occupies the centre, while a wealthy elderly gentleman sits swollen out on a 'gout table'. An inset portrait shows Death attempting to lead away a younger turbaned man, but futilely. In the main scene Death stands on a time glass, his conventional violin announcing his message. Antiquarian coins and an open book cover the man's table, signifying learning and piety. A

HISTORIA
PODAGRAE

EMINENTISSIMI CARDINALIS

PHILIPPI LVDOVICI

NATI COMITIS

A

SINZENDORFF

S. R. E. PRESBYTERI,

EPISCOPI WRATISLAVIENSIS,

SERENISSIMIQVE NISSENSIVM

ET

GROTKAVIENSIVM DVCIS,

*REGII BORVSSICI ORDINIS AQVILAE
NIGRAE EQVITIS,*

CONSCRIPTA

AB IPSIVS MEDICO,

IOANNE GODOFR. de HAHN,

CONSILIARIO REGIO AVLICO,
ACADEM. IMPERIAL. NAT. CVRIOSOR. SOCIO, ET
COLLEGII MEDICI ET SANITATIS
DECANO.

NORIMBERGÆ, IMPENSIS W. M. ENDTERI CON-
SORTIVM, ET VID. B. IVL. ARNOLD. ENGELBRECHTI.
M D C C L I.

16. Title page of *Historia podagrae*
by Ioanne Godofr. de Hahn.
Published by Arnold Engelbrechti,
1751.

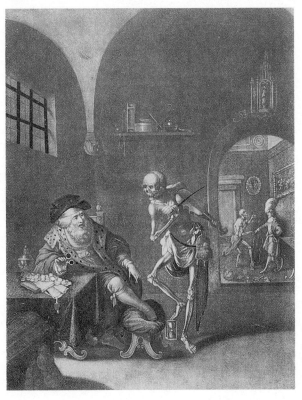

17. Anonymous print,
'Gichtkranker Und Tod'.
c. 1600. Illustration in an
undated volume entitled
*Bildersammlung aus der
Geschichte der Medizin.*

miniature Christian temple adorns the arcade door, endorsing the patient's God-fearing piety. The older man's imprecation pleads for time – to no avail. The collection of silver, paintings and costume suggests gentility; a wooden chest abundant goods and chattels to purchase time. 'Gout Patient with Death' may have been inserted by a later editor, but this time the malady is fatal. Why should this be so? The ludic tradition of Beham (plate 9) and the early Menippean satirists entirely lack such gouty gravitas.

The title pages of most published works and broadsides touting panaceas and miracle potions were unillustrated. Their rhetoric is humorous, even risible, suggesting that one function of the title page as a discrete unit was to amuse and delight. We have already discussed in Chapter 11 whimsical caricatures and astrological representations such as the Restoration 'Wipe for the Iter-Boreale' and Robert Witty's *Gout Raptures*, robustly subtitled *Astromaxia. Or an Historical Fiction of a War among the Stars: Wherein are mentioned the 7 Planets, the 12 signs of the Zodiack, and the 50 Constellations of Heaven mentioned by the Ancients, Also several eminent Stars, and the most principal parts and lines of the Celestial Globe with their Natures and Uses are pointed at. Useful for such as apply themselves to the Study of Astronomy, and the Celestial Globe.*

Gout was diagnosed to gullible audiences according to the 'stars', and these sheets cost a penny a piece. The curious aspect is that we have found no equivalents for other maladies; diagnosers and patients alike construed these diagnoses with a less than scrupulous eye. The erotic element is also absent, even in amorous predictions during the 'twelve moons'. Such broadsides and short pamphlets continued to be produced in the seventeenth and eighteenth centuries, as in *A Caribbee Medicine for the Gout, Rheumatism and various other Disorders. Communicated to the Count de Noziers, By the King's Attorney at Martinicio. Translated from the French* (plate 18), a seven-page first-person narrative that is not what it seems.[21] The account describes a New World native afflicted with gout eager to discover what it is. The naive narrator claims to have stumbled upon a herbal panacea on his Carib island, which he communicated to the 'King's' representative who relates it to the Count de Noziers. The herb is plugged – a flourishing pill trade – not the sufferer's quest. Lucrative trade could ensue between the 'Carib' islands and French court if the petition were approved.[22]

Transatlantic trade in gout remedies was vigorous. Gout flourished in North America, even if differentially diagnosed. John Hill, the remarkable jack-of-all-trades whose *Management of the Gout* has already been discussed, retained agents who peddled his bardana root.[23] As quacks proliferated, so did gouty panaceas illustrated and puffed up in pamphlets. Linnaeus' 'strawberry cure' was described both ways: quackishly and medicinally, as when Andrew Freake adopted the former and satirized it in *The Humulus Lupulus of Linnaeus: with an account of its use in Gout, and other diseases.*[24] The conjunction of

A

CARIBBEE MEDICINE

FOR THE

GOUT, RHEUMATISM

AND VARIOUS OTHER DISORDERS.

COMMUNICATED TO THE

COUNT DE NOZIERES,

BY THE KING'S ATTORNEY AT MARTINICO.

TRANSLATED FROM THE FRENCH.

BOSTON:

PRINTED AND SOLD BY EDMUND FREEMAN,
Oppofite the North-Door of the State Houfe.

M,DCC,LXXXVIII.

18. Title page of the
anonymous *A Caribbee
Medicine for the Gout,
Rheumatism And various
other Disorders*. Boston,
1788.

pharmacy and botany was particularly strong, even genderized for women.
William Stephens touted a 'milk diet' under the name 'Dolaeus': *Dolaeus upon
the Cure of the Gout*.[25] Building on John Arbuthnot's diet theories, whose
pathbreaking essay on diet had appeared a year earlier (1731), Stephens
proclaimed that natural milk – goat's, calf's or kid's – was best. Earlier Joseph
Addison recounted that when he saw 'a fashionable Table set out in all its
Magnificence, I fancy that I see Gouts and Dropsies . . . with other innumerable Distempers lying in Ambuscade among the Dishes'.[26] Again
in 1731 the valetudinarian Alexander Pope removed himself to St John
Bolingbroke's farm at Dawley, in Hampshire, to drink directly from the
lactating teat itself.[27] Such visitations prescribed by the most competent

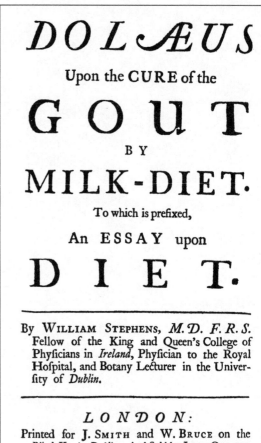

DOLÆUS

Upon the CURE of the

GOUT

B Y

MILK-DIET.

To which is prefixed,

An ESSAY upon

D I E T.

By WILLIAM STEPHENS, *M. D. F. R. S.*
Fellow of the King and Queen's College of
Phyſicians in *Ireland*, Phyſician to the Royal
Hoſpital, and Botany Lecturer in the Univer-
ſity of *Dublin*.

LONDON:
Printed for J. SMITH and W. BRUCE on the
Blind-Key in *Dublin*: And Sold by JOHN OSBORN
and THOMAS LONGMAN in *Pater-noſter Row*.
MDCCXXXII.

19. Title page of *Dolaeus
upon the Cure of the Gout
by Milk-Diet.* By William
Stephens. London, 1732.

doctors of the epoch must give us pause today about the authenticity of such
treatments.

The *visual* 'invisible made visible' neglected certain objects, while favouring
other gouty landscapes. We wonder why the infinitesimal particles of
chalkstone lodged in the joints – those white-haired Hermes-of-pain about
which the doctors pronounced and about which memoirists like Horace
Walpole generated their best coinages – were not drawn. They were certainly
captured in words, as when Walpole, rickety with age, complained to Lady
Ossory of 'constant chalky rills running from his fingers'.[28] Walpole
prognosticated in this letter to milady of Berkeley Square that the raffish
Duchess of Devonshire could dictate a revolution by making gout fashionable
among *women*. Why exclude them from its glorious insulations? Walpole

pecked on: the ladies 'recall their chins, and thrust out a shoe wadded with flannel'.[29]

Painterly images like these, white if barely feline, should have been grist for the caricaturist's quill in a satiric ambience in which the sexes were being regulated more rigidly than at any time since the moral inquisitions of the 1690s. Were gouty women never painted or drawn despite their refusals to be remembered this way? 'Recalled chins' and swollen calves among a cultural mind-set so self-conscious of its ladylike curves that every curl of the head was measured should have lent themselves to colour far more than words. Even the great Dutch anatomist Leeuwenhoek had described Walpole's 'chalky rills' in medical narrative more appropriate for the palette than the quill.[30] Leeuwenhoek comically recounted a relation whose chalk 'broke out of his heel'. Leeuwenhoek examined the chalk under his new microscope where it appeared like the finest horse-hairs: polka-dotted white and red flaming daggers of pain to 'something sharp at both ends'. A chalky, wave-crested, white matter mixed with particles of blood – almost a work of modern art. 'These figures I judged so thin, that more than a 1000 of them lying close together, would not make out, the thickness of a hair of our head.' Yet no paintings known survive to capture these miniatures of the seventeenth-century lens.

If joints pouring forth 'chalk lava' were not bared to the artist, neither were gouty feet in an Oriental mode during the Georgian peak of chinoiserie. Tightly bound Chinese feet, we might think, should have struck the fancy of the gouty as entailing the analogue of their own fettered condition. So it seemed to Edward Young, the melancholic poet of *Night Thoughts*, who unctuously consoled the Duke of Portland and his rheumatic Duchess, Young's constant correspondent, to whom he revealed that gout's chronic insulations had prolonged him (Young) into a dreadful longevism.[31] The Duke was gouty himself and had made a financial killing in 'Portland powders'. 'Madam,' Young imprecated, 'That my Ld Duke may before this be on better than a Chinese foot, & yt ye Little ones may long trip it with ye foot of Fairies on Mrs Delanys Light phantastick Toe before they know wt Pain means is ye hearty Prayr of their humble sevt & Admirer.'[32]

Historically, the hand had been almost as cramped and swollen as the legendary foot, despite obvious differences in the trajectory of their eroticization.[33] Painters had visualized the 'afflicted hand' more than the impaired foot. Engels and the anthropologists explained why: the hand, especially its dextrous index finger, had been responsible for man's mammalian superiority. The history of painting abounds with figures composing at their writing desks, few of whom suffer from the 'writer's cramp' about which Jonathan Goldberg has written so eloquently.[34] Edward Young himself (by then an octogenarian) descanted on these anxieties to the young *Sturm und Drang* poet Friedrich Gottlieb Klopstock in a 'postcard' message:

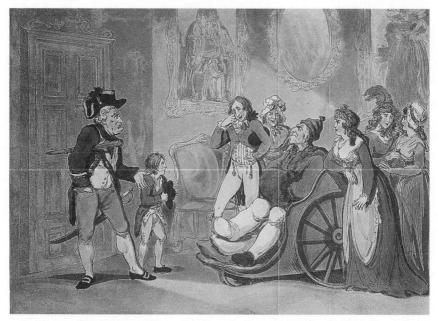

20.   Thomas Rowlandson, 'Lieut. Bowling pleading the cause of young Rory to his Grandfather'. Illustration from an 1805 edition of Tobias Smollett's *Roderick Random*.

'Rheumatism robbed me of the use of my Pen, which I can but very ill hold now.'[35] Was it the painters or their sitters who were uninterested in this admittedly unflattering pose through which both could have immortalized themselves?[36]

Technology and machinery also played a role in gout's visual heritage. Moving gadgets – especially gout-chairs and moveable stools – had existed from the era of the Spanish and Italian Renaissance. Philip II, the multi-wived Spanish King contemporaneous with Shakespeare, provided 'monarchical proof' that gout insulated the great. He lived to a ripe age but was so ravaged by disease that his court invented a new 'chair', still on view in his court in the Escorial. His last years were confined strapped to his sedentary invention. Eventually he designed 'gout chairs' for commercial transport that were widely used throughout Europe by 1700.[37] The 'gout' or 'sedan chair' took hold in Britain, especially at the spas, as illustrations to early English novels make evident. The gout chair initiated a new sense of space and motion in relation to the 'enlarged self' whose sign system must be decoded if we are to understand Horace Walpole's Monty Pythonesque hallucination that he saw a member of Parliament and his wife kissing in their wheelchairs;[38] or Gibbon's comic descriptions of being wheeled about in one.

He felt 'like Merlin' in the newfangled vehicle, his sense of visual presence altered by the new physical capability.[39]

A Rowlandson print entitled 'Lieut. Bowling pleading the cause of young Rory to his Grandfather'[40] had appeared in an 1800 reprint of Tobias Smollett's bestselling novel *The Adventures of Roderick Random* (1748), displaying 'the gouty grandfather' in such a chair, surrounded by a group of four women: two chatty young girls and two adults uninterested in the valetudinarian before them. Grandson Rory holds a monocle to his eye and his hat in the other hand as he comforts his grandfather, the centre of attention. This is the old man's final plea: a setpiece to enshrine physical debility. The aesthetics of longevism cry out to be understood in the eighteenth-century world; and even here the mechanical vehicle commands attention.

Lieutenant Bowling implores the old man to provide for his flesh and blood. A rejected plea: 'My grandfather (who was laid up with the *gout*) received this relation . . . with that coldness of civility which was peculiar to him.'[41] The caricature abounds with the art of contrast: in Rowlandson's comic noses, in the parodied pedigree of the chap on the wall, in 'the young ladies, who thought themselves too much concerned to contain themselves any longer, [who] set up their throats altogether against my protector . . . the scurvy Companion – saucy tarpaulin – rude, impertinent fellow – did he think to prescribe to grandpapa?'[42] Even the gout chair features prominently as rather more than the proverbial sofa. It was the ultimate status symbol in an era when the cost of its purchase was high, as in many other gout caricatures by Rowlandson and Cruikshank.

Running throughout these visual satires as a well-developed leitmotif is the protagonist's constant sang-froid: whether as cold civility, irritability or anger. The English novelists after Fielding captured and developed this mood; Scott and Thackeray commented upon it – the latter frequently dramatizing it in his novels, as in his quarrelling males in *The Adventures of Philip* . . . (1862). For the afflicted gout was, of course, no laughing matter, as Cruikshank and other cartoonists noted: a Cruikshank print is titled as such. Many reasons were offered, a main one being the victim's perpetual immobility. Motion and movement had been intrinsic to these verbal and visual traditions, as James Joyce sensed when he sustained the usage of 'Dollard': his term to describe a certain type of throwing motion made by gouty figures like Bloom in old age, Kilmainham the inmate of Simpson's Hospital and 'Ben Dollard' himself.[43]

Motion and mobility were so crucial that progress and advancement were said to be occurring when gout chairs were introduced at the end of the seventeenth century and soon produced in different styles and woods. Varieties were customized according to the purse of the buyer (by the 1760s the poet–scholar Thomas Gray thought they had become massively expensive),[44] some studded with bejewelled handles and gilt edges. They had two

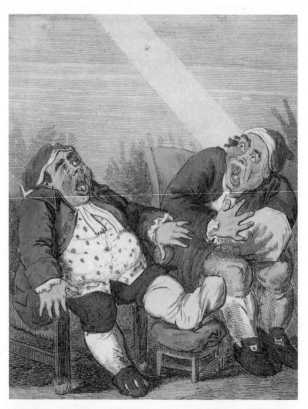

21. William Cruikshank.
'Lords of the Creation'.
Print. 1796.

22. William Cruikshank.
'Pain and Champage'.
Print. 1826.

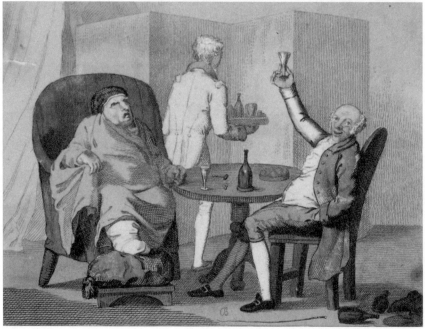

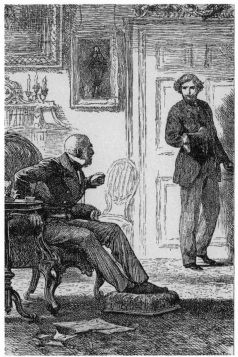

23. 'A Quarrel'. Illustration in the *Cornhill Magazine* for Thackeray's *The Adventures of Philip*.

24. Isaac or George Cruikshank. 'Nobody laughs at a touch of the gout'. Cartoon, early nineteenth century.

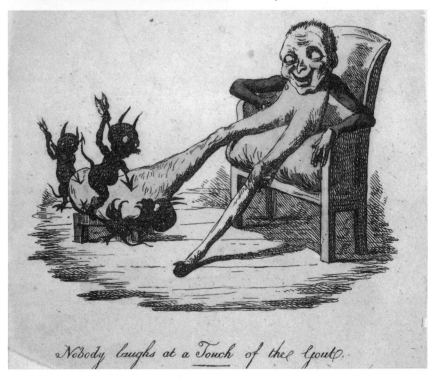

Nobody laughs at a Touch of the Gout.

wheels, their size indicative of the quality and ease with which the chair was manoeuvred around a house and gardens.[45] Evelyn the diarist commented of Lord Clarendon's gout chair that it was of monstrous size.[46] The ever attentive Pepys noted in 1668: 'Thence after dinner to the office and there did a little business; and so to see Sir W. Penn, who I find still very ill of the goute [sic], sitting in his great chair, made on purpose for persons sick of that disease, for their ease; and this very chair he tells me was made for my Lady Lambert'[47] – General John Lambert's depressive rheumatic wife who built numbers of them.[48] To what end remains unclear; she fetishistically collected them.[49] By approximately 1800 the purchasers of these chairs were selective, so common was their use and now reduced price. In Rowlandson's print the chair is drawn symmetrically and parallel to the portraits and mirrors on the walls to indicate the Randoms' status and pedigree.

To these technologies of the wheel were added the 'air pump' and 'vapour bath' patented and manufactured by 1800 on both sides of the Atlantic by enterprising businessmen. Ralph Blegborough, the doctor we discussed in Chapter 6, touted his 'air-pump vapour bath', a water cure based on hot steam with blown-in hot air.[50] He marketed it in the colonies, as did H. O. Hebert, for whom Benjamin Jones drew prints.[51] A sketch of other gout instruments is found in a colonial reprint of Heberden's *Commentaries* dated 1802 in the Burney–Fraser Collection of Gout and Arthritis in Houston, Texas, the world's largest repository of this material.[52] These examples merely indicate the range of devices from special stools and chairs to pulleys and ropes.

The simple crutch itself was transformed: turned stronger and sturdier, bejewelled and hewn out of embossed woods. Its iconography challenges a clandestine phallic symbolism lodged in swollen legs. Dozens of popular novels illustrated in the Georgian period featured it as an emblem commanding attention and eliciting guarded comic response. Illustrated editions of the early novelists thrived on scenes of invalids clinging to their sticks and using them to beat others. These were stock and often grotesque images in the early illustrated editions of Sterne's *Tristram Shandy*, serially published in two volumes every few years from 1760 forward, one of the most highly illustrated novels of the second half of the eighteenth century. Hogarth himself drew at least four scenes, bringing out the gouty line in the construction of bellies and calves. Later caricaturists from Rowlandson through Cruikshank captured an essential flavour of the Shandy parlour – its hearth and sofa – by beefing up the presence of bloated legs lopped over gout stools, with gouty cats soaking up the warmth and parodying their masters through their own well-fed enormity. Peter Maverick (1780–1831), for example, drew these for American audiences, as in Colonel Trim's handing over a crutch to his gouty compatriot Uncle Toby, an immortal set piece of the benevolent pair.[53] By the mid nineteenth century the proverbial Uncle Toby wheeled about in a 'gout chair' with disproportionately huge wheels would not have

FACTS AND OBSERVATIONS

RESPECTING THE

AIR-PUMP VAPOUR-BATH,

IN

GOUT, RHEUMATISM, PALSY,

AND

OTHER DISEASES.

BY RALPH BLEGBOROUGH, M. D.

MEMBER OF THE ROYAL COLLEGE OF SURGEONS,
LONDON.

'Αλλὰ τό μέν θέρμόν, μή πρόσω καίειν, κρίνει δέ αυτός.

Hippoc. De Usu Liquid.

London:

PRINTED FOR LACKINGTON, ALLEN, AND CO.

TEMPLE OF THE MUSES, FINSBURY-SQUARE,

By J. D. Dewick, Aldersgate-Street.

MDCCCIII.

25. Title page of *Facts and Observations respecting the Air-Pump Vapour-Bath, in Gout, Rheumatism, Palsy, and other Diseases*. By Ralph Blegborough. London, 1803.

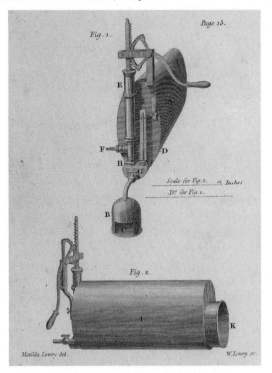

26. Sketch of medical devices used in treatment of gout from a book dated 1802.

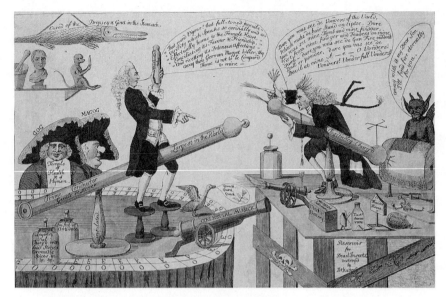

27.   Anonymous print, 'The Quacks'. London, 1783.

appeared unduly grotesque. So far had the tradition of the Shandean podagra
conceit gone.

Crutches also embellished the 'spectacular routines' of those societies. The
doctors waved their golden-headed canes in public spaces as status symbols,
imitated by ardent quacks and empirics parading their less expensive versions.
We have seen these factions warring in British novels, especially in that most
gouty of comic works, *Humphry Clinker*.[54] Politicians and patients displayed
them as cultural icons, as when gouty Edward Gibbon crawled around Bath
on them after his second 'English' gout attack.[55] When Sir John Tyrell, an
MP from Essex, histrionically waved his crutch in the House of Commons in
1838 to punctuate his point about Peel, he actually claimed to be 'fashionably
gouty'.[56] Earlier, poets scribbled couplets about Pitt on crutches; and the
outrageous John Hill, Cadogan's foe, paraded his cane in St James's, was then
beaten with it at Ranelagh, and finally appeared on crutches to cull sympathy:
all three events setting ablaze a wave of 'caning-caricatures' aimed to confirm
Hill's status.[57]

Crutches were a visual insignia of rank as well as an inherently comic
artefact to contrast with their user's deformity or size. 'The Quacks' shows
two warring empirics standing at the side of a wooden table, hoisting themselves on to its precipice.[58] The erotic – almost pornographic – component
speaks for itself. The 'English' quack is buttressed by numerous vials of
potions, a dead alligator and other stuffed animals – 'Gog' and 'Magog' – who
run the 'Temple of Health and Hymen', allusions to James Graham's noto-

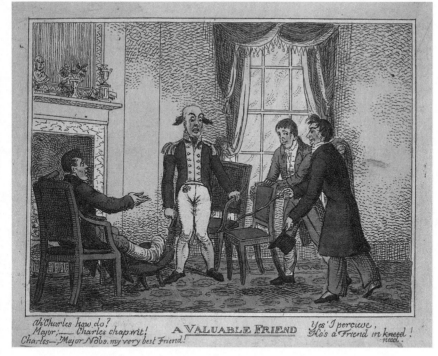

28. Anonymous print. 'A Valuable Friend'.

rious 'Temple' where rites of sexual intercourse were celebrated.[59] Note also the English quack's large, phallic telescope occupying a central position. The other 'doctor', a 'German' like Smollett's corrupt Dietrich van Linden in *Humphry Clinker*, speaks in a thick accent and also possesses his own phallic telescope appropriately reading 'Positively Charg'd'. The English quack's 'instrument' is longer and capped with 'cream' at the tip – so risible that the portion in front of the English doctor's crotch reads: 'LARGEST IN THE WORLD'.

What is 'Positively Charg'd'? The gadgets and paraphernalia are merely playful diminutive emblems. The alligator and other animals display a sign that reads 'cured of the dropsy and gout in the stomach'. A dark, devil-like figure stands behind the foreign doctor threatening to vanquish the English doctor by 'sending eternal fire to him'. The print is cluttered with figures (people), standing objects (vials, medicines and inscriptions) and technologies (telescopes). Its thrust projects to the curers of gout, and the satirist makes plain the sequitur between warring quacks and the power at stake in their feuds. Both are aggressive males whose phallic motif unifies the caricature, especially for viewers who had become depressed or impotent.

Rehabilitation of those wishing to restore their sex urge was so widespread it was recognized as a topic for narrative in pictures.[60] In each drawing or canvas a 'story' is narrated, as in 'gout in the stomach' in 'The Quacks', which suggests the public's familiarity with medical terminology. In 'A Valuable Friend' another 'gout narrative' is coloured in.[61] The setting includes a posh drawing-room adorned by four males, one reclining in a chair, his swollen right leg bandaged with 'proud gout'. He remains anonymous while 'Major Nobs' stands upright appearing desperate: knees bowed in, wet pants revealing evacuations. Charles Chapwrit is the literary type whose name appropriately alliterates: slender, haggard, holding out his hat and cane to assist his 'good friend'. A rhymed couplet-caption reads: 'Yes, I perceive / He's a friend in kneed.' Rowlandson's print omits the *k*, preposterously rewritten in the next line with an *n*. A fourth figure buttresses his friend – the third – while peering in amazement at the pissing Major. The four playful characters of this urinatory irony are social peers. Here podagra's old ludic vintage surfaces, nor did it quickly disappear from the visual heritage.

The gouty protagonist is marvellously fluent despite his stretched-out pose, the master of ceremonies arranging his guests:

Ah Charles, how do?
Major; – Charles Chapwrit!
Charles, Major Nobs's my very best friend!

Is this badinage or some coded babble of an Old Boy system? The clues lie in Chapwrit's fashionable rank and Nobs's colonial grandeur. A larger-than-life virile Major Nobs is also revealing, as he appears on the verge of ejaculatory relief. Chapwrit is a town beau: sedentary hack, hard up, yet still in this affluent company. Slender, he has no gout – yet! – nor has his friend. Of the four, urinating Major Nobs is the ruddiest and the prize for incongruity goes to him: knock-kneed, bow-legged, asymmetrical limbs. He contrasts best with the invalid who is better off in every way: secure, insulated, enjoying life. If there is a 'moral' here it is this: go with the gouty chap. This may be why Rowlandson visualized profiles in the various stages of gout: we see only the protagonist's silhouette, his gesturing hand, and hear his words.

Ludos (play) and Eros (desire) mix here through micturition, in the friendship encoded in the plate's caption ('my very best friend'), and in light of gout's common metaphors of male fraternity. The iconic story seizes on the fraternal speech-act: 'my very best friend'. Each is a candidate for the 'honour of the gout'; each occupies a stage of its acquisition. The print is thus a 'progress piece' in the metaphoric sense gout itself was, as we saw in 'Goutometries'. One character afflicted (clearly gouty), a second on the verge (Major Nobs), a third still unafflicted but expectant (Charles Chapwrit), a minor fourth. Among these patricians – the 'club,' as in Johnson's or the

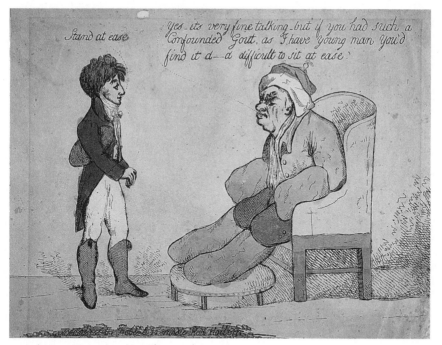

29. Anonymous print, 'A Military Salutation'. *c.* 1770.

Quadruple Alliance of Walpole, Gray *et al.* whom Cole expected *all* to end up gouty[62] – always lurked the expectation of acquisition. Such 'expectations' formed the essence of the podagra conceit.

Rowlandsonian caricatures were drawn throughout the nineteenth century; indeed they constitute a major segment of gout's visual heritage. A similarly incongruous scene lends meaning to the comic narrative in 'A Military Salutation' (*c.* 1770).[63] Here are only two figures: old-gouty, young-healthy. 'Stand at Ease,' the young soldier commands. The elder replies that, if the soldier were as sick as he is, he would not even talk. 'Yes – it's very fine talking, but if you had such a Confounded Gout, as I have young man, you'd find it d——d difficult to sit at ease.' Would viewers have thought the moral of this iconography clear? A right or wrong message? The description is threadbare: no backdrop, slight detail, two men, armchair, proverbial gout stool. The costume is equally simple: victim wrapped in grey flannels prescribed by the doctors; soldier lithe, ruddy, young, no trace of swollen limbs, an effective contrast.

Tension is established between the two morals of right and wrong. No attentive viewer could have overlooked the insensitivity of military personnel when confronted squarely with such illness, nor, secondly, the severity of the

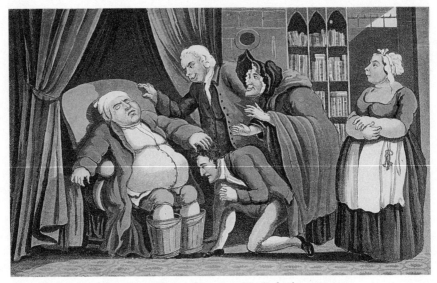

30.   Anonymous print, 'Quae Genus Discovers His Father'. *c.* 1770.

pain itself, as the patient's reply cuts to the quick of his pain. Other ironies
abound: the gap in age, youth's lack of empathy, the pedigree conceit in light
of implicit military barbarism ('Stand at Ease'). Considering the events of the
1770s the military message may have usurped the youthful one. But there
were no recorded military discharges for gout – gout was not a disease of the
young – and the caricaturist seems not to be commenting on war and illness
generally. A definitive meaning is even more difficult to pinpoint if the
caricature was one in a series. Besides, such ambiguities were routinely
inherent in the complex visual caricature of this period.

   In another caricature of the same decade entitled 'Quae Genus Discovers
His Father'[64] – 'the type who discovers his father' – the four characters resume
the symmetries of 'A Valuable Friend'. Here the 'podagra conceit' itself is on
trial: dynasties, legacies, fathers and sons and their sons. The bookshelves
demonstrate the knight's comfort, the drapes behind his gout chair his upper-
class status, no less than among the Brambles and Dedlocks of pictorial
caricature. The gouty father cannot be close to death: his robust, protruding
stomach is too fulsome for that despite legs immersed in pails of water. His
anguished son kneels at his side as his father holds his left hand over his son's
head. The standing couple's function is ambiguous. The chambermaid stands
at the right, house keys dangling, and rather well clad for a servant. The
caricature derives meaning from its action: the son's return, the same crucial
leitmotif that wove its way through the eighteenth-century novel from the

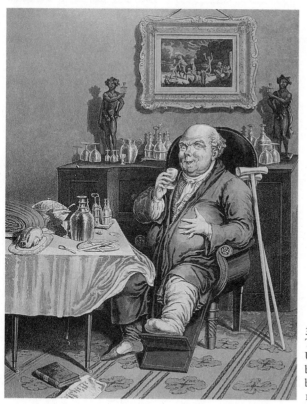

31. 'An Exquisite Taste, with an Enlarged Understanding'. Drawn by E. Y. Esq. Engraved by G. Hunt. London, 1827.

time of its appearance in Defoe's *Robinson Crusoe*.[65] Robinson's father had begged his second son not to go to sea, as he had already lost his eldest to its tempests; old and gouty, he implored Robinson to remain close to the hearth. 'Quae Genus' – the species or type – represents the other side of the trope: the son's *return* after a long time away.

The father displays no anger, despite his son's absence: time has not strained their relations. Morality here may lie in vacuum as well as in pedigree or illness: this, after all, is an upper-class father who will distribute his wealth. There is no impediment, no other son to inherit, nor does the action challenge the viewer to wonder what type of son would permit his father to linger in so chronic a condition. The focus on the represented ailment – gout – is significant as an insignia of the family's pedigree. If the intended morality centres on *absence*, then the neglected and chronically ill patriarch plays a particularly benign role in his son's return: the restoration of pedigree at all costs.

The trade in caricature developed gout for all it was worth. Themes were probed for profit, comically abused and milked until the public became

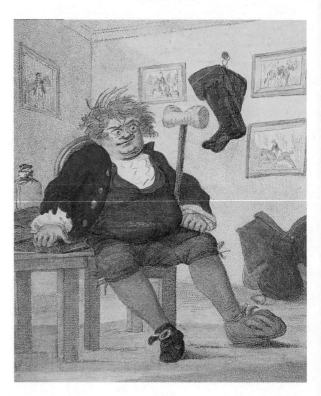

32. Anonymous print,
'Geoffrey Gambado
Esq.'. London, 1786.

cloyed and sought new ones. Not a decade passed without motifs developed
and exhausted, despite the old theme of excess remaining constant. Satire of
gourmands and gluttons continued almost *sans* interruption, gout their inevitable reward. In 'An Exquisite Taste, with an Enlarged Understanding',[66] the
gluttonous protagonist's reward is unequivocal. His life has been sedentary
and solitary. His table boasts chicken, salad dressing, a cooked casserole in a
porcelain terrine; yet he grasps for his liquor housed on his table in a large
bottle. He has tossed the proverbial crutches, hung his swollen leg on the
gout stool, avid for his bibulous sport which clutters his room. Two copper
busts of Bacchants – gods of the grape – adorn his table, as do flasks awaiting
consumption.

   The plot within the plot also requires decoding. The painting above his
table reveals a pastoral scene with naked gods imbibing the sacred fluid and
dwelling in a state of Nature. They beckon a clothed man to join in their
orgy. A large nude woman rides a horse in the centre of the painting, under
ominously gathering black clouds threatening to thunder down with rain, but
the vivants continue. Meanwhile, our gouty hedonist imbibes another drink,
his hand approvingly clutching his stomach to clinch the delight of this
gulp. The floor is littered with 'Phil Gorger's' book entitled *DOMESTIC*

COOKERY and a recipe for 'Prune Current' that commences with port, sherry and bordeaux.[67] All is in the grape. The ornate imari foot-rest has been drawn precisely in the line of the protagonist's opulent chair, every bit as ornate, its leaf adjustable to his vast leg. The moral is loud and plain: indulge in excess and suffer the consequences. If 'Quae Genus' celebrated sons and fathers, 'An Exquisite Taste' derides consumption of the economic variety through smiles and smirks.

The riding therapy Sydenham touted for gouteans continued to surface in gout's visual heritage after the late eighteenth century. Its effects rippled throughout art, not merely gouty satire, as in a favourite caricature often reprinted as 'Geoffrey Gambado Esq', published in the heyday of the steer craze when gentlemen proved their rank by riding.[68] The corpulent 'Gambado Esquire' (*gambado* as in riders' boots offering protection from horse pelts and inclement weather) suffers an acute fit of 'flying gout': his hair so wild, his eyes so accentuated, he appears unable to endure the attack. He prances and jolts, as his capering name suggests. His costume has not insulated him, suggesting that the saddle may be worse than the 'flying attack' itself.

Gambado's swollen left foot is wrapped in flannel. The instrument he employs is no cane but the crutch used by those with broken arms and legs. Riding has been his pre-eminent remedy for prevention – the virtual obsession of the great and rich at the end of the eighteenth century. Engravings of horseback riders therefore adorn his walls, and his own 'gambados' hang in full view.[69] His table reveals his book, the proverbial sign of gouty sedentary life before *and* after affliction. The irony is that sedentary pastimes, while healthy, have landed all these gambados in the prisonhouse of gout; yet, once afflicted and incarcerated, the sedentary life became the only one available, mercilessly so in view of its benign insulations. Gambado's maker, Henry William Bunbury, was particularly explicit on the sedentary malady,[70] and if there were space he would deserve more attention here.

But 'Gambado the rider' is no solitary reaper of the evils of excess; his visual brothers were many, if few his sisters, even if now lost to time – his fraternal tribe racked by gout and unimproved by horses. Gambado's caricaturist revelled in his art and was pleased to depict his scepticism about the 'riding cures'.[71] Other caricaturists were satisfied with puncturing the excesses of the table – viands of every type – through equestrian images. For example, in 'Punch Cures the Gout'[72] three saucy characters appear in a posh Regency room riotously imbibing 'punch' as their new cure. The consumptive male on the left is predictably slender; the colic woman ruddy – the colic then not thought to be gender-specific as was gout; and the merry gouty chap so far degenerated that only his right hand remains to hold up the glass.

Running like a fibre throughout these prints is fluid: as drink, water,

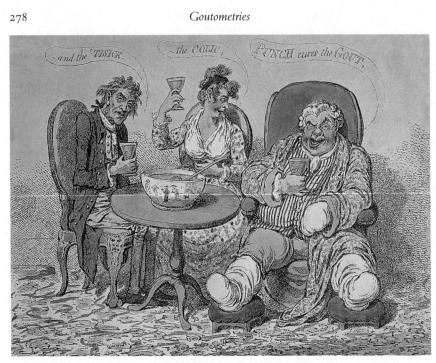

33.   Anonymous print, 'Punch Cures the Gout'. 1799.

soothing liquid. So had it been from the seventeenth-century visual heritage. An illustrated German emblem book of 1715 contains plates showing equally merry bewigged gents with both feet and hands tied to fluid:[73] hands uplifting their wine (not yet punch), their still healthy feet showered with water of some type. Is this symmetry an irony or something else? The text offers no clue but by the time punch the drink was introduced (*c.* 1800–20), gouteans were among its primary users, their pedigree already playing a role in the famous magazine of that name that commenced in 1841.[74] Unlike gin, punch was class-bound, its price too high for the common man. Fluid, not food, is the theme of both these prints: more specifically, the consequences to those who consume fluid to excess.

Gout also had a diverse political edge, even if its visual heritage was not usually so thumpingly moralistic. 'A Cure for the Gout'[75] develops two motifs: gout's psychological effects and the rapidity with which its course could alter. Here the patient receives a letter informing him that his political party has been restored to power in Parliament. Cheered, he instructs his servant to unwrap his flannels, summon his carriage and chauffeur, and convey him to town. Hosanna: he has been cured in a flash. Yet his silence about the transformation is as significant as the malady itself:

what after all *was* gout if it variegated its shapes with such rapidity? Another servant muses: 'That letter seems to have completely cured my Lord's gout, which he has had so *badly* ever since the opening of Parliament – I'd lay a wager *there is a change in the Ministry*.' No wonder 'cure' appears in the caption.

This political edge never exceeded the comic threshold of any of its manifestations. Within the history of caricature gout functioned as a type of mock-heroic equivalent in pictures. Just as nothing dire ever happens in Pope's *Rape of the Lock* or *The Dunciad*, despite dreadful consequences, so was it in this visual ephemera often hovering on the periphery of politics. Here the victim's disclaimer serves to dramatize gout's phantasmagoria: if his malady *had* been dangerous, he would not have swerved so quickly. The deflated 'political cure' tallies with the intelligence that there has been 'a change in the Ministry'.

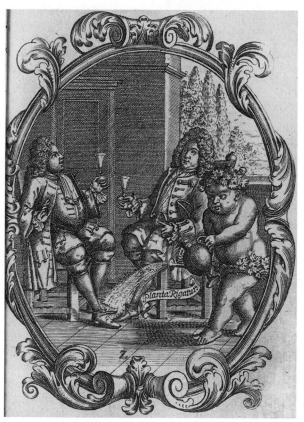

34. Anonymous,
*Dissertationes de laudibus
et effectibus podagrae.* 1715.

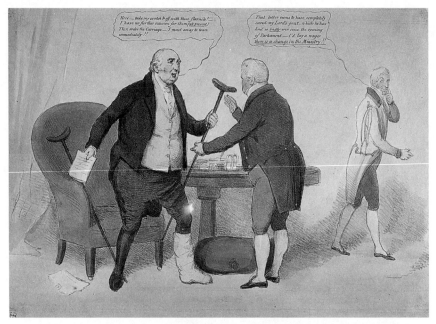

35. Anonymous print, 'A Cure for the Gout.' London, early nineteenth century.

Parliament's sway at that time extended to the regulation of drugs and the ways they could be advertised. The controls on corruption were loose and encouraged ridiculous puffery, especially in the newspapers. Jewish physician Abraham Buzaglo's 'radical gout cure' of 1778 was among the most puffed.[76] He claimed that Parliament had given him a bursary to launch his miracle medicine, and declaimed in print no less confidently than the mountebanks in Hyde Park:

> The Author has now ready for the Press, and will, as soon as he shall be enabled by a liberal Subscription, or a Grant from Parliament, to give to the Public, The GRAND SECRET, (A discovery entirely distinct from that of the *Exercise*) Which is of such admirable Efficacy, as to procure *immediate* Relief in the most violent Fit of the Gout, and *infallibly* to effect a *perfect Cure* within a Week after the first Application: The most inveterate, the most obstinate Gout, must in that short Space of Time give Way to the Power of this Discovery, which, if made public, would enable every Man to become his own Physician, banish the Gout from the World, and for ever rid Mankind of the Apprehension of its Return. FINIS

'FINIS': the rhetoric is as crashingly loud as is the visual impact of the upper cases. Other gouty texts were less brazen, others more, but always lying on the edge of the political domain. In 'Here's a dreadful situation',[77] an afflicted creature sits in his chair exclaiming to what a 'dreadful situation' his 'infernal gout' has brought him. The poker has fallen out of the fireplace, tipping over the tea kettle, whose scalding water has dropped on to the unsuspecting cat, who leaps forward for self-preservation, and on to the patient's already swollen feet. The mode can be dubbed the 'comic pathetic' – the grotesque pathetic of the comic novelists – rather than the 'sublime pathetic' of history painting or tragedy. Hence the patient's summons to 'Betty the maid' and his exclamation of grotesque horror. But who are the villains? Is it the accident, heat therapy, the nature of therapy itself? Is the satirist indicating that no amount of heat will satisfy these patients – it therefore serves them well to be

THE Author has now ready for the Prefs, and will, as foon as he fhall be enabled by a liberal Subfcription, or a Grant from Parliament, give to the Public, The

GRAND SECRET,

(A Difcovery entirely diftinct from that of the *Exercife*)

Which is of fuch admirable Efficacy, as to procure *immediate* Relief in the moft violent Fit of the Gout, and *infallibly* to effect a *perfect Cure* within a Week after the firft Application: The moft inveterate, the moft obftinate Gout, muft in that fhort Space of Time give Way to the Power of this Difcovery, which, if made public, would enable every Man to become his own Phyfician, banifh the Gout from the World, and for ever rid Mankind of the Apprehenfion of its Return.

F I N I S.

36. A. Buzaglo, *A Treatise on the gout* . . . Page 56. London, 1778.

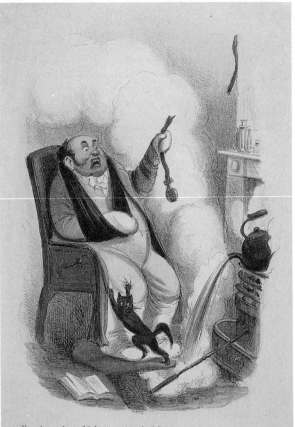

37. Anonymous print, 'Here's a dreadful situation . . .'. *c.* 1840.

Here's a dreadful situation! Murder! Betty! Here's the poker fell out! I shall be scalded to death! Oh this infernal gout!

scalded (fluid again)? The accident cannot be to blame: a scalder might have fallen out. The moralist within the caricaturist makes his point through the absurd generation of heat, but leaves the rest to the viewer's imagination.

The visual heritage we have presented is representative rather than exhaustive. We could also have demonstrated that cartoons about contemporary gout continue to appear in the media constructed in the comic and grotesque traditions surveyed here, but this would have been repetitive. These are the main varieties and they make the point about word and image in a *longue durée* in which they were intimately connected. Moreover, it would be excessive to claim that gout's visual heritage has been extraordinary within the history of art. Yet this heritage offers us much insight into the impact gout made on the observant eye. It reveals, first and foremost, its comic mode:

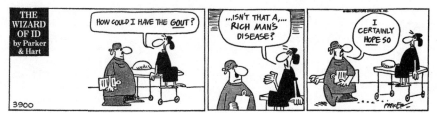

38. Parker & Hunt, 'How could I have the Gout?' *The Wizard of Id, Evening Standard*, 12 April 1996.

what struck the eye as inherently ridiculous through exaggeration and grotesque enlargement. In this sense its visual significance adumbrated discursive excess. As such it was tied, even firmly moored, to the discursive metaphoric traditions we analysed in Chapter 11, even if they were richer by virtue of their breadth.[78]

Epilogue

Ours are times when health commentators are expressing deep anxieties about the 'diseasification' of everything. All facets of human behaviour, all sides of the psyche, the critics argue, are nowadays being represented as symptomatic of some or other disease which has its own indications, diagnostic tests, experts and specialist treatments (typically complex and expensive). Newspaper accounts proliferate with exotic cases. Diagnostic handbooks mushroom.[1] This may well be, at the close of the twentieth century, a thoroughly undesirable development for patients and society alike, and there are strong reasons to be apprehensive that modern medical imperialism may, albeit inadvertently, multiply costs without enhancing health.[2]

Before accepting this blanket condemnation as true, however, we should pause for a moment. For such developments may tell us less about the overweening pretensions of the medical profession than about the post-modern proliferation of signifiers in a world dominated by images and the media. Those producing the images (TV, film, popular pulp and now the Internet and cyberspace) rather than the doctors and their paramedical assistants may be at fault. Literary theorists have come to recognize that everything is capable of representing everything else; hence we should not be surprised if there are (virtually) no limits to the ways in which disease may take on the attributes of discourse.[3]

Nor is the multiplication of disease discourse inevitably a bad thing, provided that power over the semiotics of sickness lies in the hands of sufferers or users empowered to deploy illness language in ways which are not necessarily more stigmatizing than any alternative terms of description and evaluation. This post-Foucaldian point is the nub of the matter. Why should the language of sickness *not* be available for staking out claims about the self? Might *not* there be a therapeutic value and possibly even virtual healthiness in owning one's own disorders?

This latter, we would argue, is the situation which our broadly designated 'history and philosophy of gout' has time and again disclosed, be it in an Erasmus, a Smollett or a Horace Walpole. 'Gout', it turns out, has been an irreducibly protean malady, a chameleon ailment associated with mind and body, with structures (joints) and functions (fluxes); indeed – in view of its

284

popular anchorage in the toe – a condition indexed to an extraordinary multiplicity of anatomical parts, be they extremities or innards.

Gout, moreover, has been estimable, indeed the eligible malady *par excellence*, the patrician malady to top out all others, a malaise one would *want* to possess even as it possessed one's own body. It has been the sign of distinction. It has equally been a shield, protecting the sufferer from distraction. Not least it has been a mark of mystique, in ways which, in some respects, bear comparison and share affinities (as our text has shown) with epilepsy, nervous disorders, consumption and 'good madness'. Hence one of the endeavours of this book has been to delve deeply into how people come to 'choose' to be ill and, being ill, which sickness they select and how they sell it. In this inquiry, we have explored medical writings and literary texts, journals and diaries, and, alongside this verbal testimony, visual evidence no less in view of the salutary importance of the production of images.

In so doing, we have, among other things, been offering an alternative historical and philosophical position to that set out in two books by Susan Sontag. In her *Illness as Metaphor* and *AIDS as Metaphor*, Sontag has argued, passionately and compassionately, for the desirability of demystifying disease: disease should be a scientific category not a cultural and moral sign or stigma.[4] The present book, by contrast, has suggested that the witness of history weighs heavily *against* this position – a stance which is undeniably high-minded if perhaps guilty of swallowing the propaganda of scientism. Perhaps there was more to swallow when Sontag wrote in the late 1970s and 1980s than as we approach a millenarian medicine now so complex and expensive it threatens to engulf every aspect of our lives. People and cultures always have given meaning to disease. And that is partly because disease categories have helped to articulate the experience of the body itself, and hence the project of the individual person. As is revealed by the story of gout over the long haul, there is meaning to the metaphors, images and representations of disease. It cannot have been otherwise given what humanity and human nature have amounted to in cultural history.

Notes

Page references are entered for articles and books only if attention is called to specific passages.

Chapter 1: Introduction

1. Classic is Mary Douglas (1966).
2. Nicolson and Rousseau (1968).
3. See Oppenheim (1991); Shorter (1992); *idem* (1994).
4. Charles E. Rosenberg (1989), 1–15, p. 3, and the 'Introduction' to Rosenberg and Golden, eds (1992), xiii–xxvi. For a sample of recent works on maladies and their meanings, see Gilman (1982); *idem* (1988); *idem* (1985); Sontag (1978); *idem* (1989). On hysteria, see Gilman, King, Porter, Rousseau and Showalter (1993), and Micale (1995); for leprosy, Saul Nathaniel Brody (1974).
5. Dirckx (1983); Roy Porter (1995) in a volume exploring jargon.
6. For the history and sociology of the body, see Feher, ed. (1989); Bryan S. Turner (1984); *idem* (1991); and Arthur W. Frank (1991). For the personal uses of illness, see Pickering (1976); for perceptive pathobiography, see Ober (1979).
7. Sterne, *The Sentimental Journey* (1967), 52. For Sterne's fables of disease, see D. Furst (1974); Rodgers (1978); Roy Porter (1989b).
8. Especially valuable for biographical and literary insights are the writings of G. S. Rousseau: for a beginning, see (1991b); *idem* (1993): the long

introduction to that volume gives extensive references. See also Howard Brody (1987); *idem* (1992); Kleinman (1980); *idem* (1986); *idem* (1988); Hunter (1991). A pioneering attempt to deconstruct gout from a literary-cum-psychoanalytical viewpoint is found in Gordon (1993).
9. Toothache and dentistry are traditionally comic: see Kunzle (1989). It might also be objected that the history of gout has already been written. But though Copeman's *A Short History of the Gout and the Rheumatic Diseases* (1964) has many virtues, not least the author's expertise as a rheumatologist, it is now over thirty years old; it lacks references; and it is overtly Whiggish. Moreover, its quotations are riddled with inaccuracies. We have gratefully drawn on Copeman but believe a further history is now needed. Mertz (1990) is a rather brief overview incorporating little new research.
10. See [Anon.] (1959); Philander Misaurus (1699); and for serio-comic reversal, Marten (1737). Gout meets the criteria of the grotesque: Bakhtin (1968); Paster (1993).
11. Norton, ed. (1956), ii, 239. This and other passages rework material from Roy Porter (1994).
12. Lady Holland, ed. (1855), ii, 565: Smith, letter to Countess Grey, 24

August 1841. See also Wallace (1962), and Virgin (1994), 276–7.

13. Chapman, ed. (1984), ii, 138, letter 485, 3 June 1776; J. P. W. Rogers (1986), and Wiltshire (1991), 35–6.

14. For epidemic diseases, see Crosby (1976); McNeill (1976); Charles E. Rosenberg (1962); Evans (1987); *idem* (1988). Fee and Fox, eds (1988).

15. For responses to non-lethal, painful and chronic complaints, see Roy Porter and Dorothy Porter (1988), and Dorothy Porter and Roy Porter (1989).

16. Gout of course flies around in *Pickwick Papers* and in *Bleak House*: for Dickens and medicine see Bailin (1994), 80f. Rodnan (1961) notes that gout has grown obsolete among cartoonists.

17. There are no book-length histories of rheumatism, arthritis or bronchitis, though see Brewerton (1992). As AIDS becomes viewed as a chronic condition, the history of chronic diseases will probably achieve higher profile: see Fee and Fox, eds (1992).

18. The clinical and epidemiological data offered here are largely distilled from Benedek (1993a); *idem* (1993b); Denko (1993); Duncan and Leison (1993); Estes (1993); French (1993b); Steinbock (1993b).

19. Quoted in Lady Holland (1855), i, 35.

20. Comrie (1922), 59.

21. Currie (1979). On women, see Benedek (1997).

22. Hartung (1954).

23. Rodnan and Benedek (1963).

24. Abbott *et al.* (1988).

25. [Anon.] (1967); Breckenridge (1966), i, 15–18; Montoye *et al.* (1967).

26. 'I have heard of two or three cases of the GOUT among the Indians, but it was only among those who had learned the use of rum from the white people': Rush (1947), 263–4.

27. Mody and Naidoo (1984); Beighton *et al.* (1987).

28. 'Consumption' puns on another relationship between disease and socio-economic behaviour: Roy Porter (1993c).

29. See L. Stevenson (1965); Roy Porter (1991a); *idem* (1993a). On degeneration, see Inglis (1981); Pick (1989); Chamberlin and Gilman, eds (1985); Starobinski (1992); for early medical discussions, see Tissot (1768); *idem* (1771); Thomas Trotter (1807).

30. On how disease concepts inscribe gender, see Geyer-Kordesch (1993); Jordanova (1989); Schiebinger (1989); *idem* (1993), Gilman, King, Porter, Rousseau and Showalter (1993); Micale (1995).

31. Compare dejection. In the Renaissance, upper-class depression was dignified as melancholia, among the lower orders it was stigmatized as 'mopishness': MacDonald (1981). Analysis of distinction is offered in Bourdieu (1984). For exposure of the use of maladies like hypochondriasis, hysteria, melancholy, nerves and consumption as signs of superiority, see Beddoes (1802); *idem* (1806); Roy Porter (1991a).

32. See Ellis (1927); Becker (1978); Sass (1992).

33. See Bell (1985); Vandereycken and Van Deth (1994).

34. Sontag (1978).

35. For the history of disease theory, see Riese (1953); Risse (1978); Temkin (1961); Engelhardt (1975). For the social dynamics of sickness, see Parsons (1958); Mechanic (1962).

36. See De Kruif (1926) and Greer Williams (1959).

37. See Grmek (1994); Root-Bernstein (1993).

38. Balint (1957); Watts (1992).

39. Canguilhem (1989); Bynum and Nutton, eds (1981).

40. Starobinski (1992); Bakan (1971); De Moulin (1974); Hodgkiss (1991); Keele (1957); C. S. Lewis (1940);

David B. Morris (1991); Scarry (1985); Szasz (1957); Roy Porter (1993b).

41. The following information is culled from Benedek (1993a and b); Denko (1993); Duncan and Leison (1993); Davies (1993); Estes (1993); Steinbock (1993a and b).

42. Hart (1976); Short (1959). Traditional remedies include buckthorn, burdock, centaury, chickweed, comfrey, elder, meadowsweet, restharrow, violet, wintergreen and wormwood.

43. *Agnivesa's Caraka Samhita* (1976).

44. Baillou (1940), 141–62.

45. *Ibid.*

46. Quoted in Copeman (1964), 121–2.

47. *Ibid.*, 122.

48. English (1992); Parish (1963 and 1964).

49. Alfred Garrod (1876), 498; see also the contributions by his son, Archibald Garrod (1890); *idem* (1923–4); *idem* (1897).

50. Copeman (1964), 185.

51. Archibald Garrod (1890).

52. For focal infection, see Dally (1993); Scull (1987). On arthritis treatments see Heywood (1990); Cantor (1990); *idem* (1991); *idem* (1993b); Hart (1976); Quinones (1966); Marks (1992).

53. Among other words showing similar origins is 'dripping', that is, the fat falling from roasting meat. The connotations of the term 'gout' would be interesting to pursue. In seventeenth-century vernacular parlance, 'gout' (as in 'Spanish gout' or 'Covent Garden gout') was a euphemism for venereal disease. Semantics have ruffled feathers:

> The etymology of the word *gout* is by no means clear. I myself had simply followed Garrod, who, according to the German translation of his work, regards the word *Gicht* as corresponding to the English *gout*, the French *goutte*, etc. Virchow has recently derived the word *Gicht* from the Latin *gutta*, but although this derivation agrees with the old ideas that were held as to the origin of gout, yet I cannot allow that *Gicht* comes from the same stem. According to my colleague, Professor Moritz Heyne, who is editing 'Grimm's Dictionary of the German Language', *Gicht* is the same as the Anglo-Saxon masculine *gihda* (the d in the pronunciation being the same as the English th), and the meaning is 'bodily pain in general'. *Gicht* is thus, properly speaking, a general term, and may be compared to the word *weh* = *woe*, *pain*. (Ebstein (1886), 41).

54. Duden (1991).

55. A few further introductory points should be made. This work concentrates on the period from the seventeenth to the early twentieth century: that was the time when gout interacted most fascinatingly with the culture at large. The sources studied have chiefly been English and, to a lesser degree, French-language. The German story has recently been told by Mertz (1990). On the national history of diseases, see Payer (1989).

Chapter 2: The Classical Inheritance

1. Hartung (1957). For attempts to establish the first case of gout in a historical personage: see Devries and Weinberger (1974); F. Rosner (1969). For palaeopathological and archaeological evidence, see Cockburn and Cockburn (1980), 37f.; Calvin Wells (1964); Bird (1957); Jackson (1988), 177–9; Grmek (1989), 72–3.

2. Seneca (1917–28), letter xcv, lines 16–18, pp. 66–9. Pliny the Younger held similar views: Hartung (1957).

3. Nutton (1985); Jackson (1988), 40, 166, 170, 177–9. The story, however, may be more complicated than meets the eye, since the alleged spread of gout under the empire was possibly due not to 'luxury' as such but to lead poisoning, occasioned by the use of metallic wine casks and/ or adulteration. See Wedeen (1981; 1984a; 1984b). See also Nriagu (1983); Gaebel and Nriagu (1983); Jackson (1988), 177–9.

Pliny the Elder called gout 'an ailment of foreign origins': (1949), xxvi, 100. Pliny the Younger recorded the case of a friend, Rufus, who suffered from gout for many years:

> At the age of thirty-two, I have heard him say, he developed gout in the feet, just as his father had done, for like other characteristics, most diseases are hereditary. As long as he was young and active he could keep it under control by temperate living and strict continence, and latterly when he grew worse with advancing age, he bore up through sheer strength of mind, even when cruelly tortured by unbelievable agony. ((1972, 1975), i, 12)

4. Hartung (1957); see Aretaeus (1856), 362.
5. Nutton (1993). For background and discussion, see Phillips (1973); Lloyd (1983); Grmek (1989); Edelstein (1967); Scarborough (1969). For arthritis within the empire, see Jackson (1988), 177–9.
6. 'Catarrh' also expressed the same conception of a flowing humour: French (1993b). In humoralism, much disease was attributed to a downflow of corrosive catarrh fluid from the brain through the base of the skull to various organs. In the lung it was supposed to cause abscess and phthisis, in the joints rheumatism and gout, in the legs ulceration

and decay. 'Catarrh' was thus a classic product of humoral pathology. A further linguistic parallel would be dropsy, for which see Peitzman (1992); Estes (1993); Appelboom and Bennett (1986).

7. Byl (1988) notes that the Greek 'arthron' (joint) occurs some 300 times in the *Corpus*; words denoting gout occur some twenty times.
8. Hippocrates, *On the Affections of the Parts*. See Hippocrates, *Aphorisms*, in vol. 4 of Hippocrates (1923–31).
9. Hippocrates, *Aphorisms*, in vol. 4 of Hippocrates (1923–31). The three other (non-sexual) aphorisms respecting gout are no. 25: swelling and pains in the joints, without sores whether from gout or sprains, in most cases are relieved by a copious affusion of cold water; no. 40: in gouty affections inflammation subsides within forty days; and no. 55: gout affections become active in spring and in the autumn. See also Kersley (1956); McFadzean (1965).
10. Copeman (1964), 23. Gout in males thus performed a similar function to menstruation in women, evacuating morbific matter. After menopause, such matter had to be discharged from women in some other way.
11. Galen (1821–33; 1965), xi, 275.
12. Aretaeus (1856), 363–4. See Copeman (1964), 35.
13. Aretaeus (1856), 362; Copeman (1964), 43.
14. For Celsus, see *Of Medicine in Eight Books* (1756), 227.
15. Jackson (1988), 179.
16. Phillips (1973), 35.
17. For Rufus, see Abou-Aly (1992), ch. iii. Gilbertus Anglicus, the first Englishman to write on gout, quoted freely from Rufus: Getz, ed. (1991).
18. See Paul of Aegina (1834), 354; and (1844), i, 657. The quotation comes from Book III, ch. lxxviii. Paul wrote: 'When, therefore, the humour is seated in the joints of the feet only, the complaint is called podagra; but when the cause is dif-

fused over all the joints of the body, we commonly call it arthritis': 41.

19. *Ibid.* The importance of passions of the mind was, of course, much later to be reasserted by William Cadogan. See below, Chapter 7.

20. Rodnan (1965).

21. Copeman (1964), 24–5. During the seventeenth century this method of counter-irritation was reintroduced into Europe from the Orient, using a form of cotton plant.

22. On Celsus' reservations, see (1756), 227.

23. For Galen's justification of copious and regular bloodletting, see Brain (1986).

24. Brain (1986); Ferez (1987).

25. Aretaeus (1856), 492–3; Copeman (1964), 43; Rodnan and Benedek (1963); Schnitker (1936).

26. Alexander (1933–7); Wallace (1973), 130–5; Hartung (1954), 190–200. There are hints of the use of colchicum as a gout specific in Paul of Aegina and Aetius (502–75).

27. Gunther, ed. (1934). For what follows, see Riddle (1985), 44f. *Colchicum autumnale* grows in meadows and pastures in northern Africa, middle and southern Europe, and is plentiful in southern England and Ireland. The dried bulb and seeds are powerfully diuretic, purgative and emetic. It can be fatal to animals.

    Pedacius Dioscorides (*fl.* AD 50) is believed to have been born in Anazarba, Cilicia in Asia Minor and to have been educated in Nero's army in Alexandria. His *materia medica*, assembled about AD 70, was the authoritative work on the subject for fifteen centuries.

28. Ibn Mâsawaih (Mesuë, *c.* 954–1015) followed Dioscorides' lead by making colocynth a principal gout remedy.

29. Colchicum long had its detractors, notably Haig (1901).

30. For Seneca, see *Epistulae Morales* (1917–28), letter xcv, lines 16–18, pp. 66–9. For gout in mythology, see

Rodnan (1961). Greek heroes and gods allegedly suffering from gout were listed by Stukeley (1734), 53. They included Priam, Achilles, Oedipus, Protesilaus, Ulysses, Bellerophon and Plesthemes. Doubtless Stukeley got his list from Lucian.

31. Lucian (1749), 229, quoted in Rodnan (1965), 599.

32. Lucian (1967): *Gout.* We discuss his importance to the metaphoric and visual traditions in Chapters 11 and 12.

33. *Ibid.*, 337–41. Lucian's verses were quoted by later authors; for instance Sennert (1632), Swieten (1744–73) and Sydenham (1683).

34. *Lucian* (1967), 343.

35. *Ibid.*, 347.

36. *Ibid.*, 353.

37. *Ibid.*, 353.

38. *Ibid.*, 359.

39. For the medieval background, see Cameron (1993); Cockayne (1864); Talbot (1967); Hunt (1990) – the accounts of thirteenth-century remedies presented by Hunt include references to gout; *idem* (1992); Getz, ed. (1991). The body metaphor (as plant, fortress and so on) is explored in Pouchelle (1990).

40. Gruner (1938), 479 (paragraphs 952 and 953).

41. Hartung (1957), 201.

42. Copeman (1964), 2; Lascaratos (1995).

43. See the *Oxford English Dictionary* (1989), vi, 707 (gout) and xi, 1112 (podagra): 'In his fot ane hote goute, that poudagre iclepeod is and Came a Goute In his Kneo of Anguische gret (*c.* 1290).' 'Rheumatic' is first recorded in English in 1398, in a translation from Bartholomaeus Anglicus. 'Gutta' is also an anglicized term. 'Gutta' was also a common word in pharmacy for a drop (of a medicine, for example).

44. Rodnan (1968). 'St Gervaisius' Disease became a popular name for any rheumatic affliction. Since Roman times St Gervais-les-Bains has been a well-frequented spa on the

Bon-Nant river in south-east France.
45. Saye (1934).
46. Getz, ed. (1991), 250: 'Stones ben-y-gendrid in a man-is reines and also in the bladdir.'

Chapter 3: Prometheus's Vulture: The Renaissance Fashioning of Gout

1. See Siraisi (1990); Katherine Park (1985); Slack (1979); Roy Porter, ed. (1992). For printing, see Eisenstein (1979).
2. Copeman and Winder (1969). Copeman and Winder reproduce the text in translation, and we have drawn our account from theirs. Burgawer states that 'The majority of people believe that gout [podagra] cannot be cured,' adding, 'Daily experience has convinced them of that' (A2^r). This implies that 'podagra' was a familiar condition.
3. In architectural English, 'gutta' is the word for the little drops underneath triglyphs on Doric entablatures.
4. Burgawer, A2^v; Copeman and Winder (1969), 289.
5. Copeman and Winder (1969), 289 (all these somewhat eccentric spellings are as in the translation); Benedek (1987), 186. On the non-naturals see Niebyl (1971); Rather (1968).
6. Rhazes (al-Razi, *c.* 850–932) was born in Persia. His twenty-volume masterpiece *Al-Hawi* or *El Hawi* contains medical knowledge from Greece, the Roman Empire, India, Syria and Persia, supplemented by his personal experiences.
7. Paré's works will be cited in the translation by Thomas Johnson (1634), Book xviii. See Malgaigne (1965). Following apprenticeship to a barber–surgeon, Ambroise Paré (1510–90) completed his training in

Paris. He is best known for his treatment of battle-wounds.
8. Paré (1634), 698. See the discussion in Copeman (1964), 53ff.
9. Paré (1634), 697.
10. *Ibid.*
11. *Ibid.*, 707.
12. *Ibid.*, 710.
13. Swiss-born, Paracelsus (Philippus Aureolus Theophrastus Bombastus von Hohenheim, 1493–1541) trained in medicine with his father. He travelled widely, but later went to Basel as city physician. He advocated simplicity in his recipes and his experiences in chemistry prompted him to use heavy metals. He left Basel as his teachings were considered too unorthodox. For his writings on gout, see 'Das Buch von den Tartarischen Krankheitten', in Paracelsus (1589–90). His works may be found in Sudhoff, ed. (1922–33) and Bernard Aschner, ed. (1975–7). For scholarship, see Pagel (1958a); Debus (1977); *idem* (1991); *idem* (1965).
14. See Pagel (1958a), 135.
15. *Ibid.*, 139.
16. *Ibid.*, 140.
17. *Ibid.*
18. *Ibid.*, 157.
19. The formation of stones within the human body was widely viewed as an expression of living nature. See Rudwick (1976), ch. i; Pagel (1984), 33.
20. Cited and translated in Rodnan (1965), 601, and in Pagel (1984), 33–4. See Paracelsus (1574), 28–37, which may be found in Aschner, ed. (1975–7), ii, 6–27. Paracelsus' ideas resist being translated into modern chemical equivalents. Contextualization of Paracelsus' writings within Renaissance natural philosophy is offered in Goodrick-Clarke (1990); *idem* trans. (1990b); Paracelsus (1941); *idem* (1951).
21. Théodore Turquet de Mayerne (1573–1655) was born in Geneva and studied at the University of

Heidelberg, later at Montpellier, where he graduated MD in 1597. Moving to Paris he lectured on anatomy and pharmacy and was appointed King's physician. He made use of chemical remedies, drawing condemnation from the Paris College of Physicians. Visiting England in 1606 he was appointed physician to Queen Anne of Denmark and returning in 1611 became physician to four successive monarchs. In 1618 he wrote the dedication to the King of the *Pharmacopoea Londinensis* (1618). He was knighted in 1624.

22. Turquet de Mayerne (1676), 14–15. See Debus (1965), 150–6, though this unfortunately does not mention gout; for the Paracelsian tradition, *idem* (1977); *idem* (1991); Webster (1975).

23. Boorde (1562a); *idem* (1587). See Copeman (1964), 50–1. For surveys of early-modern English medicine, see *idem* (1960); Nagy (1988); Beier (1987).

24. Boorde (1587). Andrew Boorde (1490–1549) entered the Carthusian order. He left this in 1528 and studied medicine on the Continent. He returned to England in 1542 and set up a medical practice in Winchester. His main works were: *Dyetery of Health* (1562), *Breviary of Helthe for all Manner of Syckenesses and Diseases* (1587) and a travel guide, *The First Boke of the Introduction of Knowledge* (1562).

25. Boorde (1587). Treacle is theriac, a complex opium preparation, with a multitude of ingredients: see Watson (1966). Scammony is the Syrian bindweed (*Convulvulus scammonia*). It is a strong cathartic, somewhat similar to jalap.

26. On cinchona (Jesuit's bark, Peruvian bark, the basis of quinine) see Jarcho (1993). *Fraxinus excelsior*, the bark and seeds of ash, is an astringent, its seeds an aperient.

27. Boorde's contemporary, Sir Thomas Elyot, issued warnings on that score, however, to the effect that 'Radysh rootes . . . cause to breake wynde and to pysse . . . they be unwholsome for theym, that have continually the goute or peynes in the joyntes': Elyot (1937), 28. Elyot wrote of 'reumes' as a synonym of catarrh.

28. Graham and Graham (1955).

29. Barrough (1590), 210. The 1st edn appeared in 1583; the 3rd in 1596; the 4th in 1610; the 5th in 1617; the 6th in 1624; the 7th in 1634; the 8th in 1639.

30. *Ibid.*

31. Cogan (1584), title page (in Latin). The reference to Hippocrates shows Cogan was stressing the non-naturals. See Niebyl (1971); Rather (1968). Thomas Cogan (1545?–1607) studied in Oxford and became a fellow of Oriel in 1563. His works include *The Well of Wisedome . . .* (1577), and *The Haven of Health Made for the Comfort of Students* (1584).

32. Cogan (1584), Epistle Dedicatorie (at beginning).

33. *Ibid.*, 161. The cheese-and-bacon poultice long continued popular.

34. *Ibid.*, facing p. 4 of the Epistle Dedicatorie.

35. For an overview on treatment, see Ackerknecht (1973) and Urdang (1944). For herbal cures, see Arber (1938); Foust (1992); B. Griggs (1981). For folk remedies, see W. G. Black (1883); Chamberlain (1981); Loux (1978); *idem* (1979); *idem* (1988); *idem* (1993). In twentieth-century America, folk cures for gout have included angelica, birch leaves (as a blood purifier), holly, strawberry, primrose root and various other bitters: see Crellin and Philpott (1991); Barton and Castle (1877), 108f.

36. Nash (1600), p. E.

37. Gilman (1989); Andreski (1990); Quétel (1990).

38. Joubert (1989), 260.

39. Yet I am better

Than one that's sick o' th' gout,
since he had rather
Groan so in perpetuity than be cur'd
By th' sure physician, Death,

proclaims the imprisoned Posthumus in *Cymbeline* (V.iv.4). In *Henry IV, Part 2* (I.ii.273) Falstaff declares: 'A pox of this gout! or, a gout of this pox! For the one or the other plays the rogue with my great toe.' Kail (1986), 232; see also Hoeniger (1992).

40. *Henry IV, Part 2*, I.ii.256.
41. This and the following come from Copeman (1964), 54–5; see also Appelboom and Bennett (1986).
42. Dying at fifty-three, he was succeeded by his young son, Lorenzo the Magnificent (1449–92), who, although inheriting the family gout, was less harshly afflicted than his father and grandfather, becoming the Italian Maecenas. On gout and the Medici, see Schevil (1950), ch. vii.
43. On Charles V, see Alvarez (1975).
44. See Estes (1990), 46, 92. For guaiacum, see Hutten (1536).
45. Weatherall, 'Drug Therapies', in Bynum and Porter, eds (1993).
46. The following paragraphs distil Copeman (1957).
47. *Ibid*. In ancient medicine, weird, wonderful and often repugnant treatments were standard, especially among adepts of the esoteric arts. For the arcane background, see Eamon (1994). There is little information about Nones (Nunez); he was admitted a Fellow of the College of Physicians in 1554 and was a censor in 1562 and 1563.
48. *Ibid*. Copeman is citing Lansdowne Manuscripts (British Library), no. 69, art. 60.
49. See also Alan G. R. Smith, ed. (1990); Haynes (1989). For Mayerne's views, see Turquet de Mayerne (1676).
50. For this divine pedigree, see Benedek and Rodnan (1963b).

51. *Idem* (1970).
52. Hawes (1634), 31. See Eamon (1981). The same class point was made by the preacher Henry Smith. Waving aside objections among upper-class ladies that they were not physically incapable of breast-feeding their babies, he demanded: 'But whose breasts have this perpetual drought? Forsooth it is like the goute, no beggars may have it, but citizens or Gentlewomen': Henry Smith (1598), quoted in Fildes (1985), 101.
53. Hawes (1634), 31.
54. La Fontaine (1966). Rodnan and Benedek have traced the 'gout and the spider' tale back to the ninth century. In La Fontaine's telling of 1668, when given a choice of earthly resting places, the spider first selected a palace, and the gout, to avoid physicians, chose a mean hut. They then traded places. The spider took to the peasant's shack where she could live undisturbed, while the gout, craving nourishment and attention,

went straight, as lodger,
To the palace of a bishop,
who was bedbound
Thereafter, her helpless prisoner.
(Rodnan and Benedek (1970))

55. Also personified was venereal disease, thanks to Fracastoro's poem, *Syphilis, sive morbus gallicus* (1530). In that pastoral myth, Syphilis was a shepherd.
56. For such beliefs, see Ficino (1989); Kristeller (1979); Barkan (1975). On Death teaching lessons, see Ariès (1981); Geddes (1981). For piety and sickness, see Wear (1985b); *idem* (1987).
57. Benedek and Rodnan (1963a). Francesco di Petrarch (1304–74) was the key figure in the early Italian Renaissance. He studied the humanities between 1315 and 1319 while in Montpellier. He moved to

Vaucluse in 1337 where he wrote much of his most important work. In 1347 he set up home in Parma where he pursued the vocations of a poet and idealistic politician.

58. Petrarch (1975–85), bk vi, letter 3, p. 309, cited in and discussed by Benedek and Rodnan (1963a).

59. Petrarch (1975–85), bk vi, letter 3, p. 309.

60. Petrarch (1991), 198–200, p. 198.

61. *Ibid.*, ch. 84, p. 199.

62. *Ibid.*, p. 200.

63. *Ibid.*

64. For the encomium, see Kaiser (1963); Benedek (1962), 236–42. Desiderius Erasmus (1466–1536), whom we also discuss in Chapter 11, was educated at Gouda and Deventer. He was ordained in 1492 but left his order in 1494. The remainder of his life he travelled in Europe, writing, studying and teaching. As a Humanist, he encouraged interest in learning, self-knowledge and simple devotion. His writings include *In Praise of Folly* (1519); *Encomium artis medicae* (1518); *In Novam Testamentum ab eodem denuo recognitum* (1519). See Mynors and Thomson, eds (1974–9), ii, 110–11, no. 189:

65. Erasmus to Servatus Rogerus, 1 April 1506; and Benedek (1983).

66. Allen and Allen, eds (1906–47), vi, 422–4, no. 1759: Erasmus to John Francis, October 1526. Erasmus' letters are here presented as translated by Krivasy in an excellent article: 'Erasmus's Medical Milieu' (1973).

67. Eckert and Imhoff (1971); Krivasy (1973), 134. The Humanist Willibald Pirckheimer (1470–1530) spent his youth in Munich then studied Greek in Padua and law in Pavia. He returned to Nuremberg without graduating and remained there all his life. He suffered from acute gout.

68. Eckert and Imhoff (1971); Benedek (1983).

69. Pirckheimer (1617).

70. Reicke (1930), 56: Pirckheimer to Konrad Adelmann.

71. Allen and Allen, eds (1906–47), vi, 47–8, no. 1558.

72. Erasmus, Preface to St John Chrysostom, translated in Benedek (1983), 537.

73. *Ibid.*

74. Cardano (1653). Jerome Cardan (1501–76) studied medicine at Padua and held the chairs of medicine in Pavia in 1543 and Bologna in 1562. He is remembered for his contributions to chemical thought and his work in algebra. It is believed that he gave an accurate early picture of rheumatic fever and differentiated it clearly from gout.

75. Benedek (1969): the following quotations are taken from Benedek's translation. See also *idem* (1987), 186.

76. Benedek (1969), 126.

77. *Ibid.*, 126–7.

78. *Ibid.*, 129.

79. *Ibid.*, 129–30.

80. *Ibid.*, 130.

81. Benedek and Rodnan (1963b). Gottfried Rogg of Augsburg (1669–1742) was a draftsman, publisher and engraver, working between 1704 and 1732. Most of his illustrations are views of towns; *Podagra* seems to be his only work pertaining to a disease. See also Googe (1990).

82. Benedek and Rodnan (1963b), 350–2.

83. *Ibid.*, 352.

Chapter 4: Science and Sydenham

1. For recent historiography, see Roy Porter (1986); 'Introduction' to Porter and Teich, eds (1992), 1–10. For a radical critique see Cunningham (1988).

2. For an introduction, see French (1993a).

3. On Harvey, see Pagel (1958b); *idem* (1976); Keele (1965), and, most

recently, French (1994). William Harvey (1578–1637) studied medicine in Cambridge and Padua. He became physician to James I and Charles I. His views on the heart and circulation were published in *De motu cordis* (1628).

4. Frank (1980); Webster (1975).

5. For Leeuwenhoek, see below, Chapter 5.

6. Marcello Malpighi (1628–94) studied medicine at Bologna, graduating in 1653. He held chairs of medicine at Pisa, Messina and from 1666 in Bologna. Giovanni Alphonso Borelli (1608–79) studied mathematics at Rome and became professor at the University of Messina in his early thirties. He wrote on various subjects including astronomy and physiological phenomena such as respiration, digestion and the secretion of urine.

7. Giorgio Baglivi (1668–1707) studied medicine in Naples, after which he travelled extensively among the hospitals and schools of Italy, and in 1692 Pope Innocent XII obtained for him a position in the Collegia dell Sapienza at Rome. Four years later he published *De Praxi Medica* (1696), which brought him international recognition.

8. Pagel (1982). Johannes (Joan) Baptiste van Helmont (*c.* 1579–1644) studied at Louvain and practised medicine at Vilvorde, near Brussels. He later turned to chemistry. His doctrines were assembled in the *Ortus medicinae* (1648).

9. Pagel (1982), 35.

10. Franciscus de le Boë Sylvius (1614–72) studied medicine at Leiden and received his degree at Basel in 1637. The first volume of his main work, *Praxeos medicae idea nova*, was published in 1671.

11. French and Wear, eds (1989).

12. See the convincing arguments in Wear (1989).

13. Slack (1979); Beier (1987).

14. Culpeper (1652); Archer (1671),

132–4. A 'practitioner in Physick and Chyrurgerie', Ralph Williams described treatments for plague, tertian fevers and gout, all based on herbs, roots, bark and other easily accessible ingredients. In *Physical Rarities*, 2nd edn (1652), 105f., he recommended for gout old cheese soaked in bacon broth and made into a plaster for local application: Nagy (1988), 64.

15. See Watson (1966), 133. William Salmon (1644–1713) was author, *inter alia*, of *Synopsis Medicinae* (1671); *Seplasium. The Compleat English Physician* (1693); *Botanologia. The English Herbal* (1710). His *The Country Physician, or A Choice Collection of Physick Fitted for Vulgar Use* (1703) discussed gout remedies on pp. 174, 177, 185, 204, 207, 222–3, 249, 303–6, 327–9. See also Wear (1992).

16. 'Philiatros' (1655); see Nagy (1988), 44.

17. Nagy (1988), 47.

18. *Ibid.*, 47.

19. *Ibid.*

20. *Ibid.*, 68.

21. Poynter and Bishop, eds (1956), x, xxv. John Symcotts (*c.* 1592–1662) was educated at Cambridge, settling as a physician in Huntingdon. He was the medical attendant of Oliver Cromwell and his family for many years. What the physician made of the wine-merchant's advice is not recorded. See also Nagy (1988), 45–7.

22. For Bacon and medicine, see Boss (1978).

23. Hart (1984). Various other notables suffered. It has been argued that James I had gout; Milton was a sufferer. In his near-contemporary biography, John Toland stated that 'the Distemper that troubled [Milton] most of any other was the Gout': Darbishire, ed. (1932), 193; Block (1954). An interesting account of an ordinary seventeenth-century arthritis sufferer is to be found in Gillow and Hewitson, eds (1873).

There is little reference to gout in Samuel Pepys's diary, apart from Sir William Penn, whose sufferings are mentioned, without great comment, five or six times: for example, 'Thence with W. Penn, who is in great pain of the gowte, by coach round by Hoborn home, he being at every kennel full of pain': Latham and Matthews, eds (1970–83), ix (1668–9), 246.

24. Hart (1984), 126.

25. *Ibid.*

26. *Ibid.*

27. Aubrey (1972), 131.

28. Quoted in Copeman (1964), 76. Referring back to such episodes, William Falconer observed that 'such facts are, however, rather matters of curiosity than utility': Falconer (1788), 48. On Boyle's views, see Barbara Beigun Kaplan (1994). A slightly earlier writer who expressed views on gout was the German Daniel Sennert (1572–1637), who studied medicine at Leipzig, Jena and Frankfurt. His *De arthritide tractatus* (1632) was translated as *A Treatise of the Gout* (1660). Sennert was one of the many physicians who termed gout the *opprobrium medicorum*.

29. Benjamin Welles became a Fellow of All Souls College and in 1650 was admitted to the practice of medicine. He practised in Greenwich, but being of morose temper attracted few patients, and he died in poverty in 1678. He wrote *A Treatise on the Gout or Joint Evil* (1669).

30. Dewhurst (1963), 10. John Locke (1632–1704) was well acquainted with Thomas Sydenham. He was educated at Oxford, and although his interests were primarily philosophical, he also practised as a doctor.

31. *Ibid.*, 128.

32. *Ibid.*, 130.

33. *Ibid.*, 149.

34. *Ibid.*, 184. See Watson (1966).

35. Dewhurst (1963), 186.

36. *Ibid.*, 189. This he got on the authority of 'Mr Kek', probably Anthony Keck, one of the Commissioners of the Great Seal.

37. *Ibid.*, 190. Here the informant was an unidentified 'Mr John Amery'.

38. *Ibid.*, 206. For the bark, see Jarcho (1993).

39. Dewhurst (1963), 254: 'In the Count of Fürstenberg it removed deposits the size of a hen's egg.'

40. *Ibid.*, 255.

41. *Ibid.*, 213.

42. *Ibid.*, 273.

43. *Ibid.*, 274.

44. For Cardano, see above, Chapter 3.

45. As emphasized in Benedek and Rodnan (1982).

46. He warned that those who suffer 'two or three times from rheumatism, unless they take care of themselves can scarcely hope to escape chronic arthritis': Baillou (1642); *idem* (1643). Guillaume de Baillou (1538–1616) studied at the University of Paris and became a skilful physician and a student of epidemics.

47. For his life, see Cunningham (1989); Dewhurst, ed. (1966). Thomas Sydenham (1624–89) was educated at Oxford, gaining his medical degree in 1648, after which he served in the Parliamentary Army. From 1655 he practised in London. His scientific approach to the natural history of disease, and his conservative attitudes to treatment, earned him the title of the 'English Hippocrates'. He was a pioneer in the use of quinine in the treatment of malaria and the first to use laudanum for pain relief. Alongside the *Tractatus de podagra* (1683), his works include *Methodus curandi febres* (1666).

48. Dewhurst, ed. (1966), 49; Cunningham (1989).

49. Sydenham, *Tractatus de podagra et hydrope* (1683); translated as *A Treatise on Gout, and Dropsy*, in *The Works of Thomas Sydenham* (1850). Quotations will generally be given from the con-

venient modern (abridged) edition: Comrie, ed. (1922), 58.

50. Comrie, ed. (1922), 70.
51. *Ibid.*, 61.
52. *Ibid.*, 61–2.
53. *Ibid.*, 58.
54. *Ibid.*, 59.
55. Sydenham states that he had intended to write broadly on chronic diseases 'but too much study and business is pernicious for me': *ibid.*, 86.
56. *Ibid.*, 75.
57. In traditional Hippocratic manner, he viewed gout as a disease of males.
58. Comrie, ed. (1922), 58.
59. *Ibid.*, 75–6.
60. *Ibid.*, 76–7.
61. The notion of a disease of un-digested humours was central to humoralism. The underlying con-cepts have been elucidated by King (1970), 131–2.
62. On opium, see Kramer (1979); Paulshock (1983). For a contempo-rary work, see J. Jones (1701). The medicinal treatment of an acute attack, according to Sydenham, entailed bed rest and the 'immediate recourse to laudanum, twenty drops of it in a small draught of plague-water . . . Of all simples the *Peruvian bark* is the best, for a few grains taken morning and evening strengthen and enliven the blood' (74). For bark, see Jarcho (1993), 46.
63. Comrie, ed. (1922), 93–4. Sydenham advocated minimal inter-ference with the acute attack as he considered that 'this pain is the dis-agreeable remedy of Nature herself'.
64. *Ibid.*, 95.
65. *Ibid.*, 78–9.
66. Sydenham (1850), ii, 161.
67. Comrie, ed. (1922), 95–6.
68. *Ibid.*, 78.
69. *Ibid.*, 67.
70. *Ibid.*
71. *Ibid.*, 94–5. Sydenham also had little faith in external applications. He mentioned moxa, but was not unduly impressed by such sympto-

matic treatments. Moxa were rec-ommended by Sir William Temple (1681); see Rosen (1970).

72. Comrie, ed. (1922), 66.
73. *Ibid.*, 72.
74. *Ibid.*, 72–3.
75. *Ibid.*, 79.
76. *Ibid.*, 79–80.
77. *Ibid.*, 86–7.
78. *Ibid.*, 77.
79. *Ibid.*
80. *Ibid.*, 85–6.
81. Copeman (1964), 62. There is of course anachronism in Copeman's judgment.
82. Comrie, ed. (1922), 72. Like others, he recognized a relation between gout and calculi.
83. *Ibid.*, 65. In the spirit of jest, Sydenham, perhaps following Sen-nert, ended his essay on gout by including, for readers who might judge he had been niggardly in sug-gesting medicines, the list from Lucian's *Tragopodagra*. In her con-cluding speech Podagra itemized some fifty useless remedies directed against her in vain (see above, Chapter 2).
84. Hull (1899), ii, 360.
85. Halsband (1965), 3, 171–2; letter of 5 September 1758 to Sir James Steuart.

Chapter 5: The Eighteenth-Century Medical Debates

1. Desault (1738); editions of 1725 and 1728 are cited in German bibliogra-phies of the history of medicine but we have found none prior to 1738. For Dover, see Strong (1955).
2. See French and Wear, eds (1989); (1970); *idem* (1978); Theodore Brown (1987).
3. Digby (1994); for patient and practi-tioner dialogues, see Dorothy Porter and Roy Porter (1989) and McKee (1994).
4. Flannagan (1981); Block (1954).

5. For diagnostic fashion, see Shorter (1992).
6. McKendrick, Brewer and Plumb (1982); Brewer and Porter, eds (1993).
7. Stokes, ed. (1931), 269. On the folklore, see Bywaters (1962); Wedeen (1981).
8. This question is further discussed in Chapter 8. On lead adulteration, see Wedeen (1984a).
9. Thomas Cadwalader (1745).
10. Baker (1785).
11. Hardy (1778; 1780).
12. *Idem* (1780), title page.
13. Only a sample of these can be discussed in this chapter. Others, for the scholar who may wish to consult them, include (in alphabetical order): [Anon.] (1731); Atkins (1694); J. Cadwallader (1721); Caverhill (1769); Thomas Dawson (1774, 1775); Dolaeus (1732); J. Douglas (1741); Drake (1758); *idem* (1771); d'Escherny (1760); Flower (1766); Gardiner (1792); Garlick (1729); Groenevelt (1691); Havers (1691); Hawkins (1826); Haygarth (1805); D. Ingram (1743); Richard Ingram (1767); James (1745); J. Johnson (1818); Kinglake (1804); Lee (1782); *idem* (1785); Lobb (1739); Mann (1784); Marshall (1770); Mooney (1757); Nelson (1727); *idem* (1728); Robinson (1753); Rowley (1792); Scot (1780); Spilsbury (1787; 1778); T. Thompson (1740); John Williams (1774); Wood (1775). See also the *Encyclopaedia Britannica* (1768, 1797), article under 'Medicine', p. 211, for the standard discussion of podagra in the period.
14. For bibliography and analysis of eighteenth-century popular medical texts, see Virginia S. Smith (1985).
15. For quacks, see Doherty (1992); Roy Porter (1989a). Also see below, Chapter 8.
16. For spas, see Hembry (1990); see also Chapter 8. For a flavour of the talk about gout in Bath, see Wagner, ed. (1989) and Mitchell and Penrose, eds (1983). Visiting Bath in 1766, the Revd John Penrose was anxious to transform his 'bastard gout' into a real attack (55). 'I hate for gouty folks to lie at home grunting when so cheap a Remedy as water is within 200 miles of them' (51).
17. 'Eighteenth century' will here be used in the 'long eighteenth century' sense, from the Restoration to the Regency. With respect to Britain, it will be used interchangeably with 'Georgian' or 'Hanoverian'.
18. Dobrée, ed. (1932), vi, 2685: letter 2391.
19. Beresford, ed. (1978–81), ii, 179. Like many of his contemporaries, Woodforde was inclined to blame all sorts of minor indispositions on gout: 'I was but poorly all day . . . I think it is some gouty humour lurking in the Constitution': iii, 209: 25 August 1790. For the views of gout sufferers, see Roy Porter and Dorothy Porter (1988), ch. 8. For the theory of disease mobility, see Malcolm Nicolson (1988).
20. Olby (1993).
21. See Bynum and Nutton, eds (1981).
22. One arguing this view was John Marten in his *A Treatise of All the Symptoms of the Venereal Disease, in both Sexes* (1708); see Roy Porter (1996).
23. Carpenter (1993); Estes (1993).
24. Gideon Harvey (1672b), 4, 8, 22; *idem* (1675). On scurvy, see Carpenter (1986). Quack doctors in particular made much of it: see Roy Porter (1989a), ch. 5. As used throughout this book, 'quack' primarily means an irregular, not necessarily a fraud.
25. Benjamin Marten (1720), 10; L. Stevenson (1965). It is important not to assume that a single, fixed, specific 'ontological' disease was implied by 'consumption' or its synonym 'phthisick'.
26. Gideon Harvey (1675), 11: smoke and pollution produced 'vitiated choler': 33.

27. Cummins (1949), 16.
28. Morton (1694). See Flick (1925), 99, 155; Trail (1970), 166–74; Keers (1982).
29. Benjamin Marten (1720), 22, 36.
30. Christopher Bennet (1720), 19; Estes (1993).
31. Christopher Bennet (1720), 33–5.
32. See Flick (1925), 134.
33. The following pages depend on the excellent discussion in Vandereycken and Deth (1994), 118f. For 'wasting', see Roy Porter (1993c); David Trotter (1988).
34. Celsus (1756).
35. Cheshire (1723), 4–5.
36. Another physician sufferer was Erasmus Darwin. See King-Hele (1977), 132.
37. Cheshire (1723), iv. He confessed elsewhere: '*My Cup of* Gouty *Bitters, has had as large a Diameter as any Man's of my Age*'. *Ibid.*, xiv–xv.
38. Andree (1778), v, i.
39. For aggressive methods, see Colbatch (1700).
40. Sydenham (1850), ii, 161. See above, Chapter 4.
41. Timotheus Bennet (1734), 34.
42. Ferdinando Warner (1768).
43. Timotheus Bennet (1734), 34.
44. Buzaglo (1778), 17.
45. *Ibid.*, 4.
46. *Ibid.*, 4–5.
47. *Ibid.*, 17.
48. *Ibid.*, 18.
49. An obvious parallel lies in the Christian doctrine of the 'fortunate fall'.
50. For these new medical philosophies see above, note 2.
51. McCarty (1970); Dobell (1960). Leeuwenhoek was not aware of the chemical nature of the crystals: uric acid was not known until Scheele's description of 'lithic acid' in urine in 1776.
52. McCarty (1970).
53. *Ibid.*
54. *Ibid.*
55. *Ibid.*
56. *Ibid.* See Leeuwenhoek (1685).
57. George Cheyne (1671–1743) studied at Edinburgh, at first favouring mathematics and natural philosophy rather than medicine. He struggled with gross obesity, and his *The English Malady* (1733) was a critique of the lifestyle of the rich.
58. For Archibald Pitcairne (1652–1713), see Guerrini (1986; 1987).
59. See Guerrini (1985), 222–45; Shuttleton (1992). For his anxieties and phobias, see Rousseau (1988). See also Cheyne (1722; 1734; 1724; 1733; 1740; 1742; 1743).
60. Cheyne (1733): see the Introduction by Roy Porter to the reprint (1990). For background, see Rousseau (1976; 1980; 1991).
61. Cheyne (1734; 1st edn 1724).
62. *Idem* (1720). A 2nd edn appeared in the same year titled *An Essay of the True Nature and Due Method of Treating the Gout* (1720). Further editions under that title appeared in 1721, 1722, 1723, 1724, 1725, 1737, 1738 and 1753.
63. *Idem* (1743), 17. This may of course be authorial flimflam.
64. *Idem* (1720), 78.
65. *Idem* (1742), 179.
66. *Idem* (1720), 7.
67. *Ibid.*, 7.
68. *Ibid.*, 10.
69. *Idem* (1743), 40–1. Bleeding haemorrhoids were widely seen, like gout, as Nature's process for the evacuation of poisonous matter: compare menstruation.
70. *Idem* (1742), 177.
71. *Ibid.*, 177–80.
72. *Ibid.* See Schnitker (1936), 89–120.
73. See below, Chapter 7.
74. Blackmore (1726), xxxvii. See also his *A Treatise of the Spleen and Vapours* (1725); Albert Rosenberg (1953); Bishop (1958), 118–211; on Blackmore's place, see Levine (1991a); Julian Martin (1988).
75. Blackmore (1726), 35; McMahan (1976).
76. Blackmore (1726), 48.
77. *Ibid.*, 118.
78. *Ibid.*, 133–4. Regarding the

personification of illness, it is worth
remembering that scrofula was actually called the King's Evil.

79. Neuburger (1932).
80. Blackmore (1726), 65, 36–7.
81. *Ibid.*, 61–2.
82. *Ibid.*, 14–15.
83. *Ibid.*, 60.
84. *Ibid.*, 2. For digestion, see McKee
     (1994).
85. Blackmore (1726), 52–3. The cri-
     tique of luxury was especially pow-
     erful: Sekora (1977).
86. Blackmore (1726), 35.
87. *Ibid.*, 38.
88. *Ibid.*, 40.
89. *Ibid.*
90. *Ibid.*
91. *Ibid.*, 74.
92. *Ibid.*
93. *Ibid.*, 84. For the confidence of
     Georgian physicians in the safety of
     opium, see Kramer (1979), 377–89;
     Paulshock (1983), 53–6.
94. Blackmore (1726), 91.
95. *Ibid.*, 99.
96. *Ibid.*, 101.
97. For the 'moral economy', see
     E. P. Thompson (1991); respecting
     gout, one may suggest that many
     physicians thought in terms of a
     medical economy, with inbuilt
     checks and sanctions. For
     Blackmore's wider commitments as
     expressed through his verse, see
     Marjorie Hope Nicolson (1946),
     57–8, 60, 66–7, 103, 104, 114; *idem*
     (1959). Blackmore's poems include
     *Creation. A Philosophical Poem. In
     Seven Books* (1712). Book V evokes
     gout (lines 28–32, 37–8):

     See, colic, gout, and stone, a cruel
       train,
     Oppos'd by all the healing race in
       vain,
     Their various racks and lingering
       plagues employ,
     Relieve each other, and by turns
       annoy,
     And, tyrant like, torment, but not
       destroy . . .

Howe'er the cause phantastic may
  appear,
Th'effect is real, and the pain
  sincere.

98. It thus bears comparison with the
     'stone of folly' so prominent in
     Renaissance representations of the
     mad.
99. William Stukeley (1687–1765) gra-
     duated MD in 1719 from London
     and became FRCP 1720, delivering
     the Gulstonian Lecture in 1722. He
     moved to Grantham in 1726 where
     he practised for many years. He was
     ordained in 1729. His writings
     include *Of the Gout* (1734) and
     *Stonehenge, A Temple Restor'd to the
     British Druids* (1740). He spent many
     of his later years in London, espe-
     cially during the 1750s, in close asso-
     ciation with John Hill (see below),
     and they may have collaborated in
     their theories of the gout. See also
     Piggott (1950); David Douglas
     (1939); Levine (1987; 1991a; 1991b).
100. The following is largely derived
     from an admirable essay: Kerin
     Fraser (1992).
101. *Ibid.*, 165. See Meade (1974); Zuc-
     kerman (1965).
102. Kevin Fraser (1992), 166.
103. *Ibid.*
104. *Ibid.*, 167.
105. *Ibid.*
106. *Ibid.*
107. *Ibid.*, 168.
108. *Ibid.*
109. *Ibid.*, 169.
110. *Ibid.*
111. *Ibid.*, 170.
112. Havers (1691).
113. Kevin Fraser (1992), 169.
114. *Ibid.* Stukeley believed the Romans
     largely escaped gout, despite luxuri-
     ous living, thanks to their habit of
     body oiling.
115. Stukeley stressed he was acting inde-
     pendently of Rogers and that 'my
     sole view was to benefit the
     publick'. See Stukeley (1734).
116. *Ibid.*, 3.
117. *Ibid.*, 3–4.

118. *Ibid.*, 10.
119. *Ibid.*, 4–5.
120. *Ibid.*, 5–6.
121. *Ibid.*, 6–7.
122. *Ibid.*, 11–13.
123. *Ibid.*, 15–16. The work is question is Walter Harris's *Pharmacologia antiempirica* (1683).
124. Stukeley (1734), 88.
125. *Ibid.*, 41.
126. *Ibid.*, 29. For Mead, see above, note 93. For poisons, see Maehle (1995). Stukeley gives no sign of being aware of Leeuwenhoek's microscopical description of the needle-shaped crystals in a gouty tophus, communicated to the Royal Society.
127. Stukeley (1734), 38.
128. *Ibid.*, 56; Kevin Fraser (1992), 176.
129. See Roy Porter (1989a).
130. Kevin Fraser (1992), 179.
131. *Ibid.*
132. For Pitt the Elder's gout, see below, Chapter 8.
133. Kevin Fraser (1992), 180.
134. *Ibid.*, 181.
135. *Ibid.*, 182.
136. Rousseau (1978a) and (1982). John Hill (1716?–75) was apprenticed to an apothecary and then set himself up in a shop in Westminster. A failure as a playwright, he continued as an apothecary. At his home in Lancaster Gate he cultivated the plants from which he made his quack medicines. His writings include *The Useful Family Herbal* (1754) and *The Management of the Gout* (1758).
137. Kerin Fraser (1992), 183.
138. The book began pseudonymously ('George Crine') as *The Management of the Gout, by a Physician From his Own Case. With the Virtues of an English Plant Bardana, Not Regarded in the Present Practice, but Safe and Effectual in Alleviating that Disease*, by George Crine (1758); 2nd, 3rd and 4th edns were published in 1758; in 1758 there appeared a 6th edn under Hill's own name as *The Management of the Gout, with the Virtues of Burdock Root,*

First Us'd in the Author's Own Case, and Since in Many Other Successful Instances; this later appeared as *The Management of the Gout in Diet, Exercise and Temper: with the Virtues of BURDOCK Root, Taken in the Manner of Tea: First Us'd in the Year 1760; in the Author's Own Case; And Since in Many Other Successful Instances, to the Present Time. By J. Hill, M. D. Member of the Imperial Academy*, 8th edn (1771). See Rousseau (1982) and Kerin Fraser (1992), 185.

139. Hill (1771), 1; restated on p. 5 of the 1771 edn.
140. *Ibid.*, 2 (p. 7, 1771 edn).
141. *Ibid.*, 3 (p. 8, 1771 edn).
142. *Ibid.*
143. *Ibid.*, 4 (p. 8, 1771 edn).
144. *Ibid.*, 6 (p. 9, 1771 edn).
145. *Ibid.*, 14 (p. 9, 1771 edn). 25. Hill cautiously subscribed to the hereditary nature of gout: 'We see by what means the gout is to be acquired: whether or not it be hereditary, tho' the appearances are strong, is less certain': pp. 5–6 (p. 9, 1771 edn).
146. *Ibid.*, 25–6 (p. 15, 1771 edn).
147. *Ibid.*, 26 (p. 15, 1771 edn).
148. *Ibid.*, 43–4 (p. 49–50, 1771 edn).
149. Cullen (1808); Doig, Ferguson, Milne and Passmore, eds (1993); Lawrence (1984); Rosner (1990).
150. Faber (1930); Bynum (1993); Lindeboom (1968; 1970; 1974).
151. Cullen (1808); see also Boissier de Sauvages (1763; 1808).
152. In a dissertation on gout to be found in vol. lvii (1807–8) of the Archives of the Royal Medical Society of Edinburgh, H. Shute stressed the value of Cullen's nosology (338), and noted, quoting Cullen, that 'it is to be feared that very many diseases commonly attributed to irregular gout, are totally independent of that disease. Thus, Hypochondriases, Asthma, Palpitations, Giddiness, Headache, Apoplexy, Palsy; in short all morbid affections of the head, Thoracic and Abdominal Viscera, occurring in a certain habit.' We

owe this reference to Dr Hannah
Augstein.
153. French (1969).
154. As, for instance, Duckworth (1889).
155. On Brown, see Risse (1988).
156. It should be added that Georgian
quacks were also developing gout
cures. There is no room to discuss
them here, but see Roy Porter
(1998).

Chapter 6: Gout and
the Georgian Gentleman

1. Digby (1994); Dorothy Porter and
Roy Porter (1989). For cartoon caricatures, see Arnold-Forster and
Tallis, comps (1989); Burnby (1989).
Self-help books included titles like
the *Family Companion for Health*
(1729); *Family Guide to Health*
(1767); Bullman (1789); Reece
(1803) – Reece is discussed below,
Chapter 8. For discussion, see Lawrence (1975); Roy Porter, ed.
(1992).
2. Andrews, ed. (1954), ii, 238.
3. The most famous philosopher–
sufferer was Immanuel Kant.
4. Ellis (1927), 162–3. See also Graham
and Graham (1957), 209; Copeman
(1964), 82.
5. Hartshorne, ed. (1905), 103.
6. Quoted in Pat Rogers (1981), 315–
16. Compare Bierce (1911), 76:
'GOUT, n. A physician's name for
the rheumatism of a rich patient'.
7. Letter to Lady Holland, 8 November 1816, in Lady Holland (1855), ii,
130–1.
8. Philander Misaurus (1735). For the
convention of the mock encomium
upon which that text draws, see
above, Chapter 3. This was, of
course, the great age of English
satire: Rawson (1994).
9. Philander Misaurus (1735), v–vi.
10. *Ibid.*, 1–2.
11. *Ibid.*, 3.
12. *Ibid.*

13. *Ibid.*
14. *Ibid.*, 6.
15. *Ibid.*, 7.
16. *Ibid.*, 7–8.
17. *Ibid.*, 9.
18. *Ibid.* For pain, see Roy Porter
(1993b).
19. Philander Misaurus (1735), 11–12.
20. Quoted in Warter, ed. (1831),
551.
21. Philander Misaurus (1735), 14.
22. *Ibid.*, 21–2.
23. *Ibid.*, 23.
24. *Ibid.*
25. *Ibid.*, 34. Was this a reference to
Sydenham?
26. *Ibid.*, 35.
27. *Ibid.*
28. *Ibid.*
29. *Ibid.*, 39–40.
30. *Ibid.*, 42–3.
31. *Ibid.*, 43.
32. *Ibid.*, 49.
33. *Ibid.*, 52.
34. The motility of the traditional body
is emphasized in Duden (1991); see
also Neuburger (1932).
35. Verney, ed. (1930), ii, 56: William
Abel to Ralph, Lord Fermanagh, 3
January. 1718.
36. Lord Herbert, ed. (1950), September
1779, 265. On luxury and alcohol,
see Healey (1975), 659–62.
37. Norton, ed. (1956), ii, 239. He later
referred to the 'decline and fall' of
his gout: 375.
38. Compare Oliver Sacks's view of
migraine today (1981).
39. Thomas Jefferson to John Jay, 1
February 1787, in Boyd, ed. (1958),
99–103.
40. Hartshorne, ed. (1905), 103. The
misquotation is from Horace, *Epistles*, 1. 10. 24.
41. Sydenham to Major William Hale,
quoted in Dewhurst, ed. (1966),
174–5.
42. W. S. Lewis, ed. (1937–83), xxvi,
597: to Sir Horace Mann, 25 July
1785.
43. King and Ryskamp, eds (1979–84),
iv, 91. Cowper wrote in *The Task*:

O may I live exempted (while I live
Guiltless of pamper'd appetite
   obscene)
From pangs arthritic that infest the
   toe
Of libertine Excess! The Sofa suits
The gouty limb, 'tis true; but
   gouty limb
Though on a Sofa, may I never feel.
          (Book I: lines 103–8)

44. Greig, ed. (1969), i, 180: letter to John Clephane, 28 October 1753. Hume added: 'I fancy one Fit of the Gout wou'd much encrease your Stock of Interjections; and render that part of Speech, which, in common Grammars, is usually the most barren, with you more copious than either Nouns or Verbs.'
45. *Ibid.*
46. Smyth, ed. (1906), viii, 161; also see Wallace (1968), 312–20.
47. The Marquis of Lansdowne, ed. (1934), 258–9.
48. Chapman, ed. (1952), iii, 81: letter 891.
49. W. S. Lewis, ed. (1937–83), xxv, 402: to Sir Horace Mann, 8 May 1783. The passage reads:

> Were the House of Commons existing the worst that ever was, still it must be acceptable to our reformers; for which House of Commons, since the Restoration, ever did more than tear two Prime Ministers from the crown in one year? In short, the constitution of the House of Commons I see in the same light as I do my own constitution. The gout raises inflammations, weakens, cripples; yet it purges itself, and requires no medicines. To quack it could kill me. Besides, it prevents other illnesses and prolongs life. Could I cure the gout, should not I have a fever, a palsy, or an apoplexy?

It is of course crucial that Horace Walpole believed he was the son of

the greatest political manager of the Commons, Sir Robert Walpole.
50. Sprigge, ed. (1968–81), ii, 207.
51. W. S. Lewis, ed. (1937–83), xxxv, 259: to Richard Bentley, 16 November 1755. See Gwynn (1932), 33, 171–3, 189, 206–7, 226, 230–1, 232, 245, 250, 252, 263, 266, 267.
52. W. S. Lewis, ed. (1937–83), xxxv, 264: to Richard Bentley, 6 January 1756. Some twenty years later he was still advising friends not to try to keep gout at bay with strong wines, for that would provoke irregular gout: xxiv, 423: to Sir Horace Mann, 27 November 1778.
53. *Ibid.*, xxxv, 303: to the Earl of Strafford, 7 August 1760.
54. *Ibid.*, xxxviii, 65: to the Hon. Henry Seymour Conway, 7 August 1760. Paul Pliant is a character in Congreve's *The Double Dealer* (1693).
55. W. S. Lewis, ed. (1937–83), ix, 291: to George Montagu, 12 August 1760. He could jokingly speak on another occasion of wearing 'the gout's livery': xxii, 348: to Sir Horace Mann, 16 October 1765.
56. *Ibid.*, xxii, 110: to Sir Horace Mann, 20 December 1762.
57. *Ibid.*, x, 159: to George Montagu, 6 July 1765.
58. *Ibid.*, xxxix, 3: to the Hon. Henry Seymour Conway, 3 July 1765.
59. *Ibid.*, xxxi, 37: to the Countess of Suffolk, 3 July 1765.
60. *Ibid.*, xxii, 311: to Sir Horace Mann, 12 July 1765.
61. *Ibid.*, xxiv, 501: to Sir Horace Mann, 4 August 1779. In the same passage the gout is also 'my old enemy'. He wrote some years later: 'I firmly believe, the gout, which I have long known for a Harlequin, that can assume any form': xxix, 89: to the Revd William Mason, 4 January 1781.
62. Toynbee, ed. (1903–25), vi, 270, letter 1038: to George Montagu, 28 July 1765. See below for the politics of liberty.

63. W. S. Lewis, ed. (1937–83), i, 95: to the Revd William Cole, 5 September 1765. The pain 'is no flea-bite': xxii, 348: to Sir Horace Mann, 16 October 1765.

64. *Ibid.*, x, 179–80: to George Montagu, 16 October 1765.

65. *Ibid.*, xiii–xiv, 143: to Thomas Gray, 19 November 1765. There is no sign that Walpole ever relented and went in for nostrums. For Gray's gout, see Ketton-Cremer (1955), 118, 260.

66. W. S. Lewis, ed. (1937–83), xxxii, 210: to the Countess of Upper Ossory, 15 October 1774.

67. *Ibid.*, xxxix, 206: to the Countess of Ailesbury, 7 November 1774. For use of the word 'mummy', see also xxxix, 229: to the Hon. Henry Seymour Conway, 26 December 1774.

68. *Ibid.*, xxiv, 67: to Sir Horace Mann, 23 December 1774.

69. *Ibid.*, xxxix, 226: to the Hon. Henry Seymour Conway, 15 December 1774.

70. *Ibid.*, xxiv, 66: to Sir Horace Mann, 23 December 1774.

71. *Ibid.*, xxv, 402: to Sir Horace Mann, 9 January 1775. Many of Walpole's letters praise the bootikins. See also for instance ii, 1: to the Revd William Cole, 26 January 1776.

72. *Ibid.*, xxiv, 70–1: to Sir Horace Mann, 9 January 1775.

73. *Ibid.*, xxiv, 184: to Sir Horace Mann, 22 March 1776.

74. *Ibid.*, xxiv, 421: to Sir Horace Mann, 30 October 1778.

75. *Ibid.*, xxiv, 423: to Sir Horace Mann, 27 November 1778.

76. 'When an ancient gentleman marries, it is his best excuse that he wants a nurse, which I suppose was the motive of Solomon, who was the wisest of mortals, and a most puissant and opulent monarch, for marrying a thousand wives in his old age when, I conclude, he was very gouty': *ibid.*, xi, 72: to Miss Mary Berry, 30 September 1789.

77. *Ibid.*, xxxiii, 120: to the Countess of Upper Ossory, 5 September 1779.

78. *Ibid.*, xxix, 7: to the Revd William Mason, 22 January 1780. See, for aesthetic background, Marjorie Hope Nicolson (1959). Repeated spectacular eruptions of Vesuvius about this time doubtless prompted the analogy.

79. W. S. Lewis, ed. (1937–83), xxxi, 237: to Lady Browne, 14 December 1785.

80. *Ibid.*, xxv, 622–3: to Sir Horace Mann, 13 February 1786. He later called the chalkstone 'worthy of a place in Mr [John] Hunter's collection of human miseries' – *ibid.*, xv, 241: to the Revd Robert Nares, 5 October 1793.

81. *Ibid.*, xi, 83: to Miss Mary Berry, 10 July 1790. For Blackmore, see above, Chapter 5.

82. *Ibid.*, xxxi, 341: to Miss Hannah More, 25 July 1790.

83. *Ibid.*, xxxi, 345: to Mrs Dickenson, 25 August 1790.

84. *Ibid.*, xi, 177: to Miss Mary Berry, 9 January 1791.

85. *Ibid.*, xi, 313: to Miss Mary Berry, 17 July 1791.

86. A fine depiction of the Enlightenment style of sickness is offered in Geyer-Kordesch (1985). The political watchword of his father, Sir Robert, was *quieta non movere*.

87. This was followed by quotations from Dr John Arbuthnot, *Cymbeline* and Dryden's translation of Juvenal. The adjective *gouty* elicited from Johnson a sentence from John Graunt's *Natural and Political Observations* (1662). The arthritis entry ('Any distemper that affects the joints, but the gout most particularly') shows that it was still being used as a generic term for joint disorders. The following account of Johnson's gout is somewhat abbreviated, since there have recently been two extremely valuable discussions: J. P. W. Rogers (1986), 133–44, and Wiltshire (1991), 35–6.

88. Pottle and Bennett, eds (1936), 168–9. For Cadogan, see below, Chapter 7.

89. Chapman, ed. (1984), ii, 84: Johnson to Mrs Thrale, letter 432, 29 August 1775.

90. *Ibid.*, 147: letter 494, 6 July 1776.

91. *Ibid.*, iii, 92: letter 894, 23 October 1783.

92. *Ibid.*, ii, 138: letter 485, 3 June 1776.

93. *Ibid.*, iii, 81: letter 891.

94. *Ibid.*, 86: letter 874, 9 October 1783.

95. 'My disorders are in other respects less than usual,' he told Mrs Thrale – *ibid.*, 38: letter 853, 21 June 1783.

96. *Ibid.*, ii, 309: letter 635, 19 October 1779.

97. Redford, ed. (1992), iii, 221: to John Taylor, 9 December 1779.

98. Balderston, ed. (1951), i, 521. It is interesting to ponder the parallel with Freud, who similarly emphasized the evils of 'repression'. The belief was widespread that the shock of cold water could bring on gout, aggravate it or cause it to become repelled. See Brownrigg (1993), 53.

99. The Marquis of Lansdowne, ed. (1934), 254. Her comment follows the conviction that cold water shrank the gouty vessels, ejecting their contents to some other, more dangerous, bodily site.

100. Quennell, ed. (1948), 121.

101. Treue (1958), 147.

102. Rannie, ed. (1898), i, 266: Wednesday, 26 June 1706. The moral is that a rash curative attempt extinguished not gout but a family.

103. Swift, 'Bec's Birthday', in Swift (1937), ii, 761; Flynn (1990). Swift's maladies included rheumatism, deafness and vertigo.

104. Smyth, ed. (1906) ('Dialogue Between Franklin and the Gout'), 154. See Pepper (1970); [Anon.] (1959), 34–5; Ronald W. Clark (1983), 150, 297, 315, 364, 368–9.

105. Smyth, ed. (1906), 155.

106. *Ibid.*

107. *Ibid.*

108. *Ibid.*, 156.

109. *Ibid.*, 157.

110. *Ibid.*, 158.

111. *Ibid.*

112. *Ibid.*, 159–60.

113. *Ibid.*, 161.

114. *Ibid.*, 152.

115. On another occasion he recorded eating 'a hearty supper, much cheese and drank a good deal of champagne': [Anon.] (1959), 34–5.

116. How far such ideas had purchase in other cultures awaits research on the medical and political contexts of France, the German principalities, Italy, Scandinavia and elsewhere.

117. David Trotter (1988); Barkan (1975); Bamborough (1952).

118. Marjorie Hope Nicolson (1960).

119. Matthew Hale, quoted in Pocock (1972), 217.

120. Walter Moyle (1796), quoted in Dickinson (1977), 81.

121. David Williams (1778), 1, quoted in Gunn (1983), 199.

122. For the political idiom, see Pocock (1972; 1975; 1985); Robbins (1959); Dickinson (1977).

123. For the Burke quotation, see Pocock (1972), 226. See also Brewer (1976), who has explored the pictorialization of such metaphors (1986). For this aspect, see also Rodnan (1961), 27–46; Atherton (1974; 1982), 3–31; George (1967a; 1967b); Helfand (1978).

124. Sekora (1977); Berry (1994).

125. Duncan Forbes (1975).

126. Mandeville (1970), 67–8; McKee (1991).

127. For 'cosmic toryism', see Willey (1962).

128. Dickinson (1977), 142.

129. Pocock (1972), 129.

130. Hume, 'Of the Original Contract', in (1963), 463.

131. *Ibid.*

132. Edmund Burke (1901), ii, 307, discussed in Pocock (1972), 211.

133. Blackmore (1726), 40.

134. Roy Porter (1992b); Marcovich (1982).

135. On political management, see Plumb (1967).
136. Grant (1779), 21.
137. Quoted in Dickinson (1977), 204.
138. *Ibid.*, 243.
139. Norton, ed. (1956); Craddock (1982; 1989); Spacks (1976), ch. iv.
140. Bonnard, ed. (1966), 40. The *Memoirs* afford a richly fantasized rendering – or rather six successive versions – of a man's relationship to his body, not least its (fortunate) infirmities.
141. Norton, ed. (1956), i, 356: to Dorothea Gibbon, letter 214, 22 December 1772.
142. *Ibid.*, ii, 50: to J. B. Holroyd (later Lord Sheffield), letter 284, 20 December 1774.
143. *Ibid.*, 54: to Dorothea Gibbon, letter 288, 7 January 1775.
144. *Ibid.*, 163: to J. B. Holroyd, letter 396, 4 November 1777.
145. *Ibid.*, 165: to Dorothea Gibbon, letter 400, 13 November 1777. Military language was ubiquitous. See Spilsbury (1775), 58–9.
146. Norton, ed. (1956), ii, 165: to J. B. Holroyd, letter 401, 14 November 1777.
147. *Ibid.*, 238: to Dorothea Gibbon, letter 468, 10 March 1780.
148. *Ibid.*, 239: to Dorothea Gibbon, letter 469, 18 March 1780.
149. *Ibid.*, 290: to Dorothea Gibbon, letter 531, 23 January 1782.
150. *Ibid.*, 322: to Dorothea Gibbon, letter 565, 19 February 1783.
151. *Ibid.*, 324: to Dorothea Gibbon, letter 568, 29 March 1783.
152. *Ibid.*, 330: to Dorothea Gibbon, letter 572, 30 May 1783.
153. *Ibid.*, 375: to Lady Sheffield, letter 607, 28 October 1783. One imagines, here and elsewhere, that the reference to his 'member' had certain sexual insinuations for Gibbon. Was he engaging in *double entendre* with Lady Sheffield?
154. *Ibid.*, 411: to Dorothea Gibbon, letter 618, 28 May 1784.
155. *Ibid.*
156. *Ibid.*, iii 18: to Dorothea Gibbon, letter 624, 17 October 1784.
157. *Ibid.*, 18: to Lord Eliot, letter 625, 27 October 1784.
158. *Ibid.*, 27–8: to Dorothea Gibbon, letter 627, 15 July 1785. The notion that gout should teach philosophy was an Augustan commonplace. Thus on 8 June 1741 Vanbrugh began a reply to a letter from the third Earl of Carlisle by expressing sympathy that 'you shou'd owe any stroaks [?] of philosophy to a fit of the Gout': Downes (1987), 385.
159. Norton, ed. (1956), iii, 41: to Dorothea Gibbon, letter 633, 3 May 1786.
160. *Ibid.*, 82: to Lord Sheffield, letter 660, 26 November 1787.
161. *Ibid.*, 190–1: to Lord Sheffield, letter 759, 15 May 1790. There is sexual banter in the reference to 'noble parts'.
162. *Ibid.*, 197: to Lord Sheffield, letter 762, 7 August 1790.
163. *Ibid.*
164. *Ibid.*, 199.
165. *Ibid.*, 264: to Dorothea Gibbon, letter 804, 1 August 1792.
166. Rodnan and Benedek (1965), 115–39; see more generally Cotton Mather (1994).

Chapter 7: Smollett, Cadogan and Controversy

1. Tierney (1989), 209.
2. *Ibid.*, 249.
3. *Ibid.*, 261.
4. *Ibid.*
5. *Ibid.*, 270.
6. *Ibid.*, 279.
7. *Ibid.*, 300–1.
8. *Ibid.*, 326.
9. *Ibid.*, 440.
10. *Ibid.*, 481.
11. For the identity of Dr William Lewis as a fictional character, see Rousseau (1982); in several signifi-

cant senses Lewis was based on the Scottish physician John Moore (1729–1802).

12. Preston, ed. (1990), 1: to Dr Lewis, 2 April. All citations to *Humphry Clinker* are from Preston.

13. *Ibid.*, 336: to Dr Lewis, 20 November.

14. *Ibid.*

15. For the critical heritage, see Kelly, ed. (1987).

16. See Rousseau (1982). Crawford (1992), ch. iv, is well worth consulting for the appropriation of the 'Scottish Smollett' as an 'English' author. Nemonianou (1989), in a chapter entitled 'Illness and Style: The Case of Bramble's Hypochondria', has written that 'gout is a chronic illness, compatible with valetudinarianism and ripe old age, neither of which disturbs the idyll as would acute illness or life-threatening diseases'. This is entirely true, but Smollett makes clear that gout, much more so than hypochondria, is the chronic condition which Bramble must overcome if he is to integrate himself with his society back home in Wales. And it is gout's comic paradoxes, an illness rather more than a mere cultural sign in Smollett, not the tedious repetitions of hypochondria – both admittedly benign – on which Smollett draws for the characterization of his hero. In this sense gout and hypochondria need to be differentiated more sharply than Nemonianou does, especially in view of the Georgian contexts of hypochondria.

17. These issues are complex and cannot be discussed here but see: Rousseau (1982); Boucé (1971); Basker (1988). We need a study of Smollett as an author in Grub Street producing a certain number of words a day according to economic and professional timetables.

18. See Bourgeois (1986); Knapp (1949); Musher (1967); Rousseau (1966);

Schuyler (1890); Sena (1975); Underwood (1937).

19. In the source where one would expect to find discussion there is only silence; see Rothfield (1987).

20. See Kelly, ed. (1987), 320–5 and 357–64.

21. See Knapp (1949); Rousseau (1966).

22. Preston, ed. (1990), 25: to Dr Lewis, 20 April.

23. *Ibid.*

24. *Ibid.*, 52: to Dr Lewis, 5 May.

25. *Ibid.*, 26: to Dr Lewis, 20 April.

26. *Ibid.*, 138: to Dr Lewis, 12 June.

27. *Ibid.*, 151: to Dr Lewis, 14 June.

28. *Ibid.*, 159: to Dr Lewis, 26 June.

29. *Ibid.*, 168: to Dr Lewis, 26 June. See also Rousseau (1991d), 41–2.

30. Preston, ed. (1990), 168: to Dr Lewis, 26 June.

31. *Ibid.*, 17: to Dr Lewis, 4 July.

32. *Ibid.*, 325: to Dr Lewis, 26 October.

33. *Ibid.*

34. Rothfield (1992), 4.

35. Rousseau (1982), 1–9.

36. Knapp, ed. (1970), 82: letter 64.

37. *Ibid.*, 106: letter 86, dated 1 June 1762.

38. *Ibid.*, 119: letter 94.

39. *Ibid.*, 107–8: letter 87.

40. *Ibid.*, 109–10: letter 88, dated 2 October 1762.

41. *Ibid.*, 119: letter 94.

42. *Ibid.*, 121: letter 95.

43. *Ibid.*, 120–1, for Dr A. Fizes, 'Systema nervosum maxime irritabile'.

44. *Ibid.*, 126: letter 97; letter to John Moore from Bath dated 13 November 1765; subsequent quotations in this paragraph are from this letter.

45. *Ibid.*

46. Smollett was right-handed; it apparently does not occur to him here that excessive overuse has caused his distress.

47. *Ibid.*, 129–31: letter 100.

48. For biography, see Mullins (1968); Ruhräh (1925a); Rendle-Short (1960b).

49. See McLure (1981). Cadogan's *An Essay upon Nursing and the*

50. Quoted in Ruhräh (1925b), 5. Cadogan's statement was probably not completely facetious.
51. Cadogan (1748), 24–5; see Rendle-Short (1960a); Fildes (1985), 398–9; *idem* (1988), 113–16, 134–5; A. Wilson (1995).
52. Cadogan (1771); Cadogan's essay (1772 edn) is reprinted in Ruhräh (1925b). Cadogan's publisher, Robert Dodsley, a close friend of Samuel Johnson, suffered acute symptoms by his mid-thirties, requiring the adoption of 'crutches and cloath shoes'. His poem *Pain and Patience* (1743) addressed the topic. After turning sixty, he could scarcely walk at all: Straus (1910), 79f., 295f.
53. Trimmer (1967); Gruman (1966).
54. Drake (1758), 35; *idem* (1771).
55. Cheyne (1722), 35. For Cheyne, see above, Chapter 5. For medical primitivism, see Roy Porter (1991a).
56. Pottle and Bennett, eds (1936), 168–9.
57. Campbell (1969; 1st edn, 1747), 37.
58. *Ibid.*, 37–8.
59. *Ibid.*, 38.
60. Wesley (1747); Rousseau (1968); Cule (1990). Later writers would reiterate these messages: Willich (1799). For discussion, consult Roy Porter (1991b), ch. vi.
61. Questions of possible plagiarism are mooted in Rendle-Short (1960b).
62. For Hill, see above, Chapter 5; see also Rousseau (1978a).
63. Kevin Fraser (1992).
64. W. Buchan (1769); Lawrence (1975); Roy Porter, ed. (1992).
65. W. Buchan (1769).
66. *Ibid.*, 484.
67. *Ibid.*
68. *Ibid.* Unlike certain popular writers, Buchan took some care to differentiate gout from rheumatism, which he noted had 'great affinity to the gout' (465–6).
69. *Ibid.*, 464.
70. *Ibid.*
71. For these connections, see Rendle-Short (1960b).
72. Cadogan (1771), 16–17. All the quotations from Cadogan are from the 1772 edn as reprinted in Ruhräh (1925).
73. Cadogan (1771), 16.
74. *Ibid.*, 13–14. The parallel with Buchan's denunciation of the quasi-conspiratorial conduct of the medical profession is here very clear.
75. *Ibid.*, 14.
76. *Ibid.*, 19–20.
77. *Ibid.*, 25.
78. *Ibid.*
79. *Ibid.*, 26.
80. *Ibid.*, 29.
81. *Ibid.*, 30.
82. *Ibid.*, 31–2. 'Nine in ten of all the chronic diseases in the world,' he stressed, 'particularly the gout, owe their first rise to intemperance' (47).
83. *Ibid.*, 35–7.
84. *Ibid.*, 44.
85. *Ibid.*, 46–7. For parallel arguments, see Roy Porter (1988; 1992a).
86. Cadogan (1771), 49–51.
87. *Ibid.*, 53, 58, 64–8.
88. *Ibid.*, 72–4.
89. *Ibid.*, 76–7.
90. *Ibid.*, 79–80.
91. *Ibid.*, 85.
92. *Ibid.*, 85–6.
93. *Ibid.*, 25.
94. *Ibid.*, 19.
95. *Ibid.*, 102.
96. Little and Kahrl, eds (1963), ii, 738: to the Revd Dr John Hoadly, letter 632, 9 May 1771.
97. Shebbeare (1772), 171.
98. *Ibid.*, 172.
99. This poem is reprinted in Ruhräh (1925b), 104.
100. *Ibid.*, 105.
101. *Ibid.*
102. *Ibid.*, 107.
103. *Ibid.*
104. *Ibid.*
105. *Ibid.*, 108.
106. *Ibid.*, 110.
107. Gilmour (1992); Brewer (1986).

108. Ruhräh (1925b), 113.
109. See Pottle and Bennett, eds (1936), 168–9.
110. John Hill (1758a); Kevin Fraser (1992).
111. Hill (1758a), 6; compare with *idem* (1771), 11.
112. *Idem* (1771), 11.
113. *Ibid.*, 49.
114. *Ibid.*, 50.
115. *Ibid.*, 23.
116. *Ibid.*, 14.
117. For instance Berkenhout (1772); William Carter (1772); Shebbeare (1772); Falconer (1772).
118. [Anon.] (1771), 16–17. Sir William De Grey was a sufferer.
119. *Ibid.*, 9.
120. *Ibid.*
121. Berdoe (1772), 63.
122. *Ibid.*, 14–15. Many used parallel arguments with respect to nerves or hypochondria.
123. *Ibid.*, 24–5.
124. *Ibid.*, 27.
125. *Ibid.*, 29.
126. *Ibid.*, 30.
127. *Ibid.*, 31.
128. *Ibid.*, 59.
129. *Ibid.*, 69.
130. *Ibid.*
131. William Carter (1772), vi.
132. *Ibid.*, 6.
133. *Ibid.*, 7.
134. *Ibid.*, 10.
135. *Ibid.*, 12.
136. *Ibid.*
137. *Ibid.*, 27–8.
138. *Ibid.*, 28.
139. *Ibid.*
140. *Ibid.*, 30–1.
141. *Ibid.* With those already suffering from gout, the priority was *relief*, not Cadogan's *lectures*: *ibid.*, 43–4.
142. *Ibid.*, 34–5. Mention of acorns suggests Mandeville's satirical *Fable of the Bees*, which, ironically, urged a return to acorn-eating as the manly way of recovering liberty and virtue.
143. *Ibid.*, 46.
144. [Anon.] (1771), 17.
145. Jay (1772), 18.

146. *Ibid.*, 2.
147. *Ibid.*, 10–11.
148. *Ibid.*, 18.
149. *Ibid.*, 25–6.
150. *Ibid.*, 43.
151. *Ibid.*, 44.
152. *Ibid.*, 21.
153. Kentish (1789), 17.
154. Sir James Mackintosh (1791), 48–9, quoted in Dickinson (1977), 243. On radicalism, see E. P. Thompson (1963).
155. Grant (1779), 1–2. This book has two paginations: all the following quotations, till noted, are from the first pagination. William Grant (d. 1786) became MD of Marischal College, Aberdeen in 1755. He practised for many years in Aberdeen.
156. *Ibid.*, 2.
157. *Ibid.*
158. *Ibid.*, 2–3.
159. Bryson (1945); Camic (1983); Roy Porter (1991a).
160. Grant (1779), 4.
161. *Ibid.*, 4–5.
162. *Ibid.*, 5–6.
163. *Ibid.*, 6. The Highlander Grant thus vindicated whisky.
164. *Ibid.*
165. *Ibid.*, 7.
166. *Ibid.*, 8.
167. *Ibid.* There are echoes here of Cheyne. Another contemporary Scot, the quackish sex-therapist James Graham, likewise blamed new comforts like soft beds for the decline in health: see Roy Porter (1989a), ch. vi.
168. Grant (1779), 9–10.
169. *Ibid.*, 10. There is an amusing echo here of the old Renaissance theory that capons were liable to gout.
170. *Ibid.*, 13.
171. *Ibid.*
172. *Ibid.*, 14–15. The ills significantly begin with the failure of the mother to give suck. Cadogan would have concurred.
173. *Ibid.*, 15.
174. *Ibid.*, 15–16.

175. *Ibid.*, 16–17.
176. *Ibid.*, 20–1.
177. *Ibid.*, 21.
178. *Ibid.*, 22–3.
179. *Ibid.*
180. *Ibid.*, 37–8.
181. *Ibid.*, 24.
182. *Ibid.*, 38–9.
183. *Ibid.*, 39.
184. *Ibid.*, 64–6.
185. *Ibid.*, 69.
186. *Ibid.*, 67–8.
187. *Ibid.*, 94.
188. *Ibid.*, 102–4.
189. *Ibid.*, 104.
190. *Ibid.*, 1 (this is from the the second pagination of the book, as are all subsequent quotations).
191. *Ibid.*, 2–3.
192. *Ibid.*, 8–9.
193. *Ibid.*, 9.
194. Grant gave the case of another Mr Grant, presumably a relative: *ibid.*
195. *Ibid.*, 10.
196. *Ibid.*, 55.
197. *Ibid.*, 55–6.
198. Beddoes (1802), ii, essay vii, 98; see Roy Porter (1991b). It might be significant that Beddoes promoted what many regarded as a quack remedy: see his contribution to A. Welles (1803) – Roy Porter (1991b), 135.
199. Beddoes (1802), ii, essay viii, 160–1.
200. Jeans (1792), 7.
201. *Ibid.*, 12.
202. *Ibid.*, 4.
203. *Ibid.*, 6–7.
204. *Ibid.*, 9.
205. *Ibid.*, 12.
206. *Ibid.*, 11.
207. *Ibid.*, 15.
208. *Ibid.*, 18.
209. *Ibid.*, 21.
210. *Ibid.*, 24.
211. William Stevenson (1779), v–vi. Stevenson (1719?–1783), an Irishman by birth, studied in Edinburgh; he practised in Coleraine for a time and then in Wells, Somerset; later he settled in Newark. He was known for his venomous pen.
212. *Ibid.*, vi–viii.

213. *Ibid.*, viii–ix.
214. *Ibid.*, ix.
215. *Ibid.*, ix–x.
216. *Ibid.*, xi–xii.
217. *Ibid.*, xii.
218. *Ibid.*, xii–xiii.
219. *Ibid.*, xviii. On popular perceptions of the alliance of death and the doctors, see Roy Porter (1989c), 77–94.
220. Stevenson (1779), xix.
221. *Ibid.*, xxii–xxii.
222. *Ibid.*, xxviii.
223. *Ibid.*, 42–3.
224. *Ibid.*, 43.
225. *Ibid.*, 44–5.
226. *Ibid.*, 48.
227. *Ibid.*, 48–9.
228. *Ibid.*, 49.
229. *Ibid.*, 50.
230. *Ibid.*, 56–7. For proof, Stevenson advised readers to 'consult the ingenious and elegant Dissertation on the gout by Dr Cadogan': 59.
231. *Ibid.*, 71.

Chapter 8: Change and Continuity, 1790–1850

1. Quoted by Pettigrew (1838–40), ii, 35.
2. Barbeau, ed. (1904); Rolls (1988), 86, 123, 142–3; Hembry (1990); Heywood (1990); Neale (1981); Wagner, ed. (1989).
3. For an instance of contemporary spa literature, see Oliver (1751); and for a bibliography, see Mullett (1946).
4. Copeman (1964), 91: grateful for his patronage, Bath made Pitt an honorary freeman in 1738. Laurence Sterne dedicated *Tristram Shandy* (1760) 'To the Right Honourable Mr. Pitt': 'I humbly beg, Sir, that you will honour this book, by taking it . . . into the country with you; where, if I am ever told it has made you smile; or conceive it has beguiled you of one moment's pain – I shall think myself as happy as a minister of state.' Pitt's grandfather and father had both had gout, and he

appears to have suffered from gout
(or at least some sort of arthritic
condition) since childhood. His gout
was responsible for long absences
from the House of Commons. In
the Commons debate over the peace
treaty with France in 1762, Pitt was
carried into the House with his
hands and feet swathed in flannel,
and hobbled to his place. He spoke
sitting for three hours: Jeremy Black
(1992), 92–3.

5. Copeman (1964), 92.
6. William Stevenson (1779), 93–4.
7. *Ibid.*, 117.
8. Heberden (1962), 51.
9. B. Griggs (1981); Fissell (1992);
   Chamberlain (1981). There is an
   extensive bibliography in Virginia S.
   Smith (1985).
10. For some of the medicines used, see
    Estes (1990).
11. For Walpole, see above, Chapter 6.
12. W. G. Black (1883), 38, 63, 184. In
    Scotland, infusions of black slugs
    were good for rheumatism, as was
    the wearing of a hare's foot or carry-
    ing a potato in the pocket: David
    Buchan, ed. (1994), 39, 106.
13. Wesley (1747), section 103, 76 and
    passim.
14. On self-help and its dangers, see
    Roy Porter (1991b); Roy Porter and
    Dorothy Porter (1988); Spilsbury
    (1780).
15. Ziemmsen, ed. (1870), xvi, 140.
16. Pat Rogers (1979), 173f.
17. Heberden (1962), 52.
18. Copeman (1964), 88–90.
19. P. S. Brown (1975), 352–69; *idem*
    (1976), 152–68.
20. Copeman (1964), 76. Atkins was a
    colourful, bewigged vendor of gout
    pills in Restoration London: C. J. S.
    Thompson (1928), 92–3.
21. Copeman (1964), 76.
22. This has been exhaustively studied
    by Doherty (1992), 34f.
23. *Ibid.*, 67.
24. Blegborough (1803), 36. Bleg-
    borough (1769–1827) was the son of
    a surgeon and studied medicine first
    as an apprentice and then at Edin-

burgh University, although he never
took a degree there. He practised in
London.

25. *Ibid.*, 39.
26. *Ibid.*, 44. See Rowbottom and
    Susskind (1984).
27. Blegborough (1803), 7–8. On mes-
    merism, see Gauld (1992).
28. Blegborough (1803), 11–12.
29. *Ibid.*, 26–7. If this can be believed, it
    implies the interesting possibility
    that ordinary lay people were
    reading medical journals (or at least
    that Blegborough thought that plau-
    sible).
30. *Ibid.*, 28.
31. Hartung (1954); Wallace (1973);
    Copeman (1964), ch. 3; Barton and
    Castle (1877), 109f.; Flückinger and
    Hanbury (1879), 699. Among the
    vernacular names for *Colchicum
    autumnale* was 'naked ladies'. The
    plant contains several toxic alkaloids,
    the chief of which is colchicine. In
    small doses, it relieves the pain of
    gout; larger doses cause diarrhoea
    and still larger doses are toxic and
    may cause death.
32. Copeman (1964), 39. Aetius (*fl.* 540
    AD) wrote a large medical encyclo-
    paedia, *Tetrabibloi*, consisting of
    excerpts from previous medical
    authors, principally Galen.
33. *Ibid.*, 41.
34. *Ibid.*, 42.
35. William Turner (1965), 60.
36. Bullein (1579), 46.
37. Gerard (1597), 131.
38. Flückinger and Hanbury (1879),
    699–700.
39. *Ibid.* (1618), 94.
40. For Sydenham and colchicum, see
    above, Chapter 4.
41. Anton von Stoerck (1731–1803)
    studied medicine in Vienna under
    van Swieten. Among his works are
    *An Essay on the Use and Effects of the
    Roots of the Colchicum Autumnale, or
    Meadow Saffron* (London: T. Becket
    and P. A. De Honte, 1764).
42. Dicker (1951) demonstrated on rats
    the water-eliminating action of
    colchicine.

43. Husson (1783; 1807).
44. A Mr Romart had brought twelve bottles to England in 1776: Ring (1811), 180–1. John Ring (1752–1821) was a great advocate of vaccination and became a lifelong friend of Edward Jenner.
45. *Ibid.*
46. For Banks and gout, see H. B. Carter (1988), 246ff.; Gascoigne (1994); Roy Porter (1998).
47. According to Scudamore, Wilson's tincture was a secret medicine composed of vegetable ingredients with certain ingredients added for disguise: 'the proprietor of the nostrum boldly asserted that it did not bear any resemblance to the *eau medicinale*, that it did not contain colchicum, and possessed equal curative powers with the *eau médicinale*, without any of its injurious influence': (1835b), 28–9. He deemed it harmful. For contemporary opinion, see Edwin Godden Jones (1810); Ring (1811), 168–71.
48. Cave, ed. (1983), 3,873.
49. *Ibid.*
50. *Ibid.*
51. Want (1814a; 1814b; 1814c; 1814d). Scudamore (1816), 161; *idem* (1817), 193, confirmed Want's analysis, but believed that Want's praise of colchicum was too extravagant. See also Scudamore (1833b). John Want was co-editor of the *Medical and Physical Journal* for six months between December and June 1814 where he published his writings on gout, stimulating strong opposition by advocating *Colchicum autumnale* in its treatment.
52. Hellman, ed. (1931), 412–38. Jenner was interested in the relations between rheumatism and the heart. He delivered to the Gloucestershire Medical Society a paper in 1789 entitled 'Remarks on a Disease of the Heart following Acute Rheumatism, illustrated by Dissections'.
53. Treue (1958).
54. Copeman (1964), 45; Bywaters (1972).
55. Scudamore (1816).
56. A. Welles (1803).
57. Haden (1820); Wallace (1973).
58. Lady Holland, ed. (1855), i, 346.
59. Lesch (1984).
60. See for example Gairdner (1849), 35.
61. Hartung (1954).
62. Scheele (1776). Scheele's essay was soon translated into English by a champion of chemical medicine and one who had his own contribution to make to the study of the gout, Thomas Beddoes: *The Chemical Essays of C. W. Scheele Translated . . . with Additions* (1786). For Beddoes on gout, see Beddoes (1793).
63. Bergman (1785).
64. Murray Forbes (1793).
65. Shute (1807–8), 337. Shute acknowledged the importance of Forbes's work.
66. Wollaston (1797).
67. For Bostock's work, see Scudamore (1816), 35.
68. Henry Bence Jones (1842), 35.
69. Copeman (1964), 102.
70. Prout (1818), 420–8.
71. Copeman (1964), 103.
72. Reece (1803), 378. See Virginia S. Smith (1985).
73. Reece (1803), 379.
74. *Ibid.*, 380. For Kinglake's belief in cold-water immersions, see below.
75. *Ibid.*, 384.
76. *Ibid.*, 385.
77. *Ibid.*
78. *Ibid.*
79. Parkinson (1805); for an account of this wide-ranging man, see Arthur D. Morris (1989). For Parkinson's popular advice on gout, see (1801), 221–33. He is best known for his *An Essay on the Shaking Palsy* (1817), now known as Parkinson's Disease.
80. Parkinson (1805), vi.
81. *Ibid.*, viii. A political radical, Parkinson also democratized.

82. *Ibid.*, 101.
83. *Ibid.*, 102–4.
84. *Ibid.*, 159.
85. *Ibid.*, 177.
86. *Ibid.*, 179.
87. Kinglake (1804).
88. Parkinson (1805), 130ff. Parkinson was supported in this respect by Ring (1816).
89. Kinglake (1807a), in which he quoted the favourable opinions of the medical press and fellow practitioners. He followed this with (1807b).
90. Parkinson (1805), 3.
91. Kinglake (1807a).
92. Parkinson (1805), 72–3.
93. *Ibid.*
94. *Ibid.*
95. Charles Scudamore (1779–1849) was an enthusiastic purger. He advocated a formidable combination of calomel, antimony and compound extract of colocynth, repeating it nightly or every second day for a time: Scudamore (1816), 185.
96. Scudamore (1816); Copeman (1964); 105f.
97. Scudamore (1833b).
98. Idem (1816), 127–8.
99. *Ibid.*, 15.
100. *Ibid.*, 7.
101. Twenty years later Garrod repeated this analysis and reported that among his hospital patients 50 per cent of gout cases were of hereditary origin, but among his private patients a convincing family history was produced in no fewer than 75 per cent: Alfred Garrod (1859).
102. Scudamore (1823), 70.
103. *Ibid.*, 25.
104. *Idem* (1833a); Copeman (1964), 105.
105. Scudamore (1816), 9–10.
106. Gairdner (1849). William Gairdner (1793–1867) held various posts at London hospitals but grew famous as a fashionable practitioner. *On Gout* (1849) reached its 4th edn in 1860. The 2nd edn will be quoted (1851).
107. *Ibid.*, 1.
108. *Ibid.*, 4.

109. *Ibid.*, 7.
110. *Ibid.*, 45.
111. For the medical debate, see E. A. Smith (1990), 323–5.
112. Gairdner (1849), 60, 62.
113. *Ibid.*, 68.
114. *Ibid.*, 70, 79. It was for such reasons that the 'facts of clinical medicine' disproved 'Liebig's theory': 87.
115. *Ibid.*, 117.
116. *Ibid.*, 184.
117. *Ibid.*, 240. In that respect even the great Sydenham was wrong: 253.
118. *Ibid.*, 260.
119. Wardrop (1851). On gouty heart, see English (1992).
120. Evan Bedford (1974). Gouty heart also interested other nineteenth-century theorists: Fothergill (1879); Balfour (1894): he regarded the senile heart as a synonym for the gouty heart. Mention should finally be made of the pioneer of the understanding of rheumatoid arthritis: Augustin-Jacob Landré-Beauvais (1772–1840); see Parish (1964).

Chapter 9: Indian Summer: Romantic and Victorian Gout

1. Henry Halford (1766–1844) was physician to four successive monarchs and had treated almost every member of the royal family; he was created a baronet in 1809.
2. Wiltshire (1991).
3. This material is cited in Halperin (1984). See especially 221, 223, 296–7, 335–8 for her last illness, and entries for 16 December 17–18 and July 1817. Halperin attributes her own death to miliary tuberculosis. For comparison of the gender arrangements for hysteria in Austen's time, see Gilman, King, Porter, Rousseau and Showalter (1993), 135–8, 328–31.
4. Disraeli (1804–81) was much younger than Jane Austen, of course, born after she had written her first

novel, but he wrote in the same decade. Unlike his father, he did not keep the apostrophe in his name.

5. Bradford (1982).

6. See Rosa (1960); Adburgham (1983).

7. For Disraeli's 'Gallomania', see Bradford (1982), 197.

8. Sara Austen had recommended in 1821 that Colburn publish Robert Plumer Ward's *Tremaine*, which he did, and she probably introduced Disraeli to the book. A few months after the publication of *Vivian Grey*, as Disraeli's health worsened, Austen whisked him away with her to the Continent for two months. See Disraeli (1926; 1826, 1st edn) and E. A. Smith (1990).

9. See Robert E. Moore's (1948) chapter on Smollett.

10. *Vivian Grey*, VIII, iii; the following passages are from this section.

11. See William Fraser (1891), *passim*.

12. See Chapter 7 above.

13. See Adburgham (1983).

14. E. Johnson (1970).

15. Sinclair (1807), which was based on deep reading in eighteenth-century medicine.

16. Daiches (1971), ch. 1.

17. See Preston, ed. (1990), 16: to Sir Watkin Phillips, 18 April.

18. See Scott 1995b. 292.

19. *Ibid.*, 294.

20. *Ibid.*, 297.

21. See Breitenberg (1996); Spector (1994).

22. Thackeray (1972), 191. Mudge and Sears (1910), 56. They suggest that Lord Lonsdale, an old nobleman, was the original of Lord Colchicum. He was perhaps also the original of Lord Eskdale in Disraeli's *Tancred*.

23. For *Punch*, see Thackeray (1886) and Wedeen (1981).

24. Gairdner (1849).

25. Timbs (1876), 320–2. Timbs states that the passage has been reprinted from *Blackwood's Magazine* (1863), but the quotation is not to be found there.

26. Dickens (1972a), 271. For a more general discussion of Dickens and disease, see Bailin (1994). Gordon (1993) offers a psychoanalytical and deconstructionist interpretation of Dickens's use of gout that appears rather forced.

27. Dickens (1972b), 355.

28. Dickens (1972a), ch. 16.

29. *Little Dorrit*, Book i, ch. 10.

30. *Ibid.*

31. See below, Chapter 12, for discussion of Dickens's metaphoric use of gouty language.

32. It was not possible to perform a blood test for gout until Emil Fischer studied the proteins of the purine group, for which he was awarded the Nobel Prize in 1902.

33. For Coleridge's complaints and documentation of the following pages, see Lefebure (1974), 46–50, 316f., 374, 375; Fruman (1971); Holmes (1989), 352. Lefebure is probably right to suggest that Coleridge suffered from chronic rheumatic pains but not from gout proper.

34. E. L. Griggs, ed. (1956–68), ii (1801–6), 974–7: to Robert Southey, letter 513, Sunday, 14 August 1803. The *Encyclopaedia Britannica* discussion of 'atonic gout' reads:

> The first is when the gouty diathesis prevails in the system, but, from certain causes, does not produce the inflammatory affection of the joints. In this case the morbid symptoms which appear are chiefly affections of the stomach, such as loss of appetite, indigestion, and its various attendants of sickness, nausea, vomiting, flatulency, and eructations, and pains in the region of the stomach . . . These affections of the alimentary canal are often attended with all the symptoms of hypochondriasis, such as dejection of mind, a constant and anxious attention to the slightest feelings,

an imaginary aggravation of these, and an appreciation of danger from them.

Encyclopaedia Britannica (1797),
xi, article 'Medicine'

It is indeed as though the author had Coleridge in mind!

35. E. L. Griggs, ed. (1956–68), ii (1801–6), 974–7: to Robert Southey, letter 513, Sunday, 15 August 1803.
36. For the altercation between Coleridge and his physician, Thomas Beddoes, who declined to sanction Coleridge's escapist plans of travelling to a warmer clime for his health, see Roy Porter (1991b), 134f.
37. See Coleby (1954); Milner (1842).
38. Kevin Knox, formally of Queens' College, Cambridge, has kindly shared his vast knowledge of this subject with us.
39. E. L. Griggs, ed. (1956–68), ii, 978–9: to Mrs S. T. Coleridge, letter 514, 2 September 1803. The tour is well covered in Holmes (1990), 342ff.
40. *Ibid.*, 980: to Mrs S. T. Coleridge, letter 515, Saturday, 3 September 1803.
41. *Ibid.*, 991: to Thomas Wedgwood, letter 520, 16 September 1803. On hysteria, see Gilman, King, Porter, Rousseau and Showalter (1993); Micale (1995) explores the complex history of male hysteria.
42. E. L. Griggs, ed. (1956–68), ii, 993: to Sir George and Lady Beaumont, letter 521, Saturday, 22 September 1803.
43. *Ibid.*, 1020–1: to Matthew Coates, letter 529, 5 December 1803.
44. *Ibid.*, 1041–2: to Mrs S. T. Coleridge, letter 537, 24 January 1804.
45. *Ibid.*, 1026–7: to Robert Southey, letter 533, 11 January 1804.
46. *Ibid.*, vi (1826–34), 764–5: to Daniel Stuart, letter 1642, 14 October 1828.
47. *Ibid.*, 767: to Gioacchino de'Prati, letter 1643, Tuesday, 14 October 1828.
48. *Ibid.*, 780: to F. A. Cox, letter 1657, Friday, 20 February 1829. The time-honoured theme is clear: only genuinely strong constitutions can resolve crises into paroxysms of gout; in weaker ones, such crises end in less healthy ways.
49. *Ibid.*, 787: to Henry Nelson Coleridge, letter 1658, 23 March 1829.
50. *Ibid.*, 788: to Thomas Allsop, letter 1659, early May 1829. Occasionally he also used other terms like 'sciatica': *ibid.*, 874: to James Gillman Jr, letter 1719, November 1831; or 'nervous rheumatism': *ibid.*, 875: to David Scott, letter 1720, 19 November 1831.
51. The following depends upon the authoritative account in R. B. Martin (1980), 83f.
52. *Ibid.*, 84.
53. *Ibid.*, 275.
54. *Ibid.*, 278–9. James Manby Gully (1808–83) was born in Jamaica, coming to England in 1814. From 1842 until his retirement in 1876, he and James Wilson settled in Malvern to practice hydropathy.
55. R. B. Martin (1980), 279.
56. *Ibid.*, 321.
57. For Carlyle, see Fred Kaplan (1986).
58. For Carlyle at Malvern, see Fred Kaplan (1986), under 'illness'.
59. Frederick's illness has been the source of great debate; see Asprey (1986), chs. i–ii.
60. Casanova, the memoirist and adventurer, interviewed Frederick during these years around 1760 but is silent on any gout or related symptoms.
61. R. B. Martin (1980), 567.
62. Hembry (1990); Janet Browne (1990).
63. Jeffrey, ed. (1907), ii, 5. Compare Elizabeth Lucy's memoirs (29 April 1876) at Droitwich taking brine baths. At lunch there were '16 rheumatic, neuralgic and gouty patients sitting round it, and some horrible looking stew at the top'. 'Sir Thomas and Lady Riddle arrived

that evening, he seemed to be a martyr to gout and had tried the brine baths before': Fairfax-Lucy, ed. (1893), 152–3.

64. For Darwin's health and his attempts at cure, see Desmond and Moore (1991), 529; Bowlby (1990), 215, 239, 258, 267, 254 – an account especially strong on the psychosomatic dimension; Janet Browne (1990), 102–13; Colp (1977), 59: this remains the most thorough account of Darwin's illness career.

65. Sir Henry Holland (1788–1873) was appointed physician extraordinary to Queen Victoria in 1837.

66. Colp (1977), 59.

67. Janet Browne (1990), 104. The book in question was Gully (1846); his fellow hydropath James Wilson published a similar work (1842); see also *idem* (1843); and Wilson and Gully (1844).

68. Janet Browne (1990), 107.

69. *Ibid.*, 108.

70. Colp (1977), 80.

71. *Ibid.*

72. *Ibid.*, 83.

73. *Ibid.*, 109.

74. *Ibid.*

75. *Ibid.*

76. *Ibid.*

77. *Ibid.*

78. *Ibid.*; Bynum (1983). On Victorian views about hereditary illness, see Olby (1993); Lopéz-Beltrán (1994; 1992).

79. Ellis (1927).

80. Osbert Sitwell (1945), 76–7. The *Evening Standard* reported on 8 March 1995 that the talented young theatre director Sam Mendes was suffering from gout, making much of the traditional associations, and juxtaposing his photo to a portrait of Samuel Johnson.

81. *Ibid.*, 77–8.

82. See Wallace (1962); Virgin (1994).

83. Nowell C. Smith, ed. (1953), ii, 637: to Lady Grey, letter 1710, 1 February 1836.

84. *Ibid.*, 636–7: to Sir George Philips, letter 709, 11 January 1836.

85. *Ibid.*, 798: to Lady Grey, letter 937, 25 September 1843. On lay physicking, see Dorothy Porter and Roy Porter (1989). Self-dosing was encouraged by home-care manuals. Mrs Beeton (1906), in 1854–5, cautioned temperance and suggested that the tincture of wine of colchicum be given every four hours.

86. Nowell C. Smith, ed. (1953), ii, 574–5: to Lady Grey, letter 641, 22 September 1833. For Smith's makeshift village doctoring activities, see Virgin (1994), 179.

87. Nowell C. Smith, ed. (1953), ii, 710: to Lady Carlisle, letter 815, 5 September 1840.

88. *Ibid.*, 591: to Mrs Meynell, letter 664, July 1834. See Virgin (1994), 276.

89. Lady Holland, ed. (1855), i, 35.

90. *Ibid.*

91. Nowell C. Smith, ed. (1953), ii, 591: to Mrs Meynell, letter 664, July 1834.

92. *Ibid.*, 710: letter 81.

93. *Ibid.*, i, 267: to Lady Holland, 8 November 1816.

94. *Ibid.*, 452–3: to John Allen, letter 487, 9 November 1926.

95. *Ibid.*, ii, 522: to John Allen, letter 565, November 1830.

96. *Ibid.*, 643–4: to Sir George Philips, letter 720, 30 July 1836.

97. *Ibid.*, 649: to Sir George Philips, letter 727, 22 December 1836.

98. *Ibid.*, 655: to Lady Grey, letter 736, 12 May 1837.

99. *Ibid.*, 776: to Harriet Martineau, letter 907, 4 January 1843. Smith clearly thought that Miss Martineau's views about illness were over the top. In 1844 he wrote to Lady Grey: 'I have just read Miss Martineau's *Sick room*. I cannot understand it. It is so sublime, and mystical that I frequently cannot guess at her meaning': *ibid.*, 826: to Lady Grey, letter 975, 9 March 1844.

100. That market is well depicted in Shorter (1992).

101. Edward Bulwer-Lytton, *A Strange Story* (London, 1875).

102. *Ibid.*, 375. Some readers will notice the story's similarity to Patrick Süskind's *Das Parfum* (1985), although there is no mention of gout in the latter.

103. Meredith (1906), 198, ch. 21.

104. George Eliot, *Silas Marner* (London, 1860), 3. Eliot had read *Bleak House* by 1858.

105. We have been especially influenced by Furst's (1993) excellent work on George Eliot, and Peterson (1978), less so by Rothfield's (1992) chapter on Lydgate, medicine and *Middlemarch* because Rothfield seems unaware of Lydgate's final retreat into a 'treatise on gout'.

106. Le Fanu (1884), 172. For Le Fanu, see McCormack (1980) and the somewhat less reliable Begnal (1971).

107. Le Fanu (1884), 164.

Chapter 10: Gout and Glory: Garrod and After

1. Peters (1991) relates Collins's diminutive size (height, hands, feet), his bulging forehead and his poor vision: 20–1. She entertains the possibility that Collins's 'gout of the eyes' may have been Reiter's disease: 149–50.

2. Dr Francis Carr Beard treated Collins for more than thirty years, from 1855 to his death: Berridge and Edwards (1981).

3. Peters (1991), 148–50.

4. Berridge and Edwards (1981); Peters (1991), 256–8.

5. Peters (1991), 268–9.

6. *Ibid.*, 68–9.

7. *Ibid.*, 292.

8. *Ibid.*, 292.

9. Kenneth Robinson (1951), 177–8. Also see William Clarke (1988).

10. Brock (1993), 153–68.

11. For information, see Copeman (1964), 107ff.; Beck (1970); Bearn (1993) – this fine study of Garrod's son illuminates the father. On the Victorian medical world, see Lawrence (1994); Peterson (1978); Digby (1994). In 1899 the French town of Aix-les-Bains named a street after Sir Alfred Garrod, who had praised the value of the waters at Aix. He does not seem to have been honoured similarly in his own country.

12. Alfred Garrod (1848).

13. Here and below the quotations are taken from the 2nd edn of 1863: 98, 316–17. Garrod's firm conviction of the role of alcohol in gout was widely accepted. '*Alcohol* is the most potent factor in the etiology of the disease': Osler (1898), 408.

14. Alfred Garrod (1854).

15. The book enjoyed a 3rd edn in 1876. Garrod's views did not substantially change from edition to edition.

16. Alfred Garrod (1863), 316.

17. *Ibid.*

18. *Ibid.*, 317. A perceptive account of the localizing strategies of scientific physicians at this time is provided in Bynum (1994).

19. Alfred Garrod (1863), 317.

20. *Ibid.*, 319.

21. *Ibid.* The evidence was adduced in Chapter 4. For Garrod on lead, see Wedeen (1984a).

22. Alfred Garrod (1863), 320–1.

23. *Ibid.*, 321.

24. *Ibid.*, 322.

25. *Ibid.*, 323–4.

26. *Ibid.*, 324–5.

27. *Ibid.*, 325–6

28. *Ibid.*, 326–7.

29. *Ibid.*, 327–8.

30. *Ibid.*, 329–30. Garrod used the term rheumatoid arthritis 'to imply an inflammatory affection of the joints, not unlike rheumatism in some of its characters, but differing materially from it'. By contrast, the homeopath Richard Epps noted that 'this disease

in many points resembles acute rheumatism': (1863), 145. Compare also Coffin (1850), 237, where it is stated that gout is 'but another name for rheumatism'.

31. Alfred Garrod (1863), 330–1.
32. *Ibid.*, 332.
33. *Ibid.*, 332–3.
34. *Ibid.*, 333–7.
35. *Idem* (1876), 292.
36. *Ibid.*, 293–4.
37. *Idem* (1876); *idem* (1861).
38. *Idem* (1863), 251. By the final edition, however, he had mellowed somewhat on the demon drink. 'It appears', he wrote, 'that all causes leading either to an increased formation of acidity, or its defective elimination and all causes suddenly lowering the nervous system, have a powerful influence in exciting an attack of gout in subjects already predisposed to it': *idem* (1876), 248.
39. Bynum (1994); Brock (1993).
40. These questions of experimental biology in humans and animals have been masterfully dealt with by Hartung (1957).
41. Edward Duke Moore (1864).
42. *Ibid.*, 3. Old-school physicians like Moore have been well characterized by Lawrence (1985).
43. Edward Duke Moore (1864), 5.
44. *Ibid.*
45. *Ibid.*, 6–7.
46. *Ibid.*, 11.
47. *Ibid.*, 12.
48. *Ibid.*, 14.
49. *Ibid.*, 16.
50. *Ibid.*, 15.
51. *Ibid.*, 16. Warner (1986) has demonstrated how the period between *c.* 1800 and 1860 was the high noon of violent purgative medicines, notably calomel.
52. Edward Duke Moore (1864), 17.
53. *Ibid.*, 8–9.
54. Ebstein (1885), 1–3. Most gouty patients belonged 'to the higher strata of society': *ibid.*, 38.
55. *Ibid.*, 2–3. Jonathan Hutchinson (1828–1913) was surgeon at the

London Hospital (1859–83) and Professor of Surgery at the Royal College of Physicians (1879–83); he was knighted in 1908. He delivered the Bowman Lecture, 'On the Relation of Certain Diseases of the Eyes to Gout,' in 1884. Defending himself against charges of 'seeing gout in everything' he affirmed: 'that the gouty constitution exists, and is very common in our English population, that it is potent in the production of disease, and that it is remarkably hereditary, are facts which no one will doubt': (1884a), 1,000.

56. Ebstein (1885), 4–8: 'It is incomprehensible to me how any one can ever again fall back on such unsatisfying theories as these.'
57. *Ibid.*, 8.
58. *Ibid.*, 8, 14–16.
59. *Ibid.*, 17–18.
60. *Ibid.*, 19–20, 30–1, 34–5, 38–9.
61. Meyers (1991), p. 115. Our analysis of Conrad's gout relies heavily on Meyers, whose account seems authoritative beyond the other studies we have consulted.
62. *Ibid.*, 130.
63. For sources, see *ibid.*, 132–40.
64. *Ibid.*, 140–1.
65. Quoted in *ibid.*, 141–2.
66. *Ibid.*, 356.
67. *Ibid.*
68. Jean-Aubry, ed. (1927), ii, 93.
69. *Ibid.*, 193.
70. *Ibid.*, 240.
71. *Ibid.*
72. Duckworth (1889), 2. Dyce Duckworth (1840–1928) served as physician and governor at St Bartholomew's Hospital for fifty-eight years. He was also censor, councillor and treasurer at the Royal College of Physicians. On neurology, see E. S. Clarke and L. S. Jacyna (1987).
73. Duckworth (1889), 3. Duckworth upheld the old ruling that gout was a rich man's disease – a club excluding the poor and women.

74. *Ibid.*, 6.

75. *Ibid.*, 7.

76. *Ibid.*, 10–12.

77. *Ibid.*, 12.

78. Jonathan Hutchinson (1884), 3, 22, 75–6. For a helpful account of Hutchinson, see Bynum (1983).

79. Duckworth (1889), 12.

80. *Ibid.*, 12–20.

81. *Ibid.*, 30–2.

82. *Ibid.*, 52–5.

83. Fothergill (1881), 2. See also *idem* (1879).

84. *Idem* (1881), 4.

85. Fothergill (1883), Part ii, 1.

86. *Ibid.*, 42.

87. *Ibid.*, 149–50.

88. *Ibid.*, 161–2.

89. *Ibid.*, 171–2.

90. Roose (1885), 1–3. Robson Roose (1848–1905) practised in Brighton for a number of years; his home was frequented by peers and politicians and he became known as an Amphitryon.

91. *Ibid.*, 4–5, 7, 49, 51.

92. *Ibid.*, 51, 52, 92–3. See Liveing (1873).

93. Roose (1885), 80–1, 91. See Buzzard (1891).

94. Wade (1893), 10, 11, 26–7, 36. Wade cited Wilhelm Erb as a modern authority.

95. Osler (1892), 408.

96. Ewart (1896), 8. See also *idem* (1894).

97. *Idem* (1896), ix: 'Aretaeus of Cappadocia has told us that "of the nature of gout none but the gods have a true understanding". This thought may allay some of the disappointment to which our present labours are doomed': *ibid.*, 310.

98. *Ibid.*, 1–3. See also, for constitutional diseases, Roy Porter (1996b).

99. Ewart (1896), 3–4.

100. *Ibid.*, 25–9, 25–7, 25–9.

101. *Ibid.*, 29.

102. *Ibid.*, 31–8.

103. *Ibid.* Alexander Haig gained his medical qualification at St Bartholomew's Hospital, qualifying in 1879. He became assistant physician to the Metropolitan Hospital in 1883 and consultant physician in 1912. He also worked at St Bart's and the Royal Waterloo Hospital. He suffered from migraine, and research suggested to him that excessive uric acid was the cause. He wrote on diet and gout, including *Diet and Food* (1902).

104. Ewart (1896), 31–5.

105. *Ibid.*, 38–41, 202, 228.

106. *Ibid.*, 267, 311, 313, 315. The notion of nutritional disorders was of course becoming prominent at this time. See Carpenter (1993).

107. Ewart (1896), 316.

108. *Ibid.*, 318.

109. Haig (1908), vi. His career is discussed in Whorton (1982), ch. viii.

110. Haig (1908), 1, 2, 4.

111. *Ibid.*, 659.

112. *Ibid.*

113. *Idem* (1903), 40.

114. *Ibid.*, 40–4.

115. Whorton (1982), 242.

116. *Ibid.*, 242–7.

117. *Ibid.*, 250.

118. Consult Dally (1996) for parallels with the later career of Arbuthnot Lane.

119. Llewellyn (1920), 6. See also Llewellyn and Jones (1915). Richard Llewellyn Jones Llewellyn (d.1934) was educated at the University of Wales and University College London, graduating as MB in 1895. After posts in University College Hospital and Durham County Asylum, he started in medical practice in Aberystwyth. Interested in arthritis and rheumatoid conditions, he moved to Bath, starting a specialist practice there, and was appointed physician to the Royal Mineral Water Hospital. Llewellyn held office in the physical medicine section of the Royal Society of Medicine and was president of the balneological and climatological section. He was a prolific writer on the subject, and his works include *Gout* (1920) and *Aspects of Rheumatism and Gout* (1927).

120. Llewellyn (1920), 21.
121. *Ibid.*, 23.
122. *Ibid.*, 23–5.
123. *Ibid.*, 28–31.
124. *Ibid.*, 36.
125. *Ibid.*, 42.
126. *Ibid.*, 42.
127. *Ibid.*, 44.
128. *Ibid.*, 50, 52, 53, 60.
129. *Ibid.*, 69–70, 304.
130. *Ibid.*, 70.
131. *Ibid.*, 332.
132. *Ibid.*
133. *Ibid.*, 8. Llewellyn's sense that gout had had its day parallels the demise of hysteria after the war. See Micale (1993), 496–526; *idem* (1995).
134. Idem (1927), 6–7.
135. *Ibid.*
136. *Ibid.*, 8–9.
137. Ryle (1949; 1994); Dorothy Porter and Roy Porter (1988).
138. Llewellyn (1927), 6–7.
139. *Ibid.*, 10.
140. *Ibid.*, 21.
141. *Ibid.*, 147–9
142. Edel (1977).
143. *Ibid.*
144. The most reliable biographer is Lynn (1987).
145. Hemingway (1963), 122.

Chapter 11: Podagra Ludens: Disease and Discourse

1. See Pauli (1901) for H. S. Beham and these works of 1607; for the iconography, see below, Chapter 12.
2. Huizinga (1949), 28. See also Ehrmann (1968); Nardo (1991); Piaget (1972); Pensky (1993); Simons (1985); Solnit, Cohen and Neubauer, eds (1993).
3. Jacobus (1990).
4. In this curious work of 1659, copies of which are found at Harvard, Oxford and London, 'political gout' becomes a category for considera-

tion despite its amorphous politico-medico elements.
5. For the 'gout' of George III, see Macalpine and Hunter (1969).
6. See Siraisi (1990); Park (1992).
7. For metaphors of pre-Newtonian gravity, see Rousseau (1978b).
8. See Antonioli (1976), 206–12.
9. We are grateful to Richard Cooper of Brasenose College, Oxford for this information.
10. Bakhtin (1968).
11. *Ibid.*, 303–55; see especially the section on 'Menippus, or the Descent into Hades', 69–70, 386–8.
12. For this heritage, see Henry Ansgar Kelly (1993).
13. The pseudonym of Johann Valentin Andraeae (1586–1654). We use the term 'Menippean' distinctly from 'Lucianic', the latter to describe traditions set in motion by Lucian whom Sydenham read; the former – 'Menippean' – to refer to non-dramatic forms inspired by this admittedly loose category; see Frye (1957).
14. See above, Chapter 2, notes 33–5.
15. Kirk (1980).
16. See Sydenham (1850), section 70, where it is clear he composes with Lucian's text beside him.
17. Biedermann (1666): Jesuit poet who wrote the lives of Catholic saints and martyrs, victims to illness and 'martyrs to the gout'; he also wrote post-Lucianic plays about man's mortality and suffering in a world racked with jest.
18. Colie (1976); Frye (1957); Kirk (1980).
19. The 1525 edition is called *In podagram concertatio . . . Adiectus est dialogus inter Podagram & Christophorum Ballistam*, without further ludic denominator and is dialogic, while the 1570 edition is entitled *De podagræ laudibus doctorum hominum lusus, etc.*
20. McKeown, ed. (1990).
21. G. S. Rousseau and N. Rudenstine, eds (1972).

22. Holquist (1981), 59.
23. Especially 90–135, 'mercury', 'the judge'. Maier's, also Mayerne and Mayerus', copy is found in the Bodleian Library, Oxford. See Craven (1910) and Jong (1965) for overviews of Maier.
24. Maier (1654), 95.
25. *Ibid.*, 96.
26. For this literary–medical yoking, especially in the context of Pope's *Epistle to Dr Arbuthnot*, see Knoepflmacher (1970).
27. See Kirk (1980) for other works conceived through the synergy of 'overthrow'.
28. Melvyn and Joan New, eds (1978).
29. War and illness as medical metaphors are discussed by Sontag (1978).
30. Spenser (1633), 105.
31. For these early newspapers, see Raymond (1993), 14–22.
32. Cited in *ibid.*
33. For 'swelling' in mid-seventeenth-century physics and chemistry, see Shapin and Schaffer (1985) and Shapin (1994), *passim*.
34. Grierson (1912), i, 51.
35. Bald (1970); Carey (1981); Walton (1927).
36. D. C. Allen (1943).
37. Wednesday, 13 August 1645.
38. For hysteria's metaphoric status, see G. S. Rousseau in Gilman, King, Porter, Rousseau and Showalter (1993).
39. Ong (1982).
40. The matter raises large questions about the epistemological status of cultural history; see P. Burke (1992); Darnton (1984).
41. Lovejoy (1948).
42. Raymond, ed. (1993), 6.
43. A copy is in the Houghton Library, Harvard University.
44. Witty (1677); expanded version (London, 1685).
45. *Poems on Affairs of State*, I, 292.
46. Copy in Houghton Library, Harvard University.
47. For Manton, see C. Hill (1975).

48. [Anon.] (1736); subsequent passages from this edition.
49. [Anon.] (1764).
50. Brownsword is the authentic name, his poem genuinely Menippean, ludic and worthy of inclusion.
51. Foxon attributes it to Allen and dates it as 1764.
52. D'Escherny (1760).
53. As in Fenton's poem (1706) which takes 'the attack' as its specific subject for versification; it was first printed in *Oxford and Cambridge Miscellany Poems*, which Fenton had edited, but was not there identified as his.
54. D. Bond, ed. (1965), ii, 442, by 'Mr Spectator' (Steele), 7 December 1711.
55. Wagner, ed. (1989), 36.
56. See Neale (1981); for print culture, Brewer and Porter (1993).
57. Strachey (1938), vii, 314.
58. Stevens (1758); the charge was made in *Monthly Review* 10 (August 1758), 145–50, which stirred further controversy in M.D.'s 'A Treatise on the Medicinal Qualities of Bath-Waters . . .', *Monthly Review* 10 (September 1758), 371–9.
59. Charles Martin (1759), 145.
60. We do not attempt to provide examples of all the points but to survey the vast undergrowth of metaphor and linguistic variety. As we indicate, another book would be necessary to provide the documentation. The point is that idiosyncrasies in linguistic patterns varied among authors, yet it is not our task, we think, in the allotted space to list examples of these diversities but to chart their types. See also P. Rogers (1981).
61. Norton, ed. (1956), i, 160, 352ff.
62. *Ibid.*
63. Sedgwick (1985); Rousseau and Porter, eds (1987).
64. See John Dryden's Hastings poem (1649), I, 81, and the discussion of the 'gouty' Dryden–Oldham poems of the old Dryden in Winn (1992),

81–2, who also discusses the homosocial stresses.

65. Ricks, ed. (1987), iii, 57, 181. For the metaphor of gout in Tennyson, see also Tennyson's 'gouty oaks' in 'Amphion' in *idem*, ii, 115–16, and the uses of it when in old age in 'Lucretius', ii, 715.

66. Rowley (1770); *idem* (1792); the quotation is found at 415. Rowley was born in London of Irish parents. His attack on William Hunter impeded his career, which ended in less than the state of perfection he had hoped for it.

67. *Encyclopaedia Britannica* (1797), xi, 213; see also Burney (1796), 325 and 940; Edward A. and Lilian D. Bloom, eds (1978), vii, 231.

68. For a popular statement of the point see T. Dawson (1771).

69. For these uses in a medical work, see Wynter (1725).

70. King and Ryskamp (1979–84), iii, 363.

71. Massachusetts Historical Society (1969), iii, 369; 'In coffin Thomas Aston, 24 June 1800'.

72. *London Magazine* (1755). Drake's metaphors in 'A Dissertation on the Gout' include gout's 'arthritic tyranny' due to life of luxury and intemperance, its lingering death and Promethean birdlike imagery, often likened to vultures 'gnawing' the patient to 'torment'.

73. Cornford (1993), 11.

74. Reynolds (1903), 32–3.

75. Described by McGovern (1992), 72–5.

76. See below, Chapter 12, for visual representations of this strain of conjugal consolation.

77. As found in Reynolds (1903).

78. Medical and herbal images – the cabbage-hearted 'colewort' and plaster-like remedy of cataplasm – are widely found in Finch's poetry ('Spleen').

79. Both Finches were well read in medicine and knew the prevalent theory that gout clings to excess and flees poverty, as in diet and exercise; but there is no reason, as McGovern (1992) suggests (237), to link these ideas with Fuller (1704) and Palmer (1696, 1984); the ideas were widespread throughout Finch's milieu.

80. W. S. Lewis, ed. (1937–83), xiii–xiv, 143 to Thomas Gray, 19 November 1765.

81. Toynbee and Whibley (1935), III.

82. *Ibid.*, 1148: 17 September 1770.

83. W. S. Lewis, ed. (1937–83), i, 234.

84. Poem in *London Magazine* (December 1734), 660.

85. See Doren (1938); Ronald W. Clark (1983); Fleming (1972).

86. Ronald W. Clark (1983), 368.

87. Nugent (1898), 225.

88. Norton (1956), iii, 83.

89. F. E. Hutchinson (1941), 195.

90. Hence the critic and social commentator Joseph Addison records in the *Spectator* for 30 July 1714 that 'Doctor Hammond reflected when he had gout he was grateful he didn't have the Stone; and that when he had Stone, that he didn't have both Destempers on him at the same time.' See D. Bond, ed. (1965), v, 564.

91. Pye (1757), i, 18.

92. William Stevenson (1779).

93. Butt *et al.* (1939–69), 3 Ep. 1.130.25.

94. *Ibid.*, 3 Ep. 1.251.37.

95. For 'flying gout', see Rowley (1792) and above, p. 230; for Mrs Thrale, see Balderston, ed. (1951), ii, 868.

96. W. S. Lewis, ed. (1937–83), xxxiii, 428.

97. Anderson, ed. (1972), 127.

98. D. Bond, ed. (1965), v, 42: no. 597, 22 September 1714.

99. *Critical Review* (1758).

100. *Ibid.* (1771).

101. Zedler (1732–50), col. 1710, Latin verses, 'podagra'.

102. Stukeley (1734), 158.

103. Balderston (1942), ii 866, 868: 23 January 1794.

104. Derry (1982), 326, n. 7.

105. D. Bond, ed. (1965), ii, 105: by Addison, 29 March 1711.

106. *Ibid.*, i, 206–7: no. 48, 18 April 1711.

107. The process is described by Berg (1974), 227; see above, Chapter 10, for 'Pain in a Plural Existence'.
108. Arbuthnot (1731), 34.
109. Macalpine and Hunter (1969), 221–2.
110. See R. Adair, manuscript on gout in the Countway Library of Medicine; and James M. Adair (1786).
111. For Gray's gout as the 'female enemy' see above, p. 235.
112. For an excellent example, see Norton (1956), iii, 27–8. Gibbon's 'enemy' could also be seductively 'arbitrary and capricious' (53) despite attempting to 'carry the war' (83).
113. *Ibid.*, ii, 411. Tissot was the only figure in all Switzerland Gibbon had known with gout.
114. Cumberland (1807), i, 23.
115. Baring-Gould, ed. (1967), ii, 478.
116. See Zeldin (1993), and for Herrick, see L. C. Martin, ed. (1963), 98 and 207.
117. Defoe (1965).
118. Phelps (1685).
119. *London Magazine* (1754), 603.
120. See Marshall (1770), 21–3 for the father's story; our search has produced nothing biographical about LeFevre.
121. *Ibid.*, 41–2 for Myers and pp. 63–4 for the convent turned into a 'gouty nunnery'.
122. *Ibid.*, 21.
123. Eland (1931), ii, 226.
124. [Anon.] (1770); see the interesting review in *Critical Review* (1770).
125. Johnston of Kidderminster was respected for his work on the nervous system. Thirty years later Marshall wrote historical fiction rather than autobiographical memoirs; see his *Edmund and Elenora: or memoirs of the Houses of Summerfield and Gretten . . . in two volumes* (London, 1797), which was translated into French.
126. [Anon.] (1770), 56.
127. W. S. Lewis, ed. (1937–83), xxxiii, 550: 22 December 1786. The idea of a subgenre of 'gout correspondences' is not fanciful and had existed for a generation by this time, as entire correspondences, like Matthew Bramble's to Dr Lewis, existed to narrate major conditions like gout and consumption.
128. *Ibid.*, ii, 286: 30 December 1781.
129. Grierson (1933), 394–5.
130. Green (1965), 682.
131. Mallam (1993), 1188.

Chapter 12: Gout: The Visual Heritage

1. Our interpretation of images has been informed by Panofsky (1974); Culler (1981); Baxandall (1985). We have also profited from Grego (1880).
2. See Nardo (1991).
3. For Renaissance emblems books, see Siraisi (1990); Panofsky (1974).
4. Titled 'The Gout', it is signed 'by Davison of Alnwick' and is uncatalogued in the Print Collection of the Huntington Library.
5. See above, p. 251, for discussion of Jeaurat's painting.
6. It first appeared on 14 May 1799, called 'The Comforts of Bath, 1798 aquatint' and is discussed by Paulson (1972), 111; see also Wagner (1985), 175.
7. Illustrated editions appeared in England and America in the early decades of the nineteenth century but are now scarce. A 1794 colour print of the recoiling woman discussed here is found in the American Antiquarian Society, Massachusetts.
8. Lépicié, 'La Vieillesse', painted by Jeaurat, Paris, 1745.
9. See Lionel Kelly, ed. (1987). Female responses are brief and few, referring to Smollett's comic genre or the form of his novel but not remarking about Bramble's moral character or personality.
10. Rowlandson, Gillray and Cruikshank all contributed their share.
11. This is found as plate 3 in William

Hayley's *The Triumphs of Temper* (Newburyport, Mass., 1794).

12. See Wendorf (1990).

13. Sotheby's Catalogue, 8 July 1969.

14. Reprinted by kind courtesy of the Huntington Library, San Marino.

15. See Klibansky *et al.* (1964).

16. See Wuttke, ed. (1994) and Glock and Meidinger-Geise, eds (1970).

17. Benedek (1983); Eckert and Imhoff (1971); Reicke (1930).

18. See Atkins (1694), now a scarce work, a copy of which is found in the Wellcome Institute for the History of Medicine.

19. Vol. i, 693. No list of his patients is known, nor have any of Atkins's papers been found.

20. Found in an anonymous, undated volume in the Countway Library entitled *Bildersammlung aus der Geschichte der Medizin.*

21. Printed and sold by Edmund Freeman, Opposite of the North-Door of the State House. Boston: Edmund Freeman, 1788. This copy in the Houghton Library appears to be unique. It is catalogued there as by 'Emerigon' whose birth date is 1712 with no known date of death; we have been unable to determine whether this attribution is correct or gain any more information about him.

22. Dr John Scat's gouty patients bought them in England; see 'Histories of Gouty, Bilious, and Nervous Cases . . . related by the Patients Themselves to John Scat, M. D.', *Critical Review* (October 1780), 318–19.

23. Hill's colonial trade was satirized by A. Camlin in *A Satisfactory Refutation of Sir Hypo Bardana's 'Circumstances'* (London, 1775).

24. Linnaeus (1772); Andrew Freake (1806) should not be confused with John Freke (1748); for an example of the strawberry puffery, see Evan Jones to Winthrop Sargent, 7 April 1804; Massachusetts Historical Society (1969), iii, 368.

25. Dolaeus (1732), Stephens had also written about the future of the gout in 1705.

26. D. Bond, ed. (1965), ii, 265: entry for 13 October 1711.

27. Nicolson and Rousseau (1968), 37–40.

28. W. S. Lewis, ed. (1937–83), xxxiii, 534: 4 November 1786.

29. *Ibid.*

30. 'An Abstract of a Letter of Mr Anthony Leeuwenhoek Fellow of the R. Society; . . . the Chalk Stones of the Gout', *Philosophical Transactions*, 15, no. 168 (23 February 1685), 891–2.

31. He lived to almost ninety in an era when that was rare; Pettit (1971), letter 460, 24 August 1762.

32. *Ibid.*, letter 255, 20 February 1749.

33. Goldberg (1990).

34. *Ibid.*, ch. 6, 'The Hand in Theory', esp. 311–16.

35. Pettit (1971), letter 406, 492, 7 February 1759.

36. For these idealizations and portraits of 'writing males', see Wendorf (1989).

37. Parker (1978), 191–2, comments: 'It was a sort of couch, with movable positions from vertical to horizontal, seven feet long and two and a half feet wide, with a horsehair mattress. The king sat, ate and slept in it, wearing loose garments that did not put pressure on his arthritic joints.'

38. W. S. Lewis, ed. (1937–83), xxxiii, 525; the unfortunate target was John Harris, MP (d. 1767), married to Anne Seymour Conway, Walpole's cousin. Lewis notes that Harris was so ridden with gout 'he was in a wheel chair at the time of their nuptials. Walpole claims grooms of chambers would have to be called to wheel him and Lady Charleville (also gouty) when they had the urge to kiss'.

39. Norton, ed. (1956), iii, 167–8, 191, 197.

40. Rowlandson's 'Lieut. Bowling pleading the cause of young Rory to

his Grandfather'. R. Ackermann's Repository of Arts, 12 May 1800: London.

41. *Roderick Random* (1748), ch. 3; the words are Smollett's.

42. *Ibid.*

43. Joyce (1946), 263, 282, 710; Lyons (1973).

44. Toynbee and Whibley (1935), iii, 788: 4 December 1762.

45. For the metaphor of the 'wheel', see Roy Porter (1986).

46. De Beer (1955), iii, 502.

47. Latham and Matthews, eds (1970–83), ix, 215: entry for 27 May 1668.

48. *Ibid.*, 213: entry for 25 May 1668.

49. W. H. Dawson (1938), 438–9.

50. See plate 25.

51. Benjamin Jones's print of 'Hebert's Air-Pump Vapour Bath' appeared in various editions, in books, in 1802, published in New York, Philadelphia and Washington. Subtitled 'An Efficacious Remedy in Gout-Rheumatism Contractions and Enlargements'.

52. See plates 25–6.

53. Peter Maverick's plate is found in the 1813 edition of *The Life and Opinions of Tristram Shandy*, published in New York: W. Durrell and Co., after which time it routinely featured as the frontispiece of popular American editions of Sterne's novel.

54. For visual caricature and *Humphry Clinker*, see Robert E. Moore (1948); for the iconography of the gold-headed cane, see Macmichael (1923).

55. Norton, ed. (1956), iii, 92. The Swiss 'attacks' were different.

56. For the vivid episode, see Strachey and Fulford (1938), iv, 33.

57. See Hill (1958a and b) and Rousseau (1978a) for the caricatures.

58. Printed by W. Humphry, 17 March 1783.

59. For the Temple of Love, see Porter (1989a). Graham is not known to have claimed to be able to rehabilitate the gouty in his 'Temple of

Love', but no doubt the gouty also applied to him.

60. Paulson (1972).

61. This colour caricature *c.* 1780–1810 in the Countway Library has no further identification than its title.

62. Cole's only caveat was that all were such 'water drinkers' and might be prevented; W. S. Lewis, ed. (1837–83) 2, 53, Cole to Walpole, 28 August 1777.

63. This coloured caricature may have been part of a series of which only scraps remain in the Countway Library of Medicine, Boston, Massachusetts.

64. This coloured caricature may be part of the same series as the others discussed in this section but we have found no evidence to substantiate the claim.

65. Secondary works recognize the theme but rarely develop it.

66. This is an anonymous, coloured caricature of 1827, drawn by E.Y. Esq., engraved by G. Hunt, printed by Thom MacLean, 26 Haymarket, London.

67. By the 1820s dozens of such books had been printed in English, despite this one's fabrication.

68. Published 1 September 1786 by W. Dickinson, Engraver and Bookseller, 158 New Bond Street, drawn by Henry William Bunbury (1750–1811).

69. See Ritvo (1987) for the social history of this development.

70. Despite the attempts of some of the figures we have discussed – especially Cheyne in the eighteenth century – not enough was made in medical theory of the sedentary dilemma for the gouty; the visual heritage was able to elicit more fully the plight and excesses of the sedentary, as these caricatures show.

71. Bunbury (1787).

72. The Countway Library dates the print as 1799.

73. No author is known for this work of 1715.

74. See Wedeen (1981); Thackeray (1886).
75. 'A Cure for the Gout' undated but probably *c.* 1810.
76. Buzaglo (1778), 56; for Buzaglo, see Roth (1938).
77. Undated but *c.* 1810–20.
78. For contrast, see hysteria's visual heritage as developed by Gilman (1993); Panofsky (1974); Benedek and Rodnan (1963b).

Epilogue

1. See for instance Kutchins and Kirk (1997).
2. Payer (1992).
3. See the discussions in Rousseau (1991b).
4. Sontag (1988); *idem* (1979).

Bibliography

John Abernethy. 1809. *Surgical Observations on the Constitutional Origin and Treatment of Local Diseases and on Aneurisms.* London: Longman, Hurst, Rees and Orme.

R. D. Abbott, *et al.* 1988. 'Gout and Coronary Heart Disease: the Framingham Study.' *Journal of Clinical Epidemiology.* xxxi, 237–42.

Amal Mohamed Abdullah Abou-Aly. 1992. 'The Medical Writings of Rufus of Ephesus'. PhD thesis, University of London.

E. H. Ackerknecht. 1973. *Therapeutics from the Primitives to the 20th Century. With an Appendix: The History of Dietetics.* New York: Hafner.

James Makitrick Adair. 1786. *Essays on Fashionable Diseases.* Bath: R. Cruttwell.

R. Adams. 1857. *Illustrations of the Effects of Rheumatic Gout or Chronic Rheumatic Arthritis.* London: John Churchill and Sons.

Alison Adburgham. 1983. *Silver Fork Society: Fashionable Life and Literature from 1814 to 1840.* London: Constable.

John Aikin, M. D. 1780. 'Some Observations on the Origin, Progress, and Method of Treating the Atrabilious Temperament and Gout.' *Monthly Review.* July: 60–2.

A. Ainger, ed. 1888. *The Letters of Charles Lamb.* London: Macmillan.

Alexander of Tralles. 1933–7. *Oeuvres Médicales*, 4 vols. Paris: Geuthner.

D. C. Allen. 1943. 'John Donne's Knowledge of Renaissance Medicine'. *Journal of English and Germanic Philology*, 422–42.

Percy S. Allen and H. M. Allen, eds. 1906–47. *Opus epistolarum Des. Erasmi Roterodami*, 11 vols. Oxford: Clarendon Press.

Manuel Fernandez Alvarez. 1975. *Charles V: Elected Emperor and Hereditary Ruler.* London: Thames and Hudson.

Hugh Amory, ed. 1981. *Bute Broadsides in the Houghton Library, Harvard University.* New York: Research Publications.

Frank J. Anderson. 1977. *An Illustrated History of the Herbals.* New York: Columbia University Press.

W. E. K. Anderson, ed. 1972. *The Journal of Sir Walter Scott.* Oxford: Clarendon Press.

Gabriel Andral. 1823–27. *Clinique Médicale.* Paris: Gabon.

Gabriel Andral. 1829–31. *A Treatise on Pathological Anatomy.* Trans. R. Townsend & W. West. Dublin: Hodges and Smith.

Gabriel Andral. 1845. *Essai d'Hématologie Pathologique.* Paris: Fortin, Masson.

John Andree. 1778, 2nd edn; 1790. *Considerations on Bilious Diseases . . . of the Liver and the Gall Bladder.* Hertford: printed for the author; London: J. Murray.

Stanislav Andreski. 1990. *Syphilis, Puritanism and Witchcraft: A Historical Explanation in Light of Medicine and Psychoanalysis.* New York: St Martin's Press.

C. B. Andrews, ed. 1954. *The Torrington Diaries*, 4 vols. London: Eyre & Spottiswoode.

[Anon.]. 1659. *Podagra politica seu tractatus podagricus. . . .* Nuremburg: Endter.

[Anon.]. 1670. *A Wipe for Iter-Boreale Wilde. Or, An Infallible Cure for the Gout.* London.

[Anon.]. 1682. *Carolina; or a Description of the Present State of that Country.* London.

[Anon.]. 1710. *Solvere membra solet Bacchus solet & Venus ipsa, solvere, & ex illis mata Podagra solet.* n.p.: n.p.

[Anon.]. 1719. *A New System of the Gout and Rheumatism.* London.

[Anon.]. 1725. *The Secret Patient's Diary: Also the Gout and Weakness Diaries Being each a Practical Journal or Scheme.* London: s.n.

[Anon.]. 1726. *An Infallible Cure for the Gout.* Dublin: s.n.

[Anon.]. 1731. *A Treatise of the Gout, by a Licentiate Practitioner in Physick.* London: A. Millar.

[Anon.]. 1736. *An Infallible Cure for the Gout.* London: n.p.

[Anon.]. 1760. *A Treatise on the Gout.* London: R. Griffiths.

[Anon.]. 1764. *Satirical Trifles: Consisting of An Ode, written on the first Attack of the Gout.* London: printed for Fletcher [occasionally attributed to Bennet Allen, 1737–82].

[Anon.]. 1770. *A Candid and Impartial State of The Evidence of a Very Great Probability, That There is Discovered by Monsieur Le Fevre . . . a Specific for the Gout.* Canterbury: Simmons & Kirkby.

[Anon.]. 1771. *Reflections on the Gout With Observations on Some Parts of Dr. Cadogan's Pamphlet, and Mr. Marshall's Evidence in Favor of Dr. Le Fevre. In a Letter to the Right Hon. Sir William De Grey.* London: William Owen.

[Anon.]. 1772. *An Essay on the Bath Waters . . .* London: Lowndes.

[Anon.]. 1778. *Structures on the Present Practice of Physick . . . a Count of the Nature and Origen of Gout.* London.

[Anon.]. 1788. *A Caribbee Medicine for the Gout, Rheumatism And various other Disorders. Communicated to the Count de Noziers. By the King's Attourney at Martinicio. Translated from the French.* Boston: Edmund Freeman.

[Anon.]. 1959. 'Bibliographical Notes on "The Honour of the Gout" (1699), reprinted by Benjamin Franklin'. In *Annual Report of the Library Company of Philadelphia.* 34–5.

[Anon.]. 1962. 'Ingenuity of the Gout Stools'. *The Times.* 14 July.

[Anon.]. 1967. 'Genetics of Hyperuricemia and Achievement'. *Journal of the American Medical Association.* ccii, 913–14.

F. E. Anstie. 1871. *Neuralgia & the Diseases that Resemble It.* London: Macmillan.

R. Antonioli. 1976. *Rabelais et la médecine.* Geneva: Dvos.

Thierry Appelboom, ed. 1987. *Art, History and Antiquity of Rheumatic Diseases* Brussels: Elsevier.

T. Appelboom and J. C. Bennett. 1986. 'Gout of the Rich and Famous'. *Journal of Rheumatology.* xiii, 618–22.

Agnes Arber. 1938. *Herbals.* Cambridge: Cambridge University Press.

John Arbuthnot, MD. 1731. *An Essay Concerning the Nature of Ailments, and the Choice of them, According to the Different Constitutions of Human Bodies. In Which the Different Effects, Advantages and Disadvantages of Animal and Vegetable Diet are Explain'd.* Dublin: n.p.

J. Archer. 1671. *Every Man His Own Doctor.* London: for the author.

Aretaeus the Cappadocian. 1856. *The Extant Works.* Ed. and trans. Francis Adams. London: Sydenham Society.

Philippe Ariès. 1974, 1976. *Western Attitudes Towards Death: From the Middle Ages to the Present.* Baltimore: Johns Hopkins University Press.

Philippe Ariès. 1981. *The Hour of Our Death.* Trans. H. Weaver. London: Allen Lane.

George Arnaud de Ronsil. 1750. *A Dissertation on Hermaphrodites.* London.

Kate Arnold-Forster and Nigel Tallis, comps. 1989. *The Bruising Apothecary: Images of Pharmacy and Medicine in Caricature.* London: Pharmaceutical Press.

Bernard Aschner, ed. 1975–7. *Paracelsus: Sämtliche Werke*, 4 vols. Leipzig: Zentralantiquariat der Deutschen Demokratischen Republik.

R. B. Asprey. 1986. *Frederick the Great: The Magnificent Enigma*. London: Ticknor & Fields.

Herbert M. Atherton. 1974. *Political Prints in the Age of Hogarth: A Study of the Ideographic Representation of Politics*. Oxford: Clarendon Press.

Herbert M. Atherton. 1982. 'The British Defend their Constitution in Political Cartoons and Literature'. *Studies in Eighteenth Century Culture*. xi, 3–31.

William Atkins. 1694. *A Discourse Shewing the Nature of the Gout*. London: for T. Fabian.

John Aubrey. 1972. *Aubrey's Brief Lives*. Ed. Oliver Lawson Dick. Harmondsworth: Penguin.

John Aubrey. 1932. 'Minutes of the Life of Mr. John Milton.' In Helen Darbishire, ed. *The Early Lives of John Milton*. London: Constable & Co.

Barbara A. Babcock, ed. 1978. *The Reversible World: Symbolic Inversion in Art and Society*. Ithaca, NY: Cornell University Press.

Giorgio Baglivi, *De Praxi Medica*. 1696. Romae: Typis D. A. Herculis. Translated as *The Practice of Physick*. 1704. London: Alexander Bell & Others.

Miriam Bailin. 1994. *The Sickroom in Victorian Fiction: The Art of Being Ill*. Cambridge: Cambridge University Press.

Matthew Baillie. 1797; 1st edn., 1793. *Morbid Anatomy*, 2nd edn. London: J. Johnson and G. Nicol.

Guillaume de Baillou. 1642. *Liber de rheumatismo et pleuritide dorsali*. Paris: J. Quesnel. Trans. C. C. Barnard. 1940. *British Journal of Rheumatism*. ii, 141–62.

Guillaume de Baillou. 1643. *Opuscula medica, de arthritide de calculo de urinarum hypostasi*. Ed. Jacobum Thévart. Paris: J. Quesnel.

D. Bakan. 1971. *Disease, Pain and Sacrifice: Towards a Psychology of Suffering*. Chicago, Ill., and Boston, Mass.: Beacon Publications.

George Baker. 1785. 'Additional Observations Concerning the Colic of Poitou'. *Medical Transactions of London*. iii, 407–47.

Herschel Baker. 1947. *The Dignity of Man*. Cambridge, Mass.: Harvard University Press.

Robert Baker, Dorothy Porter and Roy Porter, eds. 1993. *The Codification of Medical Morality*, vol. 1. Dordrecht, Boston, and London: Kluwer Academic Publishers.

Mikhail M. Bakhtin. 1968. *Rabelais and his World*. Trans. Hélène Iswolsky. Cambridge, Mass.: MIT Press.

R. C. Bald. 1970. *John Donne: A Life*. Oxford: Oxford University Press.

Katharine C. Balderston, ed. 1951. *Thraliana: The Diary of Mrs. Hester Lynch Thrale 1776–1809*, 2 vols. Oxford: Oxford University Press.

George William Balfour. 1894. *The Senile Heart*. London: Black.

M. Balint. 1957. *The Doctor, his Patient, and the Illness*. London: Pitman.

Christophorus Ballista. 1525?, 1st edn.; 1570. *In podagram concertatio . . . Adiectus est dialogus inter Podagram & Christophorum Ballistam*. n.p: n.p.

Christophorus Ballista. 1577. *The Overthrow of the Gout*. Trans. B. G. [Barnaby Googe?]. London: Abraham Veale.

J. B. Bamborough. 1952. *The Little World of Man*. London: Longman, Green.

A. Barbeau, ed. 1904. *Life and Letters at Bath in the Eighteenth Century*. Ed. A. Dobson. London: Heinemann.

Andrew Whyte Barclay. 1857. *Manual of Medical Diagnosis*. London: Churchill.

William S. Baring-Gould, ed. 1967. *The Annotated Sherlock Holmes*, vol. ii. New York: Clarkson N. Potter.

L. Barkan. 1975. *Nature's Work of Art: The Human Body as Image of the World*. New Haven, Conn.: Yale University Press.

F. J. Barker-Benfield. 1992. *The Culture of Sensibility: Sex and Society in Eighteenth Century Britain*. Chicago: University of Chicago Press.

Phillip Barrough. 1583; 1590, 2nd edn; 1596, 3rd edn. *The Method of Phisick, Conteining the Causes, Signes, and Cures of Inward Diseases in Mans Bodie from the Head to the Foote*. London: Thomas Vautroullier.

Jonathan Barry and Colin Jones, eds. 1991. *Medicine and Charity Before the Welfare State.* London and New York: Routledge.

Benjamin H. Barton and Thomas Castle. 1877. *The British Flora Medica.* London: Chatto & Windus.

James G. Basker. 1988. *Tobias Smollett: Critic and Journalist.* Newark, NJ: University of Delaware Press.

Georges Bataille. 1985. *Literature and Evil.* Trans. Alistair Hamilton. London: Marion Boyars.

Donald G. Bates. 1977. 'Sydenham and the Medical Meaning of Method,' *Bulletin of the History of Medicine.* li, 324–38.

Donald G, Bates. 1982. 'Thomas Sydenham: The Development of His Thought, 1666–1676.' Michigan: University Microfilms, Ann Arbor University.

Michael Baxandall. 1985. *Patterns of Intention: on the Historical Explanation of Pictures.* New Haven, Conn.: Yale University Press.

Edward Baynard. 1719, 2nd edn. *Health, a poem. Shewing how to procure, perserve, and restore it. To which is annex'd the Doctor's decade.* London: J. Bettenham.

Alexander G. Bearn. 1993. *Archibald Garrod and the Individuality of Man.* Berkeley, Calif.: University of California Press; Oxford: Clarendon Press.

E. M. Beck. 1970. 'The Classic – a Treatise on Gout. Alfred Baring Garrod'. *Clinical Orthopaedics.* lxxi, 3–13.

G. W. Becker. 1808, 2nd edn. *Gicht und Rheumatismus.* . . . [Leipzig].

G. Becker. 1978. *The Mad Genius Controversy.* Beverly Hills, Calif.: Sage.

Thomas Beddoes. 1793. *Observations on the Nature and Cure of Calculus, Sea Scurvy, Consumption, Catarrh, and Fever: Together with Conjectures upon Several Other Subjects of Physiology and Pathology.* London: J. Murray.

Thomas Beddoes. 1802. *Hygëia: or Essays Moral and Medical, on the Causes Affecting the Personal State of our Middling and Affluent Classes,* 3 vols. Bristol: J. Mills.

Thomas Beddoes. 1806. *Manual of Health: or, the Invalid Conducted Safely Through the Seasons.* London: Johnson.

Emmett G. Bedford. 1974. *A Concordance to the Poems of Alexander Pope.* Detroit, Mich.: Gale Research Company.

Evan Bedford. 1974. 'The Story of the Gouty Heart.' *British Heart Journal.* xxxvi, 603–6.

Isabella Mary Beeton. 1906, new edn. *The Book of Household Management.* London: Ward and Lock.

E. S. de Beer. 1955. *The Diary of John Evelyn.* 3 vols. Oxford: Oxford University Press.

Michael H. Begnal. 1971. *Joseph Sheridan Le Fanu.* Lewisburg, Pa: Bucknell University Press.

L. M. Beier. 1987. *Sufferers and Healers: The Experience of Illness in Seventeenth-Century England.* London: Routledge & Kegan Paul.

P. Beighton *et al.* 1987. 'Rheumatic Disorders in the South African Negro', pt IV: 'Gout and Hyperuricemia'. *South African Medical Journal.* li, 304–12.

R. M. Bell. 1985. *Holy Anorexia.* London: University of Chicago Press.

T. G. Benedek. 1962. 'Doctors and Patients in "The Ship of Fools"'. *Journal of the American Medical Association.* clxxxi, 236–42.

Thomas G. Benedek. 1969. 'The Gout Encomium of Georg Fleissner, 1594'. *Bulletin of the History of Medicine.* xliii, 116–37.

Thomas G. Benedek. 1983. 'The Gout of Desiderius Erasmus and Willibald Pirckheimer: Medical Autobiography and its Literary Reflections'. *Bulletin of the History of Medicine.* lvii, 526–44.

Thomas G. Benedek. 1987. 'Popular Literature on Gout in the 16th and 17th Centuries'. *Journal of Rheumatology.* xiv, 186.

Thomas G. Benedek. 1993a. 'Gout'. In Kenneth F. Kiple, ed. *The Cambridge World History of Human Disease*. Cambridge: Cambridge University Press, 763–72.

Thomas G. Benedek. 1993b. 'Rheumatic Fever and Rheumatic Heart Disease'. In Kenneth F. Kiple, ed. *The Cambridge World History of Human Disease*. Cambridge: Cambridge University Press, 970–7.

Thomas G. Benedek and Gerald P. Rodnan. 1963a. 'Petrarch on Medicine and the Gout'. *Bulletin of the History of Medicine*. xxxvii, 397–416.

Thomas G. Benedek and Gerald P. Rodnan. 1963b. '"Podagra" by Gottfried Rogg: An Illustrated Encomium on the Gout'. *Journal of the History of Medicine*. xviii, 349–52.

Thomas G. Benedek and Gerald P. Rodnan. 1982. 'A Brief History of the Rheumatic Diseases'. *Bulletin on the Rheumatic Diseases*. xxxii, 59–60.

Christopher Bennet. 1654. *Theatri Tabidorum Vestibulum*. London: S. Thomson.

Christopher Bennet. 1720. Trans of *Tabidorum theatrum: sive pthisios, a trophiae, et hecticae xenodochium or the Nature and Cure of Consumptions, Whether a Phthisick an Atrophy or an Hectick*. London: W. and J. Innys.

Timotheus Bennet. 1734. *An Essay on the Gout; in Which a Method is Propos'd to Relieve the Hereditary, and to Cure the Acquir'd*. London: R. Ford.

Marmaduke Berdoe. 1772. *An Essay on the Nature and Causes of the Gout*. Bath: S. Hazard.

J. Beresford, ed. 1978–81. *The Diary of a Country Parson: The Rev. James Woodforde, 1758–1802*, 5 vols. London: Oxford University Press.

J. H. van den Berg. 1974. *Divided Existence and Complex Society: An Historical Approach*. Pittsburgh, Pa: Duquesne University Press.

Torbern Olaf Bergman. 1784–91. *Physical and Chemical Essays*. Trans. Edmund Cullen. London: J. Murray.

Torbern Olaf Bergman. 1785. *A Dissertation on Elective Attractions. Translated by the Translator of Spallanzani's Dissertations*. Trans. Thomas Beddoes. London: J. Murray.

J. Berkenhout. 1772. *Dr. Cadogan's Dissertation on the Gout Examined and Refuted*. London: S. Bladon.

V. Berridge and G. Edwards. 1981. *Opium and the People*. London: Allen Lane.

Gian-Paolo Biasin. 1975. *Literary Diseases: Theme and Metaphor in the Italian Novel*. Austin, Tex.: University of Texas Press.

Jacob Biedermann. 1666. *Ludi theatrales . . . sive opera comica . . .* Ed. Rolf Tarot. Tübingen: Niemeyer.

Ambrose Bierce. 1911. *The Devil's Dictionary*. New York: Neale; reprinted 1967 Garden City: Doubleday.

M. W. Bird. 1957. 'Rings on their Toes. Did the Ancient Britons Suffer from Gout?' *Practitioner*. clxxix, 312–13.

P. J. Bishop. 1958. 'Blackmore on Consumption'. *Tubercle*. xxxix, 118–21.

Jeremy Black. 1992. *Pitt the Elder*. Cambridge: Cambridge University Press.

Jeremy Black and John. Gregory, eds. 1991. *Culture, Politics and Society in Britain 1660–1800*. Manchester: Manchester University Press.

W. G. Black. 1883. *Folk Medicine: A Chapter in the History of Culture*. London: Folklore Society.

Sir Richard Blackmore. 1695. *Prince Arthur. An Heroick Poem. In Ten Books*. London: A. & J. Churchill.

Sir Richard Blackmore. 1697. *King Arthur. An Heroick Poem. In Twelve Books*. London: A. & J. Churchill; Tonson.

Sir Richard Blackmore. 1700. *Paraphrase on the Book of Job*. London: A. and J. Churchill.

Sir Richard Blackmore. 1700. *A Satyr Against Wit*. London: S. Crouch.

Sir Richard Blackmore. 1705. *Eliza. An Epick Poem. In Ten Books*. London: A. & J. Churchill.

Sir Richard Blackmore. 1706. *Advice to the Poets.* London: A. and J. Churchill.

Sir Richard Blackmore. 1708. *The Kit-Cats. A Poem.* London: E. Sanger and E. Curll.

Sir Richard Blackmore. 1709. *Instructions to Vander Bank.* London: Egbert Sanger.

Sir Richard Blackmore. 1711. *The Nature of Man. A Poem. In Three Books.* London: S. Buckley.

Sir Richard Blackmore. 1712. *Creation. A Philosophical Poem. In Seven Books.* London: S. Buckley, J. Tonson.

Sir Richard Blackmore. 1721a. *Just Prejudices Against the Arian Hypothesis.* London: W. Wilkins.

Sir Richard Blackmore. 1721b. *Modern Arians Unmasked.* London: J. Clark.

Sir Richard Blackmore. 1721c. *A New Version of the Psalms of David.* London: J. March.

Sir Richard Blackmore. 1722. *Redemption: a Divine Poem, in Six Books.* London: A. Bettesworth.

Sir Richard Blackmore. 1723. *Alfred; An Epick Poem. In Twelve Books.* London: James Knapton.

Sir Richard Blackmore. 1725. *A Treatise of the Spleen and Vapours.* London: Pemberton.

Sir Richard Blackmore. 1726. *Discourses on the Gout, a Rheumatism, and the King's Evil.* London: J. Pemberton.

Ralph Blegborough. 1803. *Facts and Observations Respecting the Air-Pump Vapour-Bath in Gout, Rheumatism, Palsy and Other Diseases.* London: Lackington, Allen & Co.

Edward A. Block. 1954. 'Milton's Gout'. *Bulletin of the History of Medicine.* xxviii, 201–11.

Edward A. and Lillian D. Bloom, eds. 1978. *The Journals and Letters of Fanny Burney (Madame D'Arblay),* vol. vii: *1812–1814.* Oxford: Clarendon Press.

Herman Boerhaave. 1715. *Boerhaave's Aphorisms: Concerning the Knowledge and Cure of Diseases.* Translated from the Latin. London: B. Cowse and W. Innys.

Herman Boerhaave. 1735. *Elements of Chemistry.* Translated from the Dutch. London: J. & J. Pemberton.

François Boissier Sauvages. 1763. *Nosologica methodica sistens morborum classes, genera et species,* 3 vols. Amstelodami: Bros de Tournes.

F. Boissier de Sauvages. 1808. *A Methodical System of Nosology.* Trans. Eldad Lewis. Stockbridge: Cornelius Sturtevant, jun.

Donald F. Bond, ed. 1965. *The Spectator,* 5 vols. Oxford: Clarendon Press.

Richmond Pugh Bond. 1932. *English Burlesque Poetry, 1700–1750.* Cambridge, Massachusetts: Harvard University Press.

Théophile Bonet. 1684. *A Guide to the Practical Physician.* London: T. Flesher.

G. A. Bonnard, ed. 1966. *Edward Gibbon: Memoirs of my Life.* London: Nelson.

Andrew Boorde. 1562a. *Dyetary of Health.* London: T. Colwel.

Andrew Boorde. 1562b. *The First Boke of the Introduction of Knowledge.* London: W. Copeland.

Andrew Boorde. 1587. *Breviary of Helthe for All Manner of Syckenesses and Diseases.* London: W. Middleton.

Pierre Borel. 1676. *Historiarum et Observationum Medico-Physicarum Centuriae.* Francofurti & Lipsiae: Laur. Sigism. Cörnerum.

Giovanni Alphonso Borelli. 1734. *De Motu Animalium.* Naples: Mosca.

J. Boss. 1978. 'The Medical Philosophy of Francis Bacon (1562–1626)'. *Medical Hypotheses.* iv, 208–20.

James Boswell. 1934–50. *The Life of Samuel Johnson.* 6 vols. Ed. G. B. Hill. Oxford: Clarendon Press.

P.-G. Boucé, ed. 1971. *Les Romans de Smollett: étude critique.* Paris: Didier.

P.-G. Boucé, ed. 1982. *Sexuality in Eighteenth Century Britain.* Manchester: Manchester University Press.

Samuel Boulton. 1656. *Medicina Magica Tamen Physica: Magical, but Natural Physick.* London: T. C. for N. Brook.

P. Bourdieu. 1984. *Distinction: A Social Critique of the Judgement of Taste.* Trans. R. Nice. London: Routledge & Kegan Paul.

Susan Bourgeois. 1986. *Nervous Juyces and the Feeling Heart: The Growth of Sensibility in the Novels of Tobias Smollett.* New York: P. Lang.

Janine Bourriau, ed. 1992. *Understanding Catastrophe.* Cambridge: Cambridge University Press.

John Bowlby. 1990. *Charles Darwin: A Biography.* London: Hutchinson.

Julian Boyd, ed. 1958. *The Papers of Thomas Jefferson,* vol. xi: *1 January to 6 August 1787.* Princeton, N.J.: Princeton University Press.

Mary Boyle. 1990. *Schizophrenia; A Scientific Delusion.* London: Routledge.

Robert Boyle. 1660. *New Experiments Physico-Mechanicall.* Oxford: printed by H. Hall for T. Robinson.

Robert Boyle. 1661. *Certain Physiological Essays.* London: H. Herringman.

Robert Boyle. 1666. *Origin of Forms and Qualities.* Oxford: R. Davies.

Robert Boyle. 1712, 5th edn. *Medicineal Experiments; Or, a Collection of Choice Remedies, for the Most Part Simple, and Easily Prepared,* London, Sam. Smith.

Henry Bracken. 1737, 1st edn.; 1749, 6th edn. *Farriery Improved.* London: J. Shuckburgh & W. Johnston; in 2 vols, London: J. Clarke.

Sarah Bradford. 1982. *Disraeli.* London: Weidenfeld & Nicolson.

Peter Brain. 1986. *Galen on Bloodletting.* New York: Cambridge University Press.

A. Breckenridge. 1966. 'Hypertension and Hyperuricemia'. *Lancet.* i, 15–18.

M. Breitenberg, ed. 1996. *Anxious Masculinity in Early Modern England.* Cambridge: Cambridge University Press.

John Brewer. 1976. *Party Ideology and Popular Politics at the Accession of George III.* Cambridge: Cambridge University Press.

John Brewer. 1986. *The Common People and Politics, 1750–1790s.* Cambridge: Chadwyck Healey.

John Brewer and Roy Porter, eds. 1993. *Consumption and the World of Goods.* London: Routledge.

Derrick Brewerton, MD. 1992. *All About Arthritis: Past, Present, Future.* Cambridge, Mass.: Harvard University Press.

W. Brock. 1981. 'Liebigiana: Old and New Perspectives.' *History of Science.* xix, 210–18.

W. Brock. 1985. *From Prototyle to Proton: William Prout and the Nature of Matter, 1785–1985.* Bristol: Hilger.

W. Brock. 1993. 'The Biochemical Tradition.' In W. F. Bynum and Roy Porter, eds. *Companion Encyclopedia of the History of Medicine.* London: Routledge, 153–68.

Sir Benjamin Collins Brodie. 1818. *Pathological and Surgical Observations on Diseases of the Joints.* London: Longman, Hurst, Rees, Orme and Brown.

B. C. Brodie. 1850. *Diseases of the Joints.* London: Longman, Brown, Green and Longman.

Howard Brody. 1987. *Stories of Sickness.* New Haven, Conn.: Yale University Press.

Howard Brody. 1992. *The Healer's Power.* New Haven, Conn., and London: Yale University Press.

Saul Nathaniel Brody. 1974. *The Disease of the Soul: Leprosy in Medieval Literature.* Ithaca, N.Y.: Cornell University Press.

Een Bronnenstudie. 1977. *Mijpalen uit de geschiedenis van de reumatische ziekten.* Culemborg: Princo Offset Drukkerij b.v.

Chandler McCuskey Brooks and Paul F. Cranefield, eds. 1959. *The Historical Development of Physiological Thought.* New York: Hafner Pub. Co.

John Brown. 1780. *The Elements of Medicine.* Edinburgh: C. Elliot.

Joseph Brown. 1828. *Medical Essay on Fever, Information, Rheumatism, Diseases of the Heart etc.* London: Longman, Rees, Orme, Brown & Green.

P. S. Brown. 1975. 'The Vendors of Medicines Advertised in Eighteenth-Century Bath'. *Medical History*. xix, 352–69.

P. S. Brown. 1976. 'Medicines Advertised in the Eighteenth Century Bath Newspapers.' *Medical History*, xx, 152–68.

Theodore Brown. 1970. 'The College of Physicians and the Acceptance of Iatromechanism in England, 1665–1695.' *Bulletin of the History of Medicine*. xliv, 12–30.

Theodore Brown. 1974. 'From Mechanism to Vitalism in Eighteenth Century English Physiology.' *Journal of the History of Biology*. vii, 179–216.

Theodore Brown. 1987. 'Medicine in the Shadow of the *Principia*'. *Journal of the History of Ideas*. xli, 629–48.

Janet Browne. 1990. 'Spas and Sensibilities: Darwin at Malvern'. In Roy Porter, ed. *The Medical History of Waters and Spas*. London: *Medical History*, Supplement 10, 102–13.

Sir Thomas Browne. 1964. *Religio Medici and Other Works*. Ed. L. C. Martin. Oxford: Oxford University Press.

Robert Browning. 1937. *The Complete Poetical Works of Robert Browning*. New York: The Macmillan Company.

William Brownrigg. 1993. *The Medical Casebook of William Brownrigg, M. D., F.R.S. (1712–1800) of the Town of Whitehaven in Cumberland*, Ed. and trans. Jean E. Ward and Joan Yell. *Medical History* Supplement xiii.

William Brownsword. 1739. *Laugh and Lye Down; or, a Pleasant, but Sure, Remedy for the Gout, Without Expence or Danger . . . In a Poem Serio-comic. Humbly Inscribed to Sir Hans Sloane.* London: Lawton Gulliver.

Thomas Lauder Brunton. 1885. *Textbook of Pharmacology and Therapeutics*. London: Macmillan.

G. Bryson. 1945. *Man and Society: The Scottish Inquiry of the Eighteenth Century*. Princeton, N.J.: Princeton University Press.

David Buchan, ed. 1994. *Folk Tradition and Folk Medicine in Scotland. The Writings of David Rorie.* Edinburgh: Canongate Academic.

W. Buchan. 1769. *Domestic Medicine, or a Treatise on the Prevention and Cure of Diseases by Regimen and Simple Medicines*. Edinburgh: Balfour, Auld & Smellie.

Guilaume Budaeus. 1539. *De Curandis Articularibus Morbis Comentarius.* Paris: Regnault.

William Bullein. 1579. *Booke of Simples*. London: Thomas Marsh.

E. Bullman. 1789. *The Family Physician*. London: for the author.

Henry William Bunbury. 1787. *An Academy for Grown Horsemen*. London.

Henry Burdon. 1734. *The Fountain of Health: or a View of Nature*. London.

Edmund Burke. 1901. *Reflections on the Revolution in France* in *Works*. London: Bohn's Libraries Edition.

Peter Burke. 1992. *The Fabrication of Louis XIV*. New Haven: Yale University Press.

Peter Burke and Roy Porter, eds. 1991. *Language, Self and Society: The Social History of Language*. Cambridge: Polity Press.

Peter Burke and Roy Porter, eds. 1995. *Social History of Language*, vol. iii. Cambridge: Polity Press.

J. G. L. Burnby. 1989. *Caricatures and Comments*. Staines, Middlesex: Merrell Dow Pharmaceuticals.

J. Compton Burnett. 1895. *Gout and its Cure*. Philadelphia: Boericke and Tafel.

Frances Burney. 1796. *Camilla: Or A Picture of Youth*. Oxford: Oxford University Press.

Frances Burney. 1814. *The Wanderer; Or, Female Difficulties*. Oxford: Oxford University Press.

Frances Burney. 1904–5. *Diary and Letters of Madame d'Arblay*. 6 vols. Ed. Austin Dobson.

J. H. Burton, ed. 1860. *The Autobiography of Alexander Carlyle*. Edinburgh: W. Blackwood.

J. B. Bury. 1920. *The Idea of Progress: an inquiry into its origin and growth*. New York: Dover and London: Constable and Co., Ltd.

Hermann Busschof. 1676. *Two Treatises, the one Medical, of the Gout, etc.* London.

Abraham Buzaglo. 1778, 3rd edn. *A Treatise on the Gout: Wherein the Efficacy of the Usual Treatment in That Dreadful Disorder is Demonstrated and the Facility of a Speedy and Radical Cure*. London: T. Bensley.

Thomas Buzzard. 1891. *The Simulation of Hysteria by Organic Disease*. London: J. A. Churchill.

S. Byl. 1988. 'Rheumatism and Gout in the Corpus Hippocraticum'. *Antiquité Classique*. lvii, 89–102.

Jerome J. Bylebyl, ed. 1978. *William Harvey and His Age: The Professional and Social Context of the Discovery of the Circulation*. Baltimore: Johns Hopkins University Press.

W. F. Bynum. 1981. 'Cullen and the Study of Fevers in Britain 1760–1820.' In W. F. Bynum and Vivian Nutton, eds. *Theories of Fever from Antiquity to the Enlightenment*. London: *Medical History*. Supplement 1, 135–48.

W. F. Bynum. 1983. 'Darwin and the Doctors: Evolution, Diathesis, and Germs in 19th-century Britain'. *Gesnerus*. xl, 43–53.

W. F. Bynum. 1993. 'Nosology'. In W. F. Bynum and Roy Porter, eds. *Companion Encyclopedia of the History of Medicine*. London: Routledge, 335–56.

W. F. Bynum. 1994. *Science and the Practice of Medicine in the Nineteenth Century*. New York: Cambridge University Press.

W. F. Bynum and Vivian Nutton, eds. 1981. *Theories of Fever, Antiquity to the Enlightenment*. London: *Medical History*, Supplement 1.

W. F. Bynum and Roy Porter, eds. 1988. *Brunonianism in Britain and Europe*. London: *Medical History*. Supplement 8.

W. F. Bynum and Roy Porter, eds. 1993. *Companion Encyclopedia of the History of Medicine*. London: Routledge.

E. G. L. Bywaters. 1962. 'Gout in the Time and Person of George IV: a Case History.' *Annals of the Rheumatic Diseases*. xxi, 325–38.

E. G. L. Bywaters. 1972. 'Gout'. *Teach-In*. v, 459–69.

William Cadogan, MD. 1748. *An Essay upon Nursing, and the Management of Children*. London: J. Roberts.

William Cadogan, MD. 1771, 3rd edn. *A Dissertation on the Gout and All Chronic Diseases*. London: J. Dodsley.

Thomas Cadwalader. 1745. *An Essay on the West-India Dry-Gripes: with the Method of Preventing and Curing that Cruel Distemper. To Which is Added, an Extraordinary Case in Physick*. Philadelphia: Franklin.

Jonathan Cadwallader. 1721. *The Physicians Outdone, or the Gout Curable*. London: Nath. Dodd.

Giulia Calvi. 1989. *Histories of a Plague Year: The Social and the Imaginary in Baroque Florence*. Trans. Dario Biocca and Bryant T. Ragan Jr, with a Foreword by Randolph Starn. Berkeley and Los Angeles: University of California Press.

Joseph Cam. 1722. *A Miscellaneous Essay on the Rheumatism, Gout, and Stone in which the Causes of Those Diseases are Proved to Arise from the Same Origin. . . .* London: John Clarke.

M. L. Cameron. 1993. *Anglo-Saxon Medicine*. Cambridge: Cambridge University Press.

Charles Camic. 1983. *Experience and Enlightenment: Socialization for Cultural Change in Eighteenth-Century Scotland*. Chicago, Ill.: University of Chicago Press; Edinburgh: Edinburgh University Press.

R. Campbell. 1969; 1747, 1st edn. *The London Tradesman*. London: David & Charles.

Georges Canguilhem. 1989. *The Normal and the Pathological*. Trans. Carolyn R. Fawcett. New York: Zone Books.

David Cantor. 1990. 'The Contradictions of Specialization: Rheumatism and the Decline of the Spa in Inter-War Britain'. In Roy Porter, ed. *The Medical History of Waters and Spas*. London: *Medical History*, Supplement 10, 127–44.

David Cantor. 1991. 'The Aches of Industry: Philanthropy and Rheumatism in Inter-War Britain'. In Jonathan Barry and Colin Jones, eds. *Medicine and Charity before the Welfare State*. London and New York: Routledge, 225–45.

David Cantor. 1993a. 'Cancer.' In W. F. Bynum and Roy Porter, eds. *Companion Encyclopedia of the History of Medicine*. London: Routledge, 561–83.

David Cantor. 1993b. 'Cortisone and the Politics of Empire: Imperialism and British Medicine, 1918–1955'. *Bulletin of the History of Medicine*. lxvii, 463–93.

Geronimo Cardano. 1639, 2nd edn. *Podagra Encomium*. Issued with J. Loesel the Elder, *De Podraga Tractatus*, Lugduni Batavorum: Ex Officina Joannis Maire.

Arthur L. Caplan, *et al*, eds. 1981. *Concepts of Health and Disease: Interdisciplinary Perspectives*. Massachusetts: Addison-Wesley.

Arthur L. Caplan. 1993. 'The Concepts of Health, Illness, and Disease.' In W. F. Bynum and Roy Porter, eds. *Companion Encyclopedia of the History of Medicine*. London: Routledge, 233–48.

J. F. I. Caplin. 1870. *The Philosophy of Rheumatism, and Gout; and a New Method of Radically Curing those Distressing Maladies, Without the Use of Internal Medicine*. London: Trübner & Co., Paternoster-Row.

Geronimo Cardano. 1639, 2nd edn. *Podagra Encomium*. Issued with J. Loesel the Elder, *De Podraga Tractatus*, Lugauni Batavorum: Ex Officina Joannis Maire.

Girolamo Cardano. 1545. *Artis Magnae, Sive Regulis Algebraicis Liber Unus*. Nuremberg: h. Petreium Excusum.

Girolamo Cardano. 1653. *In aphorismos Hippocratis commentaria*. Ed. Paulus Frambottus. Padua: Apud Paulum Frambottum.

John Carey. 1981. *John Donne: Life, Mind and Art*. Oxford: Oxford University Press.

Charles Carlton. 1992. *Going to the Wars*. London: Routledge.

Thomas Carlyle. 1916. *Frederick the Great*. Ed. A. M. D. Hughes. Oxford: Clarendon Press.

Mark C. Carnes and Clyde Griffen, eds. *Constructions of Masculinity in Victorian America*. Chicago: Univerity of Chicago Press, 1993.

K. J. Carpenter. 1986. *The History of Scurvy and Vitamin C*. Cambridge: Cambridge University Press.

K. J. Carpenter. 1993. 'Nutritional Diseases'. In W. F. Bynum and Roy Porter, eds. *Companion Encyclopedia of the History of Medicine*. London: Routledge, 463–82.

Vincent Carretta. 1983. *The Snarling Muse: Verbal and Visual Political Satire from Pope to Churchill*. Philadelphia: University of Pennsylvania Press.

Vincent Carretta. 1991. *George III & Satirists from Hogarth to Byron*.

H. B. Carter. 1988. *Sir Joseph Banks: 1743–1820*. London: British Museum, Natural History.

William Carter. 1772. *A Free and Candid Examination of Dr. Cadogan's Dissertation on the Gout, and Chronic Diseases*. Canterbury: Simmons and Kirkby.

Kathryn Cave, ed. 1983. *The Diary of Joseph Farington*, vol. xi. New Haven, Conn., and London: Yale University Press.

John Caverhill. 1769. *A Treatise on the Cause and Cure of the Gout*. London: G. Scott.

Louis Cazamian. 1973. *The Social Novel in England 1830–1850: Dickens, Disraeli, Mrs. Gaskell Kingsley*. London: Routledge and Kegan Paul.

Celsus. 1756. *Of Medicine in Eight Books*. Trans. with notes critical and explanatory by James Greive. London: D. Wilson and T. Durham.

Mary Chamberlain. 1981. *Old Wives' Tales: Their History, Remedies and Spells*. London: Virago.

J. E. Chamberlin and Sander L. Gilman, eds. 1985. *Degeneration: The Dark Side of Progress*. New York: Columbia University Press.

R. W. Chapman, ed. 1984. *The Letters of Samuel Johnson*, 3 vols. Oxford: Clarendon Press.

Walter Charleton. 1661. *Exercitationes Pathologicae*. London.

Louis Chauvois. 1957. *William Harvey*. London: Hutchinson Medical Publications.

John Cheshire. 1723. *A Treatise upon the Rheumatism*. London: Rivington.

John Cheshire. 1747. *The Gouty Man's Companion, or a Dietetical and Medicinal Regimen: As Well On the Approach, as in the State, and In the Declination of the Gout: With Preventative Directions, in the Intervals of the Paroxysms*. Nottingham: G. Ayscough.

G. Cheyne. 1720. *Observations Concerning the Nature and Method of Treating the Gout; For the Use of my Worthy Friend, Richard Tennison, Esq.: Together with an account of the Nature and Qualities of the Bath Waters*. London: G. Strahan.

G. Cheyne. 1722. *An Essay on the True Nature and Due Method of Treating the Gout*. London: G. Strahan.

G. Cheyne. 1733; 1990. *The English Malady; or, A Treatise of Nervous Diseases*. London: G. Strahan; London: Routledge.

G. Cheyne. 1724, 1st edn. 1734, 8th edn; *An Essay on Health and Long Life*. London: Strahan & Leake.

G. Cheyne. 1742. *The Natural Method of Cureing Diseases of the Body and the Disorders of the Mind*. London: G. Strahan.

G. Cheyne. 1743. *Dr Cheyne's Own Account of Himself and his Writings, Faithfully Extracted from his Various Works*. London: J. Wilford.

G. Cheyne. 1770. *Rules and Observations for the Enjoyment of Health and Long Life*. Leeds: G. Wright.

John Christie and Sally Shuttleworth, eds. 1989. *Nature Transfigured*. Manchester: Manchester University Press.

John Willis Clark. 1904. *Endowments of the University of Cambridge*. Cambridge: Cambridge University Press.

Ronald W. Clark. 1983. *Benjamin Franklin: A Biography*. London: Weidenfeld & Nicolson.

E. S. Clarke and L. S. Jacyna. 1987. *Nineteenth Century Origins of Neuroscientific Concepts*. Berkeley, Calif.: University of California Press.

William M. Clarke. 1988. *The Secret Life of Wilkie Collins*. London: Alison & Busby.

Richard Cobbold. 1865. *Geoffrey Gambado: or, A Simple Remedy for Hypochondriacism and Melancholy Splenetic Humours. By a Humouralist Physician*. London: printed by Dean.

Rev. Thomas Oswald Cockayne, ed. 1864. *Leechdoms, Wortcunning and Starcraft of Early England*. London: Holland Press.

Aidan Cockburn and Eve Cockburn. 1980. *Mummies, Disease, and Ancient Cultures*. Cambridge and New York: Cambridge University Press.

A. I. Coffin. 1850. *Botanic Guide to Health, and the Natural Pathology of Disease*. Manchester: British Medico-Botanic Press.

Thomas Cogan. 1577. *The Well of Wisedome, Conteining Chiefe and Chosen Sayinges . . . Gathered out of the Five Bookes of the Olde Testament*. London: T. Vstroullier.

Thomas Cogan. 1584. *The Haven of Health Made for the Comfort of Students*. London: Henrie Midleton for William Norton.

Henry Cohen. 1961. 'The Evolution of the Concept of Disease.' In Brandon Lush, ed. *Concepts of Medicine*. Oxford: Pergamon Press, 159–69.

I. Bernard Cohen. 1985. *Revolution in science*. Cambridge, Massachusetts: Belknap Press of Harvard University Press.

John Colbatch. 1695. *Novum Iumen Chirurgicum*. London: D. Brown.

John Colbatch. 1697. *A Treatise of the Gout: Wherein both its Cause and Cure are Demonstrably Made Appear. To which are Added, Some Medicinal Observations Concerning the Cure of Fevers, &c. by the Means of Acids*. London: Roger Clavel.

John Colbatch. 1700, 1st edn. *A Collection of Tracts, Chirurical and Medical*. London: D. Brown.

L. J. M. Coleby. 1954. 'Isaac Milner and the Jacksonian Chair of Natural Philosophy'. *Annals of Science*. 234–57.

Rosalie L. Colie. 1976. *Paradoxia Epidemica: The Renaissance Tradition of Paradox*. Hampden, Conn.: Archon Books.

Wilkie Collins. 1890; 1866, 1st edn. *Armadale*. London: Chatto & Windus.

Wilkie Collins. 1966; 1862, 1st edn. *No Name*. London: Anthony Blond, Limited.

Wilkie Collins. 1990; 1860, 1st edn. *The Woman in White*. New York and London: Bantam Books.

R. Colp. 1977. *To Be an Invalid: The Illness of Charles Darwin*. Chicago, Ill.: Chicago University Press.

John D. Comrie, ed. 1922. *Selected Works of Thomas Sydenham MD With a Short Biography and Explanatory Notes*. London: John Bale, Sons & Danielsson.

Lawrence Conrad, Michael Neve, Vivian Nutton, Roy Porter and Andrew Wear. 1995. *The Western Medical Tradition: 800BC to AD1800*. Cambridge: Cambridge University Press.

Harold J. Cook. 1986. *The Decline of the Old Medical Regime in Stuart London*. Ithaca, NY: Cornell University Press.

W. S. C. Copeman. 1957. 'The Gout of William Cecil – First Lord Burghley (1520–98)'. *Medical History*. i, 262–4.

W. S. C. Copeman. 1960. *Doctors and Disease in Tudor Times*. London: William Dawson & Sons.

W. S. C. Copeman. 1964. *A Short History of the Gout and the Rheumatic Diseases*. Berkeley, Calif.: University of California Press.

W. S. C. Copeman, ed. 1964, 3rd edn. *Textbook of the Rheumatic Diseases*. Edinburgh and London: Livingstone.

W. S. C. Copeman and Marianne Winder. 1969. 'The First Medical Monograph on the Gout'. *Medical History*. xiii, 288–93.

George W. Corner and Willard E. Goodwin. 1953. 'Benjamin Franklin's Bladder Stone.' *Journal of the History of Medicine*. October: 363–77.

F. M. Cornford. 1993. *Microcosmographia Academica: Being a Guide for the Young Academic Politician*. Cambridge, Mass.: Main Sail.

M. Coste. 1768, 3rd edn. *Traité-Pratique de la Goutte, Ou l'on Indique les Moyens de Guerir Cette Maladie*, Paris: Herissant fils.

Patricia B. Craddock. 1982. *Young Edward Gibbon: Gentlemen of Letters*. Baltimore, Md, and London: Johns Hopkins University Press.

Patricia B. Craddock. 1989. *Edward Gibbon: Luminous Historian 1772–1794*. Baltimore, Md, and London: Johns Hopkins University Press.

J. B. Craven. 1910, 1968. *Count Michael Maier: Doctor of Philosophy and of Medicine, Alchemist, Rosicrucian, Mystic, 1568–1622: Life and Writing*. Kirkwall: W. Peace; reprinted London: Dawsons.

Thomas Crawford. 1992. *The Devolution of English Literature*. Oxford: Oxford University Press.

John K. Crellin and Jane Philpott. 1991. *Herbal Medicine Past and Present*, 2 vols. Durham, NC: Duke University Press.

George Crine. 1758, 3rd edn. *The Management of the Gout . . .* London: Baldwin.

Critical Review. 1758. 'Review of the Management of the Gout'. April: 347.

Critical Review. 1768. 'Remarks on the Rev. Dr. Warner's Full and Plain Account of the Gout.' September: 226–7.

Critical Review. 1770. 'A Pamphlet: A Candid and Impartial State of the Evidence of the very great Improbability that there is discovered by M. Le Fevre from Liege in Germany, a Specific for the Gout'. June: 479.

Critical Review. 1771. 'A Dissertation on the Gout, and all Chronic Diseases . . .' May: 398.

Critical Review. 1771. 'Review of Cadogan's *A Dissertation on the Gout*'. May: 398.

Critical Review. 1771. 'An Address to Doctor Cadogan.' August: 159.

Critical Review. 1780. 'Histories of Gouty Bilious, and Nervous Cases . . . related by the Patients Themselves to John Scat, M. D.' October: 318–19.

T. Crofton Croker. 1848. *Autobiography of Mary Countess of Warwick*, vol. xxii. London: for the Percy Society.

Maurice Croiset. 1882. *La Vie et les oeuvres de Lucien*. Paris: Hachette.

A. C. Crombie. 1961. *Scientific Change*. London: Heinemann.

A. W. Crosby Jr. 1976. *Epidemic and Peace 1918*. Westport, Conn., and London: Greenwood Press.

Bryan Crowther. 1797. *Practical Observations on the Diseases of the Joints, Commonly called White-swelling*. London.

Jean Cruveilhier. 1829–35, vol. 1; 1835–42, vol. 2. *Pathological Anatomy of the Human Body*, 2 vols. Paris: J. Ballière.

John Cule. 1990. 'The Rev. John Wesley: The Naked Empiricist and Orthodox Medicine'. *Journal of the History of Medicine*. xlv, 41–63.

William Cullen. 1769. *Synopsis Nosologiae Methodicae*. Edinburgh: s.n.

William Cullen. 1776–84. *First Lines of the Practice of Physic*. Edinburgh: W. Creech.

William Cullen. 1785. *Institutions of Medicine*. London: T. Cadell.

William Cullen. 1808. *A Methodical System of Nosology*. Trans. Eldad Lewis. Stockbridge: Cornelius Sturtevant, for the translator.

Jonathan Culler. 1981. *The Pursuit of Signs*. Ithaca, N.Y.: Cornell University Press.

Nicholas Culpeper. 1652. *The English Physician; or An Astro-Physical Discourse of the Vulgar Herbs of this Nation*. London: P. Cole.

Nicholas Culpeper. 1789. *Culpeper's English Physician; and Complete Herbal*. London: P. McQueen.

Richard Cumberland. 1807. *Memoirs of Richard Cumberland*. London: Lackington, Allen & Co.

S. L. Cummins. 1949. *Tuberculosis in History from the 17th Century to our Own Times*. London: Baillière, Tindall & Cox.

Andrew Cunningham. 1987. 'William Harvey: The Discoverer of the Circulation of the Blood.' In Roy Porter, ed. *Man Masters Nature*. London: BBC Publications, 65–76.

Andrew Cunningham. 1988. 'Getting the Game Right: Some Plain Words on the Identity and Invention of Science'. *Studies in History and Philosophy of Science*. xix, 365–89.

Andrew Cunningham. 1989. 'Thomas Sydenham: Epidemics, Experiment and the "Good Old Cause"'. In Roger French and Andrew Wear, eds. *The Medical Revolution of the Seventeenth Century*. Cambridge: Cambridge University Press, 164–90.

Peter Cunningham, ed. 1900. *The Works of Oliver Goldsmith, Illustrated*. New York: Harper and Brothers.

Caroline Currer and Meg Stacey, eds. 1986. *Concepts of Health, Illness and Disease: A Comparative Perspective*. Leamington Spa, Hamburg and New York: Berg.

W. J. Currie. 1979. 'Prevalence and Incidence of the Diagnosis of Gout in Great Britain'. *Annals of Rheumatic Diseases*. xxxviii, 101–6.

Lewis Perry Curtis, ed. 1967. *Letters of Laurence Sterne*. London: Oxford University Press.

J. C. Dagnall. 1971. 'A Gout Stool'. *British Journal of Chiropody*. xxxvi, 76.

Ann Dally. 1993. 'Fantasy Surgery with Special Reference to Sir William Arbuthnot Lane'. MD thesis. University of London.

Helen Darbishire, ed. 1932. *The Early Lives of Milton*. London: Constable.

Robert Darnton. 1984. *The Great Cat Massacre*. New York: Basic Books.

Erasmus Darwin. 1791. *The Botanic Garden*. London: J. Johnson.

Scott F. Davies. 1993. 'Histoplasmosis'. In Kenneth F. Kiple, ed. *The Cambridge World History of Human Disease*. Cambridge: Cambridge University Press, 779–83.

Lloyd Davis, ed. 1993. *Virginal Sexuality and Textuality in Victorian Literature*. Albany State University of New York Press.

Thomas Dawson, MD. 1771. 'Review of A Dissertation on the Gout and all Chronic Diseases . . .' *Monthly Review*. August: 124–30.

Thomas Dawson, MD. 1774; 1775, 2nd edn. *Cases in the Acute Rheumatism and the Gout*. London: J. Johnson.

W. H. Dawson. 1938. *Cromwell's Understudy: Life and Times of General John Lambert*. London: William Hodge and Co.

Vinton A. Dearing, ed. 1974. *John Gay: Poetry and Prose*. 2 vols. Oxford: Clarendon Press.

Allen G. Debus. 1965. *The English Paracelsians*. London: Oldbourne.

Allen G. Debus. 1977. *The Chemical Philosophy: Paracelsian Science and Medicine in the Sixteenth and Seventeenth Centuries*. New York: Science History Publications.

Allen G. Debus. 1991. *The French Paracelsians: The Chemical Challenge to Medical and Scientific Tradition in Early Modern France*. Cambridge: Cambridge University Press.

Daniel Defoe. 1965. *The Life and Adventures of Robinson Crusoe*. Ed. Angus Ross. Baltimore, Md: Penguin Books.

Paul De Kruif. 1926. *Microbe Hunters*. New York: Harcourt, Brace & Company.

D. De Moulin. 1974. 'A Historical–Phenomenological Study of Bodily Pain in Western Medicine'. *Bulletin of the History of Medicine*. xlviii, 540–70.

Charles W. Denko. 1993. 'Osteoarthritis'. In Kenneth F. Kiple, ed. *The Cambridge World History of Human Disease*. Cambridge: Cambridge University Press, 906–8.

Warren Derry, ed. 1982. *The Journals and Letters of Fanny Burney (Madame D'Arblay)*. Oxford: Clarendon Press.

Pierre Desault. 1738. *Dissertation sur la Goutte, et la methode de la guérir radicalement; avec un Recueil d'observations sur les maladies dépendantes du défaut de la perspiration . . .* Paris: J. Guerin.

Adrian Desmond and James Moore. 1991; 1992. *Darwin*. London: Michael Joseph; London: Penguin Books.

André Devries and Abraham Weinberger. 1974. 'King Asa's Presumed Gout.' *Koroth*. vi, 561–7 (Hebrew); cxcv–cciii (English).

K. Dewhurst. 1963. *John Locke (1632–1704), Physician and Philosopher*. London: Wellcome Historical Medical Library.

Kenneth Dewhurst, ed. 1966. *Dr. Thomas Sydenham (1624–1689): His Life and Original Writings*. Berkeley, Calif.: University of California Press.

Charles Dickens. 1972a. *Bleak House*. Ed. Robert L. Patten. Harmondsworth: Penguin.

Charles Dickens. 1972b. *Pickwick Papers*. Ed. Robert L. Patten. Harmondsworth: Penguin.

S. E. Dicker. 1951. 'Renal Effects of Urethan and Colchicine in Adult Rats'. *British Journal of Pharmacology*. vi, 169–81.

H. T. Dickinson. 1977. *Liberty and Property. Political Ideology in Eighteenth Century Britain*. London: Weidenfeld & Nicolson.

James C. Dickinson. 1873. *Suppressed Gout: Its Dangers, Varieties, and Treatment; With an Appendix of the Medicinal Uses of the Vals Waters in Gout*. London: Baillière, Tindall & Cox.

Dictionnaire Encylopédiques des Sciences Médicales. 1864–89. Paris: Asselin.

Anne Digby. 1994. *Making a Medical Living: Doctors and Patients in the English Market for Medicine, 1720–1911*. Cambridge: Cambridge University Press.

J. H. Dirckx. 1983. *The Language of Medicine: Its Evolution, Structure, and Dynamics*. New York: Praeger.

Benjamin Disraeli. 1926; 1826, 1st edn. *Vivian Grey*. London: Peter Davies.

Isaac D'Israeli. 1795. *An Essay on the Manners and Genius of the Literary Character*. London: T. Cadell, Junr., and Paul Davies.

Isaac D'Israeli. 1812. *Calamities and Quarrels of Authors; including some inquiries respecting their moral and literary characters*. London: John Murray.

C. Dobell. 1960. *Anthony van Leeuwenhoek and his 'Little Animals'*. New York: Dover.

Bonamy Dobrée, ed. 1932. *The Letters of Philip Dormer Stanhope, 4th Earl of Chesterfield*. 6 vols. London: Eyre & Spottiswoode.

Robert Dodsley. 1743. *Pain and Patience*. London: R. Dodsley.

Francis Doherty. 1992. *A Study in Eighteenth-Century Advertising Methods: The Anodyne Necklace*. Lewiston, Me: E. Mellen Press.

A. Doig, J. P. S. Ferguson, I. A. Milne and R. Passmore, eds. 1993. *William Cullen and the Eighteenth Century Medical World*. Edinburgh: Edinburgh University Press.

Johann Dolaeus. 1684. *Encyclopaedia Medicinae Theoretico-Practicae*. Francof. ad Moenum, F. Knochii.

Johann Dolaeus. 1732. *Upon the Cure of the Gout by Milk Diet: & An Essay upon Diet by William Stephens*. London: Smith & Bruce.

John Donne. 1959. *Devotions upon Emergent Occasions, together with Death's Duel*. Ann Arbor, Mich.: University of Michigan Press.

Carl Van Doren. 1938. *Benjamin Franklin*. New York: The Viking Press.

David Douglas. 1939. *English Scholars, 1660–1730*. London: Cape.

J. Douglas. 1741. *A Short Dissertation on the Gout*. London: for the author.

Mary Douglas. 1966. *Purity and Danger: An Analysis of Concepts of Pollution and Taboo*. Harmondsworth: Penguin.

Thomas Dover. 1732. *The Ancient Physician's Legacy to his Country*. London: Bettesworth.

Kerry Downes. 1987. *Sir John Vanbrugh: a Biography*. London, Sidgwick & Jackson.

Arthur Conan Doyle. 1986. *Letters to the Press*. London: Secker and Warburg.

R. Drake. 1758. *An Essay on the Nature and Manner of Treating the Gout*. London: for the author.

R. Drake. 1771. *A Candid Account of the Probability that there is Discovered a Specific for the Gout*. London: for the author.

F. Drinka. 1984. *The Birth of Neurosis: Myth, Malady, and the Victorians*. New York: Simon and Schuster.

J. Dubois. 1761. *Relation de la maladie, de la confession, de la fin de M. de Voltaire*. Geneva.

Sir Dyce Duckworth. 1889. *A Treatise on Gout*. London: Charles Griffin.

Barbara Duden. 1991. *The Woman Beneath the Skin: A Doctor's Patients in Eighteenth-Century Germany*. Trans. Thomas Dunlap. Cambridge, Mass., and London: Harvard University Press.

John Duffy. 1966. *The Sword of Pestilence: The New Orleans Yellow Fever Epidemic of 1853*. Baton Rouge: Louisiana State University Press.

Howard Duncan and James C. C. Leison. 1993. 'Arthritis (Rheumatoid)'. In Kenneth F. Kiple, ed. *The Cambridge World History of Human Disease*. Cambridge: Cambridge University Press, 599–602.

William Eamon. 1981. 'The Tale of Monsieur Gout'. *Bulletin of the History of Medicine*. lv, 564–7.

William Eamon. 1994. *Science and the Secrets of Nature: Books of Secrets in Medieval and Early Modern Culture*. Princeton: Princeton University Press, 1994.

W. Ebstein. 1885. *The Regimen to be Adopted in Cases of Gout*. London: J. A. Churchill.

W. Ebstein. 1886. *Nature and Treatment of Gout*. London: Ballière Tindall & Cox.

Willebad P. Eckert and Christoph von Imhoff. 1971. *Willibald Pirckheimer: Dürers Freund im Spiegel seines Lebens, seiner Werke und seiner Umwelt*. Cologne: Wienand.

Leon Edel. 1977. *The Life of Henry James*. Harmondsworth: Penguin.

Ludwig Edelstein. 1967. *Ancient Medicine*. Ed. Owsei Temkin and C. Lilian Temkin. Baltimore, Md: Johns Hopkins University Press.

Jacques Ehrmann, ed. 1968. *Game, Play, Literature*. New Haven, Conn.: Yale University Press.

Elizabeth L. Eisenstein. 1979. *The Printing Press as an Agent of Change*, 2 vols. Cambridge: Cambridge University Press.

G. Eland. 1931. *Purefoy Letters 1735–1753*, 2 vols. London: Sidgwick & Jackson.

Norbert Elias. 1978, vol. 1; 1982, vol. 2; 1983, vol. 3. *The Civilizing Process: The History of Manners*. New York: Pantheon; *Power and Civility*. New York: Pantheon; *The Court Society*. New York: Pantheon.

Havelock Ellis. 1904; 1927, rev. edn. *A Study of British Genius*. London: Hurst & Blackett; London: Constable.

George H. Ellwanger. 1897. *Meditations on Gout*. New York: Donald Mead.

Sir T. Elyot. 1541, 1937. *The Castel of Health*. London: T. Berthelet; Reprint Ed. S. A. Tannenbaum, New York: Scholars Facsimiles and Reprints.

Antoinette Emch-Dériaz. 1992. *Tissot: Physician of the Enlightenment*. New York: Peter Lang.

Encyclopaedia Britannica. 1797, 3rd edn; 1768, 1st edn. Edinburgh: A. Bell and C. Macfarquhar.

Dietrich von Engelhardt, ed. 1989. *Diabetes. Its Medical and Cultural History: Outlines, Texts, Bibliography*. Berlin: Springer-Verlag.

H. Tristram Engelhardt. 1975. 'The Concepts of Health and Disease'. In H. T. Engelhardt and S. Spicker, eds. *Evaluation and Explanation in the Biomedical Sciences*. Dordrecht and Boston, Mass.: Reidel, 125–41.

H. Tristram Engelhardt and S. Spicker, eds. 1975a. *Explanation in the Biomedical Sciences*. Dordrecht and Boston: Reidel.

H. Tristram Engelhardt and S. Spicker, eds. 1975b. *Philosophy and Medicine*. Dordrecht and Boston: Reidel.

Peter C. English. 1992. 'Emergence of Rheumatic Fever in the Nineteenth Century'. In Charles E. Rosenberg and Janet Golden, eds. *Framing Disease: Studies in Cultural History*. New Brunswick, NJ: Rutgers University Press, 20–32.

Richard Epps. 1863. *The Homoeopathic Family Instructor*. London: James Epps and Co.

Desiderius Erasmus. 1517. *Adagia*. Strassburg: M. Schurer.

Desiderius Erasmus. 1518. *Encomium Artis Medicae*. Basel: J. Froben.

Desiderius Erasmus. 1519. *In Novam Testamentum ab Eodem Denuo Recognitum*. Basel: Froben.

Desiderius Erasmus. 1569. *In Praise of Folly*. Trans. Sir T. Chaloner. London: T. Berthle.

Hugo Erichsen. 1884. *Medical Rhymes: A Collection of Rhymes . . . Selected and Compiled from a Variety of Sources*. Chicago: Chambers.

David d'Escherny. 1760. *An Essay on the Causes and Effects of the Gout*. London: R. Griffiths.

J. Worth Estes. 1990. *Dictionary of Protopharmacology: Therapeutic Practices, 1700–1850*. Canton, Mass.: Science History Publications and Watson Publishing International.

J. Worth Estes. 1993. 'Dropsy'. In Kenneth F. Kiple, ed. *The Cambridge World History of Human Disease*. Cambridge: Cambridge University Press, 689–95.

Elizabeth W. Etheridge. 1972. *The Butterfly Caste: A Social History of Pellagra in the South*. Westport, CT.: Greenwood Press.

Elizabeth W. Etheridge. 1993. 'Pellagra.' In Kenneth F. Kiple, ed. *The Cambridge World History of Human Disease*. Cambridge: Cambridge University Press, 918–23.

Michael Ettmuller. 1699. *Ettmullerus Abridg'd: or A Compleat System of the Theory and Practice of Physic*. London: E. Harris.

M. Evans, ed. 1888. *The Letters of Richard Radcliffe and John James*. Oxford: Oxford Historical Society.

Richard J. Evans. 1987. *Death in Hamburg: Society and Politics in the Cholera Years 1830–1910*. Oxford: Clarendon Press.

Richard J. Evans. 1988. 'Epidemics and Revolutions: Cholera in Nineteenth-Century Europe.' *Past and Present*. cxx, 123–219.

W. Ewart. 1894. *Heart Studies, Chiefly Clinical*. London: Baillière, Tindall & Cox.

W. Ewart. 1896. *Gout and Goutiness: and Their Treatment*. London: Baillière, Tindall & Cox.

Knud Faber. 1930. *Nosography: A History of Clinical Medicine*. New York: Hoeber.

Alice Fairfax-Lucy, ed. 1983. *Mistress of Charlecote: The Memoirs of Mary Elizabeth Lucy*. London: Gollancz.

William Falconer. 1770. *An Essay on the Bath Waters*. London: G. G. J. & J. Robinson.

William Falconer. 1772. *Observations on Dr. Cadogan's Dissertation on the Gout*. London: T. Newbery.

William Falconer. 1788. *A Dissertation on the Influence of the Passions Upon Disorders of the Body*. London: C. Dilly.

Family Companion for Health. 1729. London: F. Fayram & Leake.

Family Guide to Health. 1767. London: J. Fletcher.

Mike Featherstone, Mike Hepworth and Bryan S. Turner, eds. 1991. *The Body. Social Process and Cultural Theory*. London: Sage.

Elizabeth Fee and Daniel M. Fox, eds. 1988. *AIDS: The Burdens of History*. Berkeley and Los Angeles, Calif., and London: University of California Press.

Elizabeth Fee and Daniel M. Fox, eds. 1992. *AIDS: The Making of a Chronic Disease*. Berkeley and Los Angeles, Calif., and London: University of California Press.

M. Feher, ed. 1989. *Fragments for a History of the Human Body*, 3 vols. New York: Zone.

Charlotte Fell-Smith. 1901. *Mary Rich, Countess of Warwick (1625–1678)*. London: Routledge.

E. M. Fenton. 1706. *On the First Fit of the Gout*. London: John Morphew.

J. A. Lopez Ferez. 1987. 'Rheumatism, Arthritis and Gout in Galen'. In Thierry Appelboom, ed. *Art, History and Antiquity of Rheumatic Diseases*. Brussels: Elsevier, 84–7.

Jean Fernel. 1678. *Select Medicinal Counsels of John Fernelius . . . Being Pick'd and Chosen Out of Four Hundred Consultations and Advices for Sick People; Of Which, These Are the Flower and Cream*. London: G. Sawbridge.

Marsilio Ficino. 1989. *Three Books on Life*. Trans. Carol V. Kaske and John R. Clark. Binghamton, NY: Renaissance Society of America.

C. N. Fifer, ed. 1976. *The Correspondence of James Boswell with Certain Members of the Club*. London: Heinemann.

Karl M. Figlio. 1977. The Historiography of Scientific Medicine: An Invitation to the Human Sciences'. *Comparative Studies in Society and History*. xix, 262–86.

Valerie Fildes. 1985. *Breasts, Bottles and Babies: A History of Infant Feeding*. Edinburgh: Edinburgh University Press.

Valerie Fildes. 1988. *Wet Nursing: A History from Antiquity to the Present*. Oxford: Basil Blackwell.

Valerie Fildes, ed. 1990. *Women as Mothers in Pre-Industrial England: Essays in Memory of Dorothy McLaren*. London & New York: Routledge.

Valerie Fildes, Lara Marks and Hilary Marland, eds. 1992. *Women and Children First: International Maternal and Infant Welfare, 1870–1995*. London: Routledge.

Anne Finch, Countess of Winchilsea. 1713. *Miscellany Poems . . . Written by a Lady*. London.

Mary E. Fissell. 1992. 'Readers, Texts and Contexts: Vernacular Medical Works in Early Modern England'. In Roy Porter, ed. *The Popularization of Medicine*. London and New York: Routledge, 72–96.

Roy Flannagan. 1981. 'Milton's Gout'. *Milton Quarterly*. xv, 123–4.

Thomas Fleming, ed. 1972. *Benjamin Franklin: A Biography in his Own Words*. New York: Newsweek.

L. F. Flick. 1925. *Development of our Knowledge of Tuberculosis*. Philadelphia, Pa: for the author.

Henry Flower. 1766. *Observations on the Gout and Rheumatism, Exhibiting Instances of Persons . . . Relieved . . . by Medicines Discovered in America*. London: E. Cooke.

Friedrich A. Flückinger and Daniel Hanbury. 1879. *Pharmacographia. A History of the Principal Drugs of Vegetable Origin Met With in Great Britain and British India*. London: Macmillan.

Carol Houlihan Flynn. 1990. *The Body in Swift and Defoe*. Cambridge, England; New York: Cambridge University Press.

Duncan Forbes. 1975. *Hume's Philosophical Politics*. Cambridge: Cambridge University Press.

Murray Forbes. 1793. *A Treatise upon Gravel and upon Gout*. London: T. Cadell.

William Forster. 1746. *A Treatise on the Causes of Most Diseases*. London.

J. Milner Fothergill. 1872; 1881, 2nd edn. *Indigestion, Biliousness, and Gout in its Protean Aspects*, pt I: *Indigestion and Biliousness*. London: H. K. Lewis.

J. Milner Fothergill. 1879, 2nd edn. *The Heart and its Diseases with their Treatment: Including the Gouty Heart*. London: H. K. Lewis.

Clifford M. Foust. 1992. *Rhubarb: The Wonder Drug*. Princeton, NJ: Princeton University Press.

Girolamo Fracastoro. 1530. *Syphilis, Sive Morbus Gallicus*. Verona: S. Nicolini da Sabbio.

Girolamo Fracastoro. 1984. *Fracastoro's Syphilis*. Introduction, text, trans and notes Geoffrey Eatough. Liverpool: F. Cairns.

Arthur W. Frank. 1991. 'For a Sociology of the Body: An Analytical Review'. In Mike Featherstone, Mike Hepworth and Bryan S. Turner, eds. *The Body: Social Process and Cultural Theory*. London: Sage, 36–102.

Robert G. Frank. 1980. *Harvey and the Oxford Physiologists: Scientific Ideas and Social Interaction*. Berkeley, Calif.: University of California Press.

Kevin Fraser. 1992. 'William Stukeley and his Regimen for Gout'. *Medical History*. xxxv, 160–86.

Sir William Fraser. 1891. *Disraeli and his Day*. London: Kegan Paul, Trench, Trübner, & Co.

James George Frazer. 1935. *The Golden Bough*. New York: The MacMillan Company.

A. Freake. 1806. *Observations and Experiments on the Humulus Lupulus of Linnaeus: With an Account of its Use in Gout, and Other Diseases. With Cases and Communications*. London: Hansard.

John Freke, Surgeon. 1748. *An Essay on the Art of Healing*. London.

Roger French. 1969. *Robert Whytt, the Soul and Medicine*. London: Wellcome Institute for the History of Medicine.

Roger French. 1993a. 'The Anatomical Tradition'. In W. F. Bynum and Roy Porter, eds. *Companion Encyclopedia of the History of Medicine*. London: Routledge, 1993, 81–101.

Roger K. French. 1993b. 'Catarrh'. In Kenneth F. Kiple, ed. *The Cambridge World History of Human Disease*. Cambridge: Cambridge University Press, 635–6.

Roger French. 1994. *William Harvey's Natural Philosophy*. Cambridge: Cambridge University Press.

Roger French and Andrew Wear, eds. 1989. *The Medical Revolution of the Seventeenth Century*. Cambridge and New York: Cambridge University Press.

Lorenz Fries. 1519. *Spiegel der Artzny*. Strassburg: J. Grieninger.

N. Fruman. 1971. *Coleridge, the Damaged Archangel*. London: Allen & Unwin.

Northrop Frye. 1957. *Anatomy of Criticism: four essays*. Ptinceton, New Jersey: Princeton University Press.

Francis Fuller. 1704. *Medicina gymnastica*. London.

D. Furst. 1974. 'Sterne and Physick: Images of Health and Disease in *Tristram Shandy*'. PhD thesis, Columbia University.

Lillian R. Furst. 1993. 'Struggling for Medical Reform in Middlemarch.' *Nineteenth-Century Literature*, 341–61.

Paul Fussell. 1969. *The Rhetorical World of Augustan Humanism: Ethics and Imagery from Swift to Burke*. London: Oxford University Press.

R. E. Gaebel and J. O. Nriagu. 1983. 'Saturnine Gout among Roman Aristocrats (Discussion)', New England Journal of Medicine, cccix, 431.

W. Gairdner. 1849; 1851, 2nd edn. *On Gout: Its History, its Causes and its Cure*. London: J. Churchill.

Galen. 1533, 1968. *De Usu Partium Corporis Humani Libri xvii*. Basle: A. Cratander and J. Bebelius; Trans. by M. T. May as *Galen on the Usefulness of the Parts of the Body*, 2 vols. Ithaca, NY: Cornell University Press.

Galen. 1821–33; 1965. *Commentary on Hippocrates' Aphorisms*. In C. G. Kühn, ed. *Claudii Galeni Opera Omnia*, 20 vols. Leipzig; reprinted Hildesheim, xi, 275.

John Gardiner. 1792. *An Inquiry Into the Nature, Cause and Cure of the Gout and of Some of the Diseases with Which it is Connected*. Edinburgh: Bell & Bradfute.

M. J. Gardner, *et al.* 1982. 'The Prevalence of Gout in Three English Towns.' *International Journal of Epidemiology*. xi, 71–5.

Thomas Garlick. 1729. *An Essay on the Gout*. London: T. Warner.

Sir Alfred Baring Garrod. 1854. 'On the Blood and Effused Fluids of Gout, Rheumatism and Bright's Disease.' *Transactions of the Medico-Chirurgical Society*, xxxvii, 49–60.

Sir Alfred Baring Garrod. 1855. *The Essentials of Materia Medica, Therapeutics and the Pharmacopoeias*. London: Walton and Maberly.

Sir Alfred Baring Garrod. 1848. 'Observations on Certain Pathological Conditions of the Blood and Urine in Gout, Rheumatism and Bright's Disease'. *Transactions of the Medico-Chirurgical Society*. xxxi, 83–98.

Sir Alfred Baring Garrod. 1859; 1863, 2nd edn; 1876, 3rd edn. *The Nature and Treatment of Gout and Rheumatic Gout*. London: Walton & Maberly; London: Walton & Maberly; London: Longmans, Green.

Sir Alfred Baring Garrod. 1861. *Die Nature und Behandlung der Gicht und der Rheumatischen Gicht*. Trans. Dr Weisenmann. Wurzburg: Richter.

Sir Alfred Baring Garrod. 1867. *La Goutte: Sa Nature, Son Traitment et le Rheumatisme Goutteux*. Trans. A. Ollivier. Paris: A. Delahaye.

Archibald E. Garrod. 1890. *A Treatise on Rheumatism and Rheumatoid Arthritis*. London: Charles Griffin.

Archibald Garrod. 1897. 'Rheumatoid Arthritis'. In T. C. Allbutt, ed. *A System of Medicine*, vol. iii. London: Macmillan, 73–102.

Archibald Garrod. 1923–4. 'Discussion on "The Aetiology and Treatment of Osteo-Arthritis and Rheumatoid Arthritis."' *Proceedings of the Royal Society of Medicine*. xvii, parts 1 and 2, pp. 1–4.

John Gascoigne. 1994. *Joseph Banks and the English Enlightenment*. Cambridge: Cambridge University Press.

Barbara T. Gates. *Victorian Suicide: Mad Crimes and Sad Histories*. Princeton: Princeton University Press.

Alan Gauld. 1992. *A History of Hypnotism*. Cambridge and New York: Cambridge University Press.

Gordon E. Geddes. 1981. *Welcome Joy: Death in Puritan New England*. Ann Arbor, Mich.: UMI Research Press.

Gentleman's Magazine. 1752. 'Extract from Dr. [William] Oliver's Practical Essay on the use and abuse of warm bathing in gouty cases.' January: 18–20.

M. D. George. 1959. *English Political Caricature 1793–1832*. Oxford: Clarendon Press.

M. D. George. 1967a. *English Political Caricature: A Study of Opinion and Propaganda*, 2 vols. Oxford: Clarendon Press.

M. D. George. 1967b. *From Hogarth to Cruikshank: Social Change in Graphic Satire*. London: Viking.

John Gerard. 1596. *Catalogus Arborum, Fruticum, ac Plantarum*. London: R. Robinson.

John Gerard. 1597. *The Herball or, Generall Historie of Plantes*. London: E. Bollifant for B. & John Norton.

Uta Gerhardt. 1989. *Ideas about Illness: An Intellectual and Political History of Medical Sociology*. New York: New York University Press.

Winifred Gérin. 1967. *Charlotte Brontë: The Evolution of Genius*. Oxford: Clarendon Press.

Faye Marie Getz, ed. 1991. *Healing and Society in Medieval England: A Middle English Translation of the Pharmaceutical Writings of Gilbertus Anglicus*. Madison, Wis.: University of Wisconsin Press.

Norman Gevitz. 1993. 'Unorthodox Medical Theories.' In W. F. Bynum and Roy Porter, eds. *Companion Encyclopedia of the History of Medicine*. London: Routledge, 603–33.

Johanna Geyer-Kordesch. 1985. 'The Cultural Habits of Illness: The Enlightened and the Pious in Eighteenth-Century Germany.' In R. Porter, ed. *Patients and Practitioners*. Cambridge: Cambridge University Press, 177–204.

Johanna Geyer-Kordesch. 1993. 'Women and Medicine'. In W. F. Bynum and Roy Porter, eds. *Companion Encyclopedia of the History of Medicine*. London: Routledge, 884–910.

Edward Gibbon. 1776–88. *The History of the Decline and Fall of the Roman Empire*, 6 vols. London: W. Strahan T. Cadell.

Sandra M. Gilbert and Susan Gubar. 1979. *The Madwoman in the Attic: The Woman Writer and the Nineteenth-Century Literary Imagination*. New Haven: Yale University Press. Chapter "Infection in the Sentence: The Woman Writer and the Anxiety of Authorship," 45–92.

G. Gilfillan, ed. 1877. *The Poetical Works of Armstrong, Dyer, Greene. With Memoirs and Critical Dissertations*. Edinburgh: James Nichol.

C. C. Gillispie. 1960. *The Edge of Objectivity: An Essay in the History of Scientific Ideas*. Princeton: Princeton University Press.

J. Gillow and A. Hewitson, eds. 1873. *The Tyldesley Diary*. Preston: A. Hewitson.

Sander L. Gilman. 1982. *Seeing the Insane*. New York: Brunner, Mazel.

Sander L. Gilman. 1985. *Difference and Pathology*. Ithaca and London: Cornell University Press.

Sander L. Gilman. 1988. *Disease and Representation: From Madness to AIDS*. Ithaca: Cornell University Press.

Sander L. Gilman. 1989. *Sexuality: An Illustrated History*. New York: Wiley.

Sander L. Gilman, Helen King, Roy Porter, G. S. Rousseau and Elaine Showalter. 1993. *Hysteria beyond Freud*. Berkeley, Calif.: University of California Press.

Ian Gilmour. 1992. *Riot, Risings and Revolution: Governance and Violence in Eighteenth-Century England*. London: Hutchinson.

Robin Gilmour. 1981. *The Idea of the Gentleman in the Victorian novel*. London: Allen and Unwin.

Robin Gilmour. 1986. *The Novel in the Victorian Age: a modern introduction*. London: Arnold.

René Girard. 1965. *Deceit, Desire and the Novel*. Trans. Yvonne Frecerro. Baltimore, Maryland: Johns Hopkins University Press.

Stephen H. Goddard. 1988. *The World in Miniature: Engravings by the German Little Masters, 1500–1550*. Exhibition catalogue. Spencer Museum of Art. University of Kansas.

Jonathan Goldberg. 1990. *Writing Matter: From the Hands of the English Renaissance*. Stanford, Calif.: Stanford University Press.

Laurence Goldstein, ed. 1994. *The Male Body: Features, Exploits, Conclusions.* Ann Arbor, Mich.: University of Michigan Press.

Nicholas Goodrick-Clarke. 1990. *Paracelsus: Artsen, Staat & Volksgezondheid in Nederland, 1840–1890.* London: Crucible.

Nicholas Goodrick-Clarke, trans. 1990. *Paracelsus: Essential Readings.* London: Crucible.

Barnaby Googe. 1990. *The Overthrow of the Gout, and A Dialogue Betwixt the Gout and Christopher Ballista.* Ed. and introduced by Simon McKeown. London: Indelible Inc.

Jan B. Gordon. 1993. '"The Key to Dedlock's Gait": Gout as Resistance'. In David Bevan, ed. *Literature and Sickness.* Amsterdam: Rodopi, 25–52.

P. Gosse. 1952. *Dr. Viper: The Querulous Life of Philip Thicknesse.* London: Cassell.

P. W. Graham and Fritz H. Oehlschlager. 1992. *Articulating the Elephant Man: John Merrick and His Interpreters.* Baltimore: Johns Hopkins University Press.

Wallace Graham and K. M. Graham. 1955. 'Men and Books. Our Gouty Past'. *The Canadian Medical Association Journal.* lxxiii, 485–93.

Wallace Graham and K. M. Graham. 1957. 'Symposium on Gout. Martyrs to the Gout'. *Metabolism.* vi, 209–17.

William Grant. 1776. *A Short Account of the Present Epidemic Cough and Fever.* London: T. Cadell.

William Grant. 1779. *Some Observations on the Origins, Progress, and Method of Treating the Atrabilious Temperament and Gout.* London: T. Cadell.

J. Mortimer Granville. 1885. *Gout in its Clinical Aspects: An Outline of the Disease and its Treatment for Practitioners. Part I. Facts and Indications. Part II. Treatment and Formulae.* London: J. & A. Churchill.

Mortimer Granville. 1894. *Notes and Conjectures on Gout.* London: Ballière, Tindall and Cox.

John Graunt. 1662. *Natural and Political Observations Made Upon the Bills of Morality.* London.

Roger Lancelyn Green, ed. 1965. *The Works of Lewis Carroll.* London: Paul Hamlyn.

Stephen Greenblatt. 1980. *Renaissance Self-Fashioning: from More to Shakespeare.* Chicago: University of Chicago Press.

Joseph Grego. *Rowlandson the Caricaturist.* 2 vols. London: n.p.

John Gregory. 1790. *Lectures on the Practice of Physic as Delivered in Edinburgh A. D. 1770.* n.p.

James Greig, ed. 1926. *The Diaries of a Duchess – Elizabeth Duchess of Northumberland (1716–1776).* London: Hodder and Stoughton Limited.

J. Y. T. Greig, ed. 1969. *The Letters of David Hume,* 2 vols. Oxford: Clarendon Press.

H. J. C. Grierson, ed. 1933. *The Letters of Sir Walter Scott: 1815–1817.* London: Constable & Co. Ltd.

H. J. C. Grierson, ed. 1935. *The Letters of Sir Walter Scott: 1823–1825.* London: Constable & Co. Ltd.

Sir Herbert Grierson. 1938. *Sir Walter Scott, Bart.: A New Life.* London: Constable and Company, Limited.

H. J. C. Grierson, ed. 1963; 1912, 1st edn. *The Poems of John Donne,* 2 vols. Oxford: Oxford University Press.

B. Griggs. 1981. *Green Pharmacy: A History of Herbal Medicine.* London: Jill Norman & Hobhouse.

E. L. Griggs, ed. 1956–68. *Collected Letters of Samuel Taylor Coleridge,* 6 vols. Oxford: Clarendon Press.

Mirko D. Grmek. 1989. *Diseases in the Ancient Greek World.* Trans. Mireille Muellner and Leonard Muellner. Baltimore, Md, and London: Johns Hopkins University Press.

Mirko D. Grmek. 1992. *Histoire du Sida: Début et Origine d'une Pandémie Actuelle.* Paris: Payot. Translated as *History of Aids: Emergence and Origin of a Modern Pandemic.*

1994. Trans. Russell C. Maulitz and Jacalyn Duffin. Princeton: Princeton University Press.

John Groenevelt. 1691. *Arthritology: Or, a Discourse of the Gout.* London: for the author.

Thomas Guidott. 1724. *The Lives and Characters of the Physicians of Bath.* London.

Gerald J. Gruman. 1966. *A History of Ideas about the Prolongation of Life: The Evolution of Prolongevity Hypotheses to 1800. Transactions of the American Philosophical Society*, n.s. 56, pt 9, Philadelphia, Pa.: American Philosophical Society.

O. Cameron Gruner. 1938. *A Treatise on the Canon of Medicine of Avicenna, Incorporating a Translation of the First Book.* London: Luzac & Co.

Anita Guerrini. 1985. 'James Keill, George Cheyne, and Newtonian Physiology, 1690–1740'. *Journal of the History of Biology.* xviii, 247–66.

Anita Guerrini. 1986. 'The Tory Newtonians: Gregory, Pitcairne and their Circle'. *Journal of British Studies.* xxv, 288–311.

Anita Guerrini. 1987. 'Archibald Pitcairne and Newtonian Medicine'. *Medical History.* xxxi, 70–83.

Anita Guerrini. 1989. 'Isaac Newton, George Cheyne, and the "Principia Medicinae."' In Andrew Wear and Roger French, eds. *The Medical Revolution of the Seventeenth Century.* Cambridge: Cambridge University Press, 222–45.

Anita Guerrini. 1993. '"A Club of Little Villains": Rhetoric, Professional Identity and Medical Pamphlet Wars.' In Marie Mulvey Roberts and Roy Porter, eds. *Literature and Medicine during the Eighteenth Century.* London: Routledge, 226–44.

James Manby Gully. 1846. *The Water Cure in Chronic Disease.* London: J. Churchill.

J. A. W. Gunn, *et al*, eds. 1982–7. *Benjamin Disraeli Letters: 1815–1841.* 3 vols. Toronto: University of Toronto Press.

J. A. W. Gunn. 1983. *Beyond Liberty and Property: The Process of Self-Recognition in Eighteenth-Century Political Thought.* Kingston: McGill-Queen's University Press.

Robert T. Gunther, ed. 1928. *Further Correspondence of John Ray.* London: The Ray Society.

Robert T. Gunther, ed. 1934. *The Greek Herbal of Dioscorides.* Oxford: J. Johnson.

S. L. Gwynn. 1932. *The Life of Horace Walpole.* London: Butterworth.

E. T. Haden. 1820. *Practical Observations on the Colchicum Autumnale as a General Remedy of Great Power, in the Treatment of Inflammatory Diseases.* London: Burgess & Hill.

Alexander Haig. 1901. *Causation, Prevention and Treatment of Gout.* London: John Bale, Sons & Co.

Alexander Haig. 1902. *Diet and Food.* London: Churchill.

Alexander Haig. 1903. 'The Causation, Prevention and Treatment of Gout'. *The Practitioner.* lxxi, 40–60.

Alexander Haig. 1908. *Uric Acid as a Factor in the Causation of Disease: A Contribution to the Pathology of High Blood Pressure, Headache, Epilepsy, Nervousness, Mental Disease, Asthma, Hay Fever, Paroxysmal Haemoglobinuria, Anaemia, Bright's Disease, Diabetes, Gout, Rheumatism, Bronchitis, and Other Disorders.* London: J. & A. Churchill.

Gordon S Haight. 1968. *George Eliot: A Biography.* Oxford: Clarendon Press.

B. Haley. 1978. *The Healthy Body and Victorian Culture.* Cambridge, Mass.: Harvard University Press.

Sir Henry Halford. 1831. *Essays and Orations, Read and Delivered at the Royal College of Physicians.* London: J. Murray.

L. A. Hall. 1991. "Forbidden by God, Despised by Men: Masturbation, Medical Warnings, Moral Panic, and Manhood in Great Britain," 1850–1950.' *Journal of the History of Sexuality*, 2, 365–87.

Mark Haller. 1984. *Eugenics: Hereditarian Attitudes in American Thought.* New Brunswick: N. J., Rutgers University Press.

John Halperin. 1984. *The Life of Jane Austen.* Brighton: Harvester Press.

Robert Halsband, ed. 1965. *The Complete Letters of Lady Mary Wortley Montagu*, 3 vols. Oxford: Clarendon Press.

Sir David Hamilton. 1975. *The Diary of Sir David Hamilton*. Ed. and Intro. Philip Roberts. Oxford: Clarendon Press.

C. Hannaway. 1993. 'Environment and Miasmata.' In W. F. Bynum and Roy Porter, eds. *Companion Encyclopedia of the History of Medicine*. London: Routledge, 292–334.

O. B. Hardison. 1962. *The Enduring Monument: a Study of the Idea of Praise in Renaissance Literary Theory and Practice*. Westport: Conn. 1962.

James Hardy. 1778. *A Candid Examination of what has been Advanced as the Colic of Poitou and Devonshire, with Remarks on the Most Probable Causes and Experiments Intended to Ascertain the True Cause of Gout*. London: T. Cadell.

James Hardy. 1780. *An Answer to the Letter Addressed by Francis Riollay, Physician of Newbury to Dr. Hardy, on the Hints Given Concerning the Origin of the Gout, in his Publication on the Colic of Devon*. London: T. Cadell.

M. Hardy. 1860. *Lecons sur les Maladies de la Peau. . . .* Paris: Delahaye.

David Harley. 1993. 'Ethics and Dispute Behaviour in the Career of Henry Bracken of Lancaster: Surgeon, Physician and Manmidwife.' In Robert Baker, Dorothy Porter and Roy Porter, eds. *The Codification of Medical Morality*, vol. 1. Dordrecht, Boston and London: Kluwer Academic Publishers, 47–72.

Walter Harris. 1683. *Pharmacologia antiempirica*. London: Richard Chiswell.

Walter Harris. 1689. *De morbis acutis infantum*. London: Samuel Smith.

F. Dudley Hart. 1976. 'History of the Treatment of Rheumatoid Arthritis'. *British Medical Journal*. i, 763–5.

F. Dudley Hart. 1984. 'William Harvey and his Gout'. *Annals of Rheumatic Diseases*. xliii, 125–7.

A. Hartshorne, ed. 1905. *Memoirs of a Royal Chaplain, 1729–1763: The Correspondence of Edmund Pyle, D.D. Chaplain in Ordinary to George II, with Samuel Kerrich D.D., Vicar of Dersingham, Rector of Wolferton and Rector of West Newton*. London and New York: John Lane, Bodley Head.

Edward P. Hartung. 1954. 'History of the Use of Colchicum and Related Medicaments in Gout'. *Annals of Rheumatic Diseases*. xiii, 190–200.

Edward P. Hartung. 1957. 'Symposium on Gout. Historical Considerations'. *Metabolism*. vi, 196–208.

A. D. Harvey. 1994. *Sex in Georgian England*. London: Duckworth.

Gideon Harvey. 1672a. *Great Venus Unmasked*. London: N. Brook.

Gideon Harvey. 1672b. *Morbus Anglicus, or a Theoretick and Practical Discourse of Consumptions and Hypochondriack Melancholy*. London: Thackeray.

Gideon Harvey. 1675. *The Disease of London, or a New Discovery of the Scorvey*. London: Thackeray.

William Harvey. 1628. *De Motu Cordis*. Francofurti: G. Fitzen.

William Harvey. 1961. *Lectures on the Whole of Anatomy*. Trans. C. D. O'Malley, F. N. L. Poynter and K. F Russell. Berkeley, Calif.: University of California Press.

William Harvey. 1976. *An Anatomical Disputation Concerning the Movement of the Heart and Blood in Living Creatures*. Trans. G. Whitteridge. Oxford: Blackwell Scientific.

Clopton Havers. 1691. *Osteologia Nova*. London: Samuel Smith.

Richard Hawes. 1634. *The Poore-Mans Plaster-Box. Furnished with Diverse Excellent Remedies for Sudden Mischances, and Usuall Infirmities, Which Happen to Men, Women, and Children in this Age*. London: Thomas Cotes for Francis Grove.

Francis Hawkins. 1826. *Rheumatism and Some Diseases of the Heart and Other Internal Organs*. London: Burgess & Till.

John T. Hayes. 1972. *Rowlandson*. London: Phaidon.

John Haygarth. 1793. *A Sketch Plan to Exterminate the Casual Smallpox, and to Introduce General Inoculation*, 2 vols. London: J. Johnson.

John Haygarth. 1801. *A Letter to Dr Percival on the Prevention of Infectious Fevers*. London: Cadell and Davies.

John Haygarth. 1805. *A Clinical History of Diseases: Part First Being 1. A Clinical History of the Acute Rheumatism. 2. A Clinical History of the Nodosity of the Joints*. London: Cadell & Davies.

William Hayley. 1794. *The Triumphs of Temper*. Newburyport, Massachusetts.

Alan Haynes. 1989. *Robert Cecil, Earl of Salisbury, 1563–1612: Servant of Two Sovereigns*. London: Peter Owen.

L. A. Healey, M.D. 1971. 'Gout and Gluttony, Yesterday and Today.' *Medical Opinion and Review*. February: 46–55.

L. A. Healey, M.D. 1975. 'Port Wine and the Gout.' *Arthritis and Rheumatism*. xviii. 6 Supplement, 659–62.

Ernest Heberden. 1989. *William Heberden 1710–1801: Physician of the Age of Reason*. London and New York: Royal Society of Medicine Services.

W. Heberden. 1962; 1802, 1st edn. *Commentaries on the History and Cure of Diseases*. London: T. Payne; facsimile reprint, New York: New York Academy of Medicine/ Hafner Publishing.

H. O. Hebert. 1802. *Hebert's Air Pump Vapour Bath*. New York and Philadelphia.

Ferdinand Hebra. 1866–80. *On Diseases of the Skin*. London: New Sydenham Society.

W. H. Helfand. 1978. *Medicine and Pharmacy in American Political Prints (1765–1870)*. Madison, Wis.: American Institute of the History of Pharmacy.

C. D. Hellman, ed. 1931. 'An Unpublished Diary, 1810–1812, by E. Jenner'. *Annals of Medical History*. n.s. iii, 412–38.

J. Baptista van Helmont. 1648. *Ortus Medicinae*. Amsterdam: L. Elzevirium.

John Baptista van Helmont. 1662. *Oriatrike or Physick Refined*. Trans. J. Chandler. London: Lodowick Lloyd.

Phyllis Hembry. 1990. *The English Spa 1560–1815: A Social History*. London: Athlone.

Ernest Hemingway. 1963. *A Farewell to Arms*. Harmondsworth: Penguin.

Lord Herbert, ed. 1950. *Pembroke Papers*. London: Cape.

Audrey Heywood. 1990. 'A Trial of the Bath Waters: The Treatment of Lead Poisoning'. In Roy Porter, ed. *The Medical History of Waters and Spas*. London: *Medical History*, Supplement 10, 82–101.

Nathaniel Highmore. 1660. *Exercitationes duae, quarum prior de Passione Hysterica, altera de Affectione Hypochondriaca*. Oxonii.

Nathaniel Highmore. 1670. *Epistola Responsoria ad T. Willis de Passione Hysteria, et Hypochondriaca Affectione*. Londini.

Aaron Hill. 1709. *A Full and Just Account of the State of the Ottoman Empire in All its Branches*. London: John Mayo.

John Hill. 1754. *The Useful Family Herbal*. London: W. Johnston.

John Hill. 1758a, 2nd edn. *The Management of the Gout, by a Physician From his Own Case. With the Virtues of an English Plant Bardana, Not Regarded in the Present Practice, but Safe and Effectual in Alleviating that Disease, by George Crine*. London: R. Baldwin.

John Hill. 1758b, 6th edn. *The Management of the Gout, with the Virtues of Burdock Root, First Us'd in the Author's Own Case, and Since in Many Other Successful Instances*. London: R. Baldwin.

John Hill. 1771, 8th edn. *The Management of the Gout in Diet, Exercise and Temper: with the Virtues of BURDOCK Root, Taken in the Manner of Tea: First Us'd in the Year 1760; in the Author's Own Case; And Since in Many Other Successful Instances, to the Present Time. By J. Hill, M.D. Member of the Imperial Academy*. London: R. Baldwin.

Hippocrates. 1839–61. *Oeuvres Complètes d'Hippocrate*, 10 vols. Ed. E. Littré. Paris: Ballière.

Hippocrates. 1923–31. *Aphorisms*. Ed. W. H. S. Jones and E. T. Withington. In vol. 4 of *Hippocrates*. London: Heinemann, Loeb Edition.

A. D. Hodgkiss. 1991. 'Chronic Pain in Nineteenth-Century British Medical Writings'. *History of Psychiatry*. ii, 27–40.

F. David Hoeniger. 1992. *Medicine and Shakespeare in the English Renaissance*. Newark, Del.: University of Delaware Press.

Friedrich Hoffmann. 1754, 1st edn. *A Treatise of the Extraordinary Virtues and Effects of Asses Milk . . . In the Cure of Various Diseases, Particularly the Gout . . .* London: Whiston & White.

Lady Holland, ed. 1855. *A Memoir of the Reverend Sydney Smith*. 2 vols. London: Longman, Brown, Green & Longmans.

Sir Henry Holland. 1839. *Medical Notes and Reflections*. London: Longman, Orme, Brown, Green and Longmans.

Sir Henry Holland. 1852. *Chapters on Mental Physiology*. London: Longman, Brown, Green and Longmans.

Michael Hollington. 1984. *Dickens and the Grotesque*. London: Croom Helm.

Richard Holmes. 1989. *Coleridge: Early Visions*. London: Hodder & Stoughton.

Michael Holquist, ed. 1981. *The Dialogic Imagination: Four Essays by M. M. Bakhtin*. Trans. Caryl Emerson and Michael Holquist. Austin, Tex.: University of Texas Press.

Thomas Hood. 1935. 'Lieutenant Lough.' In Walter Jerrold, ed. *The Complete Poetical Works of Thomas Hood*. London: Oxford University Press, 204.

Robert Hopkins. 1969. 'The Function of the Grotesque in *Humphrey Clinker*.' *HLQ*. 32. February: 163–77.

J. Huizinga. 1949; 1944, 1st edn. *Homo Ludens: A Study of the Play-Element in Culture*. London: Routledge & Kegan Paul.

Charles H. Hull. 1899. *The Economic Writings of Sir William Petty*, 2 vols. Cambridge: Cambridge University Press.

Nathaniel Hulme, MD. 1778. *The Stone and Gout*. London.

David Hume. 1963. *Essays Moral, Political and Literary*. London: Oxford University Press.

Tony Hunt. 1990. *Popular Medicine in Thirteenth-Century England*. Cambridge: D. S. Brewer.

Kathryn Montgomery Hunter. 1991. *Doctor's Stories: The Narrative of Medical Knowledge*. Princeton, NJ: Princeton University Press.

N. Husson. 1783. *Collection de faits et recueil d'expériences sur le spécifique et les effets de l'eau médicinale*. Bouillon: J. Brasseur.

N. Husson. 1807, 2nd edn. *Recit Historique de la decouverts, du progrès et publicité de l'eau medicinale . . . Proces-verbal de l'analyse . . . faite par MM. Cadet et Parmentier*. Paris: J. Grafiot.

F. E. Hutchinson, ed. 1941. *The Works of George Herbert*. Oxford: Clarendon Press.

Jonathan Hutchinson. 1884a. 'On the Relation of Certain Diseases of the Eyes to Gout'. Bowman Lecture. *British Medical Journal*. ii, 995–1000.

Jonathan Hutchinson. 1884b. *The Pedigree of Disease*. London: Churchill.

Jonathan Hutchinson. 1891. 'Gout and Longevity.' *Archives of Surgery*. III: 363.

Robert Hutchinson, M.D. 1934. 'Medcine in Horace Walpole's Letters.' *Annals of Medical History*. vi: 57–61.

Ulrich von Hutten. 1536, 2nd edn. *Of the Wood Called Guaiacum, that Healeth the Frenche Pocks, and also Helpeth the Goute in the Feet, the Stoone, the Palsey and Other Dyseases*. Londoni: Berthelet.

B. Inglis. 1981. *The Diseases of Civilisation*. London: Hodder & Stoughton.

D. Ingram. 1743. *An Essay on the Cause and Seat of the Gout*. Reading: J. Newbery.

Richard Ingram. 1767. *The Gout: Extraordinary Cases in the Head, Stomach, and Extremities*. London: Vaillant.

Ralph Jackson. 1988. *Doctors and Diseases in the Roman Empire.* London: British Museum Publications.

E. G. Jaco, ed. 1958. *Patients, Physicians and Illness.* Glencoe, Ill.: The Free Press.

M. Jacobus, ed. 1990. *Body/Politics: Women in the Discourses of Science.* London: Routledge.

Robert James. 1745, 1st edn. *A Treatise on Gout and Rheumatism Wherein a Method is Laid Down of Relieving in an Eminent Degree Those Excruciating Distempers.* London: T. Osborne and J. Roberts.

Saul Jarcho, trans. and ed. 1984. *The Clinical Consultations of Giambattista Morgagni.* Boston: Countway Library of Medicine.

Saul Jarcho. 1993. *Quinine's Predecessor: Francesco Torti and the Early History of Cinchona.* Baltimore, Md: Johns Hopkins University Press.

Sir James Jay. 1772. *Reflections and Observations on the Gout.* London: Kearsly.

G. Jean-Aubry, ed. 1927. *Joseph Conrad: Life and Letters,* 2 vols. New York: Doubleday, Page & Co.

Thomas Jeans. 1792. *A Treatise on the Gout, Wherein is Delivered a New Idea of its Proximate Cause and Consequent Means of Relief.* Southampton: T. Baker.

R. W. Jeffery, ed. 1907. *Dyott's Diary,* 2 vols. London: Archibald Constable.

N. D. Jewson. 1974. 'Medical Knowledge and the Patronage System in Eighteenth Century England.' *Sociology,* viii, 369–85.

James Johnson. 1818. *Practical Researches on the Nature, Cure and Prevention of Gout.* London: Highley & Son.

Samuel Johnson. 1827, 2nd edn. *A Dictionary of the English Language. . . .* London: Longman, Rees, Orme, Brown, and Green.

Samuel Johnson. 1971. 'A Review of Soame Jenyns' *A Free Enquiry into the Nature and Origin of Evil.*' In B. Bronson, ed. *Samuel Johnson, Rasselas, Poems and Selected Prose.* San Francisco: Rinehart Press, 219–28.

Edwin Godden Jones. 1810, 2nd edn. *An Account of the Remarkable Effects of the Eau Médicinale d'Husson in the Gout.* London: White & Cochrane.

Greta Jones. 1980. *Social Darwinism and English Thought: the Interaction between Biological and Social Theory.* Brighton: Harvester Press.

Greta Jones. 1986. *Social Hygiene in Britain.* London: Croom Helm.

Henry Bence Jones. 1842. *Gravel, Calculus and Gout.* London: Taylor and Walton.

Henry Bence Jones. 1870. *Life and letters of Faraday,* 2 vols. London: Longmans, Green and Co.

J. Jones. 1701. *The Mysteries of Opium Reveal'd.* London: R. Smith.

H. M. E. Jong. 1965. 'Michael Maier's Atalanta Fugiens.' *Janus.* 52: 81–112.

Ludmilla Jordanova. 1989. *Sexual Visions: Images of Gender in Science and Medicine between the Eighteenth and Twentieth Centuries.* Madison, Wis.: University of Wisconsin Press.

Laurent Joubert. 1989. *Popular Errors.* Trans. and ed. Gregory David de Rocher. Tuscaloosa, Ala., and London: University of Alabama Press.

James Joyce. 1946. *Ulysses.* New York: Random House.

Aubrey C. Kail. 1986. *The Medical Mind of Shakespeare.* Balgowlah, NSW: Williams & Wilkins.

W. Kaiser. 1963. *Praisers of Folly.* Cambridge, Mass.: Harvard University Press.

Barbara Beigun Kaplan. 1994. '*Divulging of Useful Truths in Physick': The Agenda of Robert Boyle.* Baltimore, Md: Johns Hopkins University Press.

Fred Kaplan. 1975. *Dickens and mesmerism: the hidden springs of fiction.* Princeton, N.J.: Princeton University Press.

Fred Kaplan. 1983. *Thomas Carlyle: A Biography.* Cambridge: Cambridge University Press.

Frederick R. Karl. 1979. *Joseph Conrad: The Three Lives.* New York: Farrar, Straus and Giroux.

Robert S. Karsh, M.D. 1960. 'Archeology and Arthritis.' *A. M. A. Archives of Internal Medicine.* vol. 105. April: 640–4.

Wolfgang Kayser. 1963. *The Grotesque in art and literature.* Trans. Ulkrich Weisstein. Bloomington: Indiana University Press.

M. Kearns 1987. *Metaphors of Mind in Fiction and Psychology.* Lexington, Ky: University Press of Kentucky.

Kenneth D. Keele, MD. 1957. *Anatomies of Pain.* Oxford: Blackwell Scientific Publications.

Kenneth D. Keele. 1965. *William Harvey: The Man, the Physician, and the Scientist.* London: Nelson.

R. Y. Keers. 1982. 'Richard Morton (1637–98) and his "Physiologia"'. *Thorax.* xxxvii, 26–31.

Henry Ansgar Kelly. 1993. *Ideas and Forms of Tragedy from Aristotle to the Middle Ages.* Cambridge: Cambridge University Press

Lionel Kelly, ed. 1987. *Tobias Smollett: The Critical Heritage.* London: Routledge; New York: Kegan Paul.

Richard Kentish. 1787. *An Essay on Sea-Bathing.* London: J. Murray.

Richard Kentish. 1789, 1791. *Advice to Gouty Persons.* London: J. Murray.

Charles Kerby-Miller, ed. 1988. *The Memoirs of the Extraordinary Life, Works, and Discoveries of Martinus Scriblerus.* Oxford: Oxford University Press.

Alvin B. Kernan. 1959. *The Cankered Muse: Satire of the English Renaissance.* New Haven: Yale University Press.

G. D. Kersley. 1956. 'Eunuchs Do Not Take the Gout'. *Medical Journal of the Southwest.* lxxi, 136–7.

R. W. Ketton-Cremer. 1955. *Thomas Gray: A Biography.* Cambridge: Cambridge University Press.

Geoffrey Keynes, ed. 1928. *The Collected Works of Sir Thomas Browne.* London: Faber.

Geoffrey Keynes. 1966. *The Life of William Harvey.* Oxford: Clarendon Press.

J. King and C. A. Ryskamp, eds. 1979–84. *The Letters and Prose Writings of William Cowper,* 4 vols. Oxford: Clarendon Press.

Lester S. King. 1958. *The Medical World of the Eighteenth Century.* Chicago: University of Chicago Press.

Lester S. King. 1970. *The Road to Medical Enlightenment, 1650–1695.* London: Macdonald; New York: American Elsevier.

Lester S. King. 1978. *Medical Philosophy, the Early Eighteenth Century.* Cambridge, Mass.: Harvard University Press.

D. King-Hele, ed. 1963. *Erasmus Darwin.* London: Macmillan.

D. King-Hele, ed. 1968. *The Essential Writings of Erasmus Darwin.* London: MacGibbon & Kee.

D. King-Hele. 1977. *Doctor of Revolution: The Life and Genius of Erasmus Darwin.* London: Faber.

D. King-Hele, ed. 1981. *The Letters of Erasmus Darwin.* Cambridge: Cambridge University Press.

Robert Kinglake. 1804, 1st edn. *A Dissertation on Gout.* London: J. Murray.

Robert Kinglake. 1807a. *Strictures on Mr Parkinson's Observations on the Nature and Cure of Gout.* Taunton: J. Poole.

Robert Kinglake. 1807b. *Additional Cases of Gout in Farther Proof of the Efficacy of the Cooling Treatment.* Taunton: J. Poole.

Kenneth F. Kiple, ed. 1993. *The Cambridge World History of Human Disease.* Cambridge: Cambridge University Press.

Eugene P. Kirk. 1980. *Menippean Satire.* New York: Garland.

James Kirkpatrick, M.D. 1758. A Review of George Crine's 'The Management of the Gout.' *Monthly Review.* June: 531–32

Arthur Kleinman. 1980. *Patients and Healers in the Context of Culture: An Exploration of the Borderline between Anthropology, Medicine and Psychiatry*. Berkeley, Calif.: University of California Press.

Arthur Kleinman. 1981. 'The Meaning Context of Illness and Care: Reflections on a Central Theme in the Anthropology of Medicine.' In E. Mendelsohn and Y. Elkana, eds. *Science and Cultures*. Dordrecht: Kluwer, 161–76.

Arthur Kleinman. 1986. *Social Origins of Distress and Disease: Depression, Neurasthenia, and Pain in Modern China*. New Haven, Conn.: Yale University Press.

Arthur Kleinman. 1988. *Illness Narratives: Suffering, Healing and the Human Condition*. New York: Basic Books.

James R. Klinenberg, M.D. 1969. 'Current Concepts of Hyperuricemia and Gout.' *California Medicine*. 10(3). March: 231–43.

Lewis M. Knapp. 1949. *Tobias Smollett: Doctor of Men and Manners*. Princeton, NJ: Princeton University Press.

Lewis M. Knapp, ed. 1970. *The Letters of Tobias Smollett*. Oxford: Clarendon Press.

U. C. Knoepflmacher. 1970. 'The Poet as Physician: Pope's *Epistle to Dr Arbuthnot*'. *Modern Language Quarterly*. xxxi, 440–9.

Owen Knowles. 1989. *A Conrad Chronology*. London: MacMillan.

Wayne Koestenbaum. 1989. *Double Talk: The Erotics of Male Literary Collaboration*. London: Routledge.

John C. Kramer. 1979. 'Opium Rampant: Medical Use, Misuse and Abuse in Britain and the West in the 17th and 18th Centuries'. *British Journal of Addiction*. lxxiv, 377–89.

Paul Kristeller. 1979. *Renaissance Thought and its Sources*. New York: Columbia University Press.

Peter Krivasy. 1973. 'Erasmus's Medical Milieu'. *Bulletin of the History of Medicine*. xlvii, 113–54.

Paul de Kruif. 1959. 'They've Taken the Agony Out of Gout.' *Today's Health*. August: 24–76.

Milan Kundera. 1995. *Testaments Betrayed*. London: Faber.

David Kunzle. 1989. 'The Art of Pulling Teeth in the Seventeenth and Nineteenth Centuries: From Public Martyrdom to Private Nightmare and Political Struggle.' In M. Feher, ed. *Fragments for a History of the Human Body*, vol. 3. New York: Zone, 28–89.

A Lady. 1925. 'The Doctor Dissected: or Willy Cadogan in the Kitchen.' Reprinted in J. Ruhräh. *William Cadogan (His Essay on Gout)*. New York: P. B. Hoeber, 104–14.

P. Laigel-Lavastine. 1937. 'La Goutte a Byzance.' *Annales Internationales de medicine physique et physio-biologie*. vol. 30: 49–57.

Jean de La Fontaine. 1966. *Fables*. Ed. Antoine Adam. Paris: Flammarion.

The Marquis of Lansdowne, ed. 1934. *The Queeney Letters*. London: Cassell.

John Latham. 1796, 1st edn. *On Rheumatism and Gout. . . .* London: Longman.

Peter Wallwork Latham. 1895–97. *Lectures on Pharmacology for Practitioners and Students*. London: New Sydenham Society.

Robert Latham and William Matthews, eds. 1970–83. *The Diary of Samuel Pepys*. London: Bell & Hyman.

Christopher J. Lawrence. 1975. 'William Buchan: Medicine Laid Open'. *Medical History*. xix, 20–35.

Christopher J. Lawrence. 1984. 'Medicine as Culture: Edinburgh and the Scottish Enlightenment'. PhD thesis, University of London.

Christopher J. Lawrence. 1985. 'Incommunicable Knowledge: Science, Technology and the Clinical Art in Britain, 1850–1914.' *Journal of Contemporary History*. xx, 503–20.

Christopher J. Lawrence. 1988. 'Cullen, Brown and the Poverty of Essentialism.' In W. F. Bynum and Roy Porter, eds. *Brunonianism in Britain and Europe*. London: *Medical History*, Supplement 8, 1988, 1–21.

Christopher J. Lawrence. 1994. *Medicine in the Making of Modern Britain, 1700–1920*. London and New York: Routledge.

Thomas Laycock. 1840. *A Treatise on the Nervous Diseases of Women*. London: Longman, Orme, Brown, Green and Longmans.

Thomas Laycock. 1857–58 'Clinical Observations on a Characteristic of the Urine in Rheumatism and Gout.' *Edinburgh Medical Journal*. iii, 107–21.

Thomas Laycock. 1869, 2nd edn. *Mind and Brain*, London: Simkin Marshall.

John Lee. 1782. *A Narrative of a Singular Gouty Case, with Observations*. London: the author and T. Evans.

John Lee. 1785, 2nd edn. *A Narrative of a Singular Gouty Case, with Observations*. London: Debrett.

[Antoni van Leeuwenhoek]. 1685. 'An Abstract of a Letter of Mr Anthony Leeuwenhoek Fellow of the R. Society, Concerning the Parts of the Brain of Severall Animals; the Chalk Stones of the Gout; the Leprosy; and the Scales of Eeles'. *Philosophical Transactions*. xv, 883–95.

Joseph Thomas Sheridan Le Fanu. 1884. *In a Glass Darkly*. London: Richard Bentley & Son.

M. Lefebure. 1974. *Samuel Taylor Coleridge: A Bondage of Opium*. London: V. Gollancz.

J. A. Leo Lemay and G. S. Rousseau. 1978. *The Renaissance Man in the Eighteenth Century*. Los Angeles: William Andrews Clark Library.

John E. Lesch. 1984. *Science and Medicine in France: The Emergence of Experimental Physiology 1790–1855*. Cambridge, Mass.: Harvard University Press.

J. Levine. 1987. *Humanism and History: Origins of Modern English Historiography*. London: Oxford University Press.

J. Levine. 1991a. *The Battle of the Books: History and Literature in the Augustan Age*. Ithaca, NY, and London: Cornell University Press.

J. Levine. 1991b. *Dr Woodward's Shield: History, Science, and Satire in Augustan England*. Ithaca, NY: Cornell University Press.

F. J. Levy, ed. 1972. *Francis Bacon, The History and the Reign of King Henry the Seventh*. Indianapolis: The Bobbs-Merrill Company.

C. S. Lewis. 1940. *The Problem of Pain*. London: Centenary Press.

W. S. Lewis, ed. 1937–83. *The Yale Edition of Horace Walpole's Correspondence*, 48 vols. New Haven, Conn.: Yale University Press.

M. Charles Luis Liger, M.D. 1760. 'A Treatise on the Gout: from the French of M. Charles Luis Liger.' *Critical Review*. April: 283–8.

David C. Lindberg and Robert S. Westman, eds. 1990. *Reappraisals of the Scientific Revolution*. Cambridge: Cambridge University Press.

G. A. Lindeboom. 1968. *Herman Boerhaave: The Man and his Work*. London: Methuen.

G. A. Lindeboom, ed. 1970. *Boerhaave and his Time*. Leiden: E. J. Brill.

G. A. Lindeboom. 1974. *Boerhaave and Great Britain*. Leiden: E. J. Brill.

Carl Linnaeus. 1772. *Fraga vesca dissertatione botanica . . . Præside . . . Carolo Linné . . . die XXVI. maji a. MDCCLXXII . . . publicæ ventilationi proposita a . . . Sevone Andr. Hedin, &c.* Uppsalae: Typis Edmannianis.

D. Little and G. Kahrl, eds. 1963. *The Letters of David Garrick*, 3 vols. London: Oxford University Press.

Edward Liveing. 1873. *On Megrim, Sick-Headache, and Some Allied Disorders*. London: Churchill.

Llewellyn Jones Llewellyn. 1927. *Aspects of Rheumatism and Gout: Their Pathogeny, Prevention and Control*. London: William Heinemann Medical Books.

Llewellyn Jones Llewellyn and A. B. Jones. 1915. *Fibrositis (Gouty, &c.)*. London: W. Heinemann.

R. L. J. Llewellyn. 1920. *Gout.* London: W. Heinemann.

G. E. R. Lloyd. 1983. *Science, Folklore, and Ideology.* Cambridge: Cambridge University Press.

Theophilus Lobb. 1739. *A Treatise on Dissolvents of the Stone . . . and on Curing the Stone and Gout.* London: Buckland.

Peter M. Logan. 1992. *Nerves and Narrative: The Body in Nineteenth-Century British Prose.* Unpublished Ph.D. dissertation. University of Michigan.

London Magazine. 1734. 'On the Gout.' December: 660.

London Magazine. 1735. 'On the First Fit of the Gout.' September: 506.

London Magazine. 1739. 'A Cure for the Gout.' June: 298.

London Magazine. 1748. 'Several Methods of Curing the Gout.' 228.

London Magazine. 1753. 'For the Gout or Rheumatism. 396.

London Magazine. 1754. 'To a Man of Quality and Great Riches Confined by the Gout'. December: 603.

London Magazine. 1755. 'A Dissertation on the Gout'. Letter from R. Drake to Editor. October: 611–13.

The London Magazine. 1756. 'Purging in the Gout.' Letter from Sir Richard Steele: 586.

The London Magazine. 1758. 'The Management of the Gout.' From Dr Crines pamphlet. April: 190–1.

The London Magazine. 1758. 'Boerhaave's Remedy for the Gout.' December: 639.

Morris Longstreth, M.D. 1962. *Rheumatism, Gout, and Some Allied Disorders.* New York: William Wood and Company.

Carlos Lopéz-Beltrán. 1992. 'Human Heredity 1750–1870: The Construction of a Domain'. PhD dissertation. King's College, London.

Carlos Lopéz-Beltrán. 1994. 'Forging Heredity: From Metaphor to Cause. A Reification Story'. *Studies in the History and Philosophy of Science.* xxv, 211–35.

Françoise Loux. 1978. *Sagesse du Corps: Santé et maladie dans les proverbs réginaux franÿaises.* Paris: Maisonneuve et Larose.

Françoise Loux. 1979. *Practiques et savoirs populaires: le corps dans la société traditionelle.* Paris: Berger-Levrault.

Françoise Loux. 1988. 'Popular Culture and Knowledge of the Body: Infancy and the Medical Anthropologists'. In R. Porter and A. Wear, eds. *Problems and Methods in the History of Medicine.* London: Croom Helm, 81–97.

Françoise Loux. 1993. 'Folk Medicine'. In W. F. Bynum and Roy Porter, eds. *Companion Encyclopedia of the History of Medicine.* London: Routledge, 661–75.

A. O. Lovejoy. 1948. *Essays in the History of Ideas.* Baltimore, Md: Johns Hopkins University Press.

Richard Lower. 1932. *De Corde* (1669); *Treatise on the Heart.* Intro. and Trans. K. J. Franklin. Oxford: the subscribers.

E. V. Lucas, ed. 1935. *The Letters of Charles Lamb to Which are Added Those of his Sister Mary Lamb.* London: J. M. Dent & Sons Ltd.

Lucian. 1749. *The Triumphs of the Gout,* in *Odes of Pindar.* trans. Gilbert West. London: Dodsley.

Lucian. 1967. 8 vols. Trans. A. M. Harmon, N. Kilburn and M. D. Macleod. London: W. Heinemann.

A. P. Luff. 1898. *Gout: Its Pathology and Treatment.* London: Cassell.

Brandon Lush, ed. 1961. *Concepts of Medicine.* Oxford: Pergamon Press.

Tom Lutz. 1991. *American Nervousness, 1903: An Anecdotal History.* Ithaca: Cornell University Press.

Lady Luxborough. 1775. *Letters Written to William Shenstone.* n.p: n.p.

Kenneth S. Lynn. 1987. *Hemingway.* New York: Simon & Schuster.

J. B. Lyons. 1973. *James Joyce and Medicine.* Dublin: Dolmen Press.

Jean-Francois Lyotard. 1984. *The Postmodern Condition: a report on knowledge.* Minneapolis University of Minnesota Press.

The Right Hon. Lord Lytton. *A Strange Story.* 1875. London: Routledge and Sons.

Ida Macalpine and Richard Hunter. 1969. *George III and the Mad-Business.* London: Allen Lane.

Daniel J. McCarty. 1970. 'A Historical Note: Leeuwenhoek's Description of Crystals from a Gouty Tophus'. *Arthritis and Rheumatism.* xiii, 414–18.

W. J. McCormack. 1980. *Sheridan Le Fanu and Victorian Ireland.* Oxford: Clarendon Press.

Maurice and Lewis Sawin McCullen. 1977. *A Dictionary of the Characters in George Meredith's Fiction.* New York: Garland Publishing, Inc.

Michael MacDonald. 1981. *Mystical Bedlam: Madness, Anxiety and Healing in Seventeenth Century England.* Cambridge: Cambridge University Press.

A. J. S. McFadzean. 1965. 'A Eunuch Takes the Gout'. *British Medical Journal.* i, 1038–9.

Barbara McGovern. 1992. *Anne Finch and her Poetry: A Critical Biography.* Athens, Ga: University of Georgia Press.

Francis McKee. 1991. 'The Earlier Works of Bernard Mandeville, 1685–1715'. PhD thesis, Glasgow University.

Francis McKee. 1994. 'Honeyed Words: Bernard Mandeville and Medical Discourse'. In Roy Porter, ed. *Medicine and the Enlightenment.* Amsterdam: Rodopi, 223–55.

Neil McKendrick, John Brewer and J. H. Plumb. 1982. *The Birth of a Consumer Society: The Commercialization of Eighteenth-Century England.* London: Europa.

James Mackenzie. 1958. *The History of Health.* Edinburgh.

T. McKeown. 1965. *Medicine in Modern Society.* London: George Allen & Unwin.

T. McKeown. 1976. *The Modern Rise of Population.* London: Edward Arnold; New York: Academic Press.

T. McKeown. 1979. *The Role of Medicine: Dream, Mirage or Nemesis?* Oxford: Blackwell.

T. McKeown. 1988. *The Origins of Human Disease.* Oxford: Basil Blackwell.

Sir James Mackintosh. 1791. *Vindiciae Gallicae.* Dublin: Corbet.

Natalie McKnight. 1993. *Idiots, Madmen, and Other Prisoners in Dickens.* New York: St. Martin's Press. pp. 1–29.

George MacLennan. 1993. *Lucid Interval: Subjective Writing and Madness in History.* Rutherford/Madison/Teaneck: Fairleigh Dickinson University Press.

R. K. McLure. 1981. *Coram's Children: The London Foundling Hospital in the Eighteenth Century.* New Haven, Conn.: Yale University Press.

C. E. McMahan. 1976. 'The Role of Imagination in the Disease Process: Pre-Cartesian History'. *Psychological Medicine.* vi, 179–84.

R. D. McMaster. 1991. *Thackeray's Cultural Frame of Reference.* Montreal: McGill University Press.

W. H. McNeill. 1976. *Plagues and Peoples.* Oxford: Anchor Press.

Andreas-Holger Maehle. 1995. 'Experimental Research on the Effects of Opium in the Eighteenth Century'. In Roy Porter and Mikuláö Teich, eds. *Drugs and Narcotics in History.* Cambridge: Cambridge University Press, 52–76.

Michael Maier. 1654. *Lusus Serius: Or, Serious Passe-time. A Philosophical Discourse Concerning the Superiority of Creatures under Man.* London: Humphrey Moseley.

J. F. Malgaigne. 1965. *Surgery and Ambroise Paré.* Trans. W. B. Hamby. Norman, Okla.: University of Oklahoma Press.

Mallam. 1993. *Mallam's Auction Catalog.* Manuscript lot 362. Oxford.

Marcello Malpighi. 1661. *De Pulmonibus.* Bologna: Io. Baptiste Ferronij.

Bernard Mandeville. 1970. *The Fable of the Bees.* Ed. Philip Harth. Harmondsworth: Penguin.

Robert M. Maniquis. 1969. 'The Puzzling *Mimosa*: Sensitivity and Plant Symbols in Romanticism.' *Studies in Romanticism.* viii: 129–55.

T. A. Mann. 1784. *The Extraordinary Case and Perfect Cure of the Gout by the Use of Hemlock and Wolfsbane*. London: J. Stockdale.

A. Marcovich. 1982. 'Concerning the Continuity between the Image of Society and the Image of the Human Body: An Examination of the Work of the English Physician J. C. Lettsom (1746–1815)'. In Peter W. G. Wright and A. Treacher, eds. *The Problem of Medical Knowledge*. Edinburgh: Edinburgh University Press, 69–87.

Harry M. Marks. 1992. 'Cortisone, 1949: A Year in the Political Life of a Drug'. *Bulletin of the History of Medicine*. lxvi, 419–39.

Hilary Marland. 1987. *Medicine and Society in Wakefield and Huddersfield*. Cambridge: Cambridge University Press.

Thomas Marryat, M.D. 1798. *Therapeuties or, the Art of Healing to Which Is Added, a Glossary of the More Difficult Words*. Bustal.

Edmund Marshall. 1770, 2nd edn. *A Candid and Impartial State of the Evidence of a Very Great Probability, That there is discovered By Monsieur Le Fevre, A Regular Physician, Presiding and Practicing at Liege in Germany, A Specific for the Gout. Containing the Motives which induced the Authors to listen to the Pretensions of the Liege Medicine; with an Account of its Operations and Effects in his own Case. To which is Added, A Narrative of the Cases of several other Patients, Persons of Rank and Reputation, who have been cured, or are now in the Course of a Cure of the Gout, by the Efficacy of Dr LeFevre's Powders, communicated by themselves to the Author, during his Residence at Liege. In an Appendix is given An Account of a House fitted up at Liege, for the Reception of the English only; with a Table of the Expence of the different Accommodations. Also a Detail of the best and most approved Inns upon the Road to Liege, either by the Rout of Calais or Ostend*. Canterbury: printed for the author by Simmons and Kirby.

Benjamin Marten. 1720. *A New Theory of Consumptions, More Especially of a Phthisis, or Consumption of the Lungs*. London: Knaplock.

John Marten. 1706. *A Treatise of the Safe, Internal Use of Cantharides in Physick . . . To Which Are Added Observations . . . of the . . . Doctor [J. Groenevelt] . . . Likewise a Letter to the Doctor of the Effects of Cantharides in the Gout*. London: J. Wale & J. Isted.

John Marten. 1708, 6th edn. *A Treatise of All the Symptoms of the Venereal Disease, in Both Sexes*. London: Crouch.

John Marten. 1713. *The Attila of the Gout, Being a Peculiar Account of That Distemper . . . And an Infallible Method to Cure It*. London. Printed for the Author and sold by N. Crouch.

John Marten. 1737, 4th edn. *The Dishonour of the Gout: or, A Serious Answer to a Ludicrous Pamphlet, Lately Publish'd Entitled, The Honour of the Gout; Shewing, I. That the Gout is One of the Greatest Misfortunes that Can Happen . . . II. That All Those Afflicted . . . Would Gladly be Rid of It. And III. That There is a Safe and Sure Cure for It*, corr. and enl. London: J. Isted.

John Marten. 1738, 4th edn. *A Treatise of the Gout*. London: J. Torbuck & E. Torbuck.

Charles Martin, MD. 1759. 'A Treatise on the Gout'. *Critical Review*, March: 281–2.

Julian Martin. 1988. 'Explaining John Freind's *History of Physick*'. *Studies in the History and Philosophy of Science*. xix, 399–418.

L. C. Martin, ed. 1963. *The Poetical Works of Robert Herrick*. Oxford: Clarendon Press.

R. B. Martin. 1980. *Tennyson: The Unquiet Heart*. Oxford: Clarendon Press.

Edwine M. Martz, ed. 1983. *Horace Walpole's Correspondence: Additions and Corrections*. New Haven: Yale University Press.

Massachusetts Historical Society. 1969. *Catalogue of Manuscripts of the Massachusetts Historical Society*, 9 vols. Boston, Mass.: G. K. Hall.

Cotton Mather. 1994. *The Christian Philosopher*, Intro., Ed., and Notes Winton U. Solberg. Urbana and Chicago: University of Illinois Press.

Samuel Mather. 1729. *The Life of the Very Reverend and Learned Cotton Mather, D.D. & F.R.S.* Boston: Samuel Gerrish.

O. Mayr. 1986. *Authority, Liberty and Automatic Machines in Early Modern Europe.* Baltimore: Johns Hopkins University Press.

Pauline M. H. Mazumdar. 1992. *Eugenics, Human Genetics and Human Failings. The Eugenics Society, its Sources and its Critics in Britain.* London: Routledge.

Richard Mead. 1702. *Mechanical Accounts of Poisons.* London: Ralph Smith.

Richard Mead. 1721. *A Discourse on the Plague.* London: J. Darby.

Richard H. Meade. 1974. *In the Sunshine of Life: A Biography of Dr Richard Mead 1673–1754.* Philadelphia, Pa: Dorrance & Company.

David Mechanic. 1962. 'The Concepts of Illness Behavior'. *Journal of Chronic Diseases.* xv, 189–94.

J. Melling and J. Barry, eds. 1992. *Culture in History.* Exeter: Exeter Studies in History.

Ronald Melzack and Patrick D. Wall. 1983. *The Challenge of Pain.* New York: Basic Books.

E. Mendelsohn and Y. Elkana, eds. 1981. *Science and Cultures.* Dordrecht: Kluwer.

Sara Haller Mendelson. 1987. *The Mental World of Stuart Women.* Amherst, Mass.: University of Massachusetts Press.

Alex Mercer. 1990. *Disease, Mortality and Population in Transition: Epidemiological-demographic Change in England Since the Eighteenth Century as Part of a Global Phenomenon.* Leicester: Leicester University Press.

Mercurius Pragmaticus. 1649. 30 January. Full run: September 1647–May 1649.

George Meredith. 1906, rev. edn. *The Adventures of Harry Richmond.* New York: Scribner's.

Linda E. Merians, ed. 1996. *Venereal Disease in the Eighteenth Century.* Kentucky: University of Kentucky Press.

E. S. Merton. 1969. *Science and Imagination in Sir Thomas Browne.* New York: Octagon.

Dieter Paul Mertz. 1990. *Geschichte der Gicht: Kultur- und Medizinhistorische Betrachtungen.* Stuttgart and New York: Thieme Verlag.

Jeffrey Meyers. 1991. *Joseph Conrad: A Biography.* New York: Charles Scribner's Sons.

Mark S. Micale. 1993. 'On the "Disappearance" of Hysteria: A Study in the Clinical Deconstruction of a Diagnosis.' *Isis.* lxxxiv, 496–526.

Mark S. Micale. 1995. *Approaching Hysteria: Disease and its Interpretations.* Princeton, NJ: Princeton University Press.

H. C. Erik Midelfort. 1994. *Mad Princes of Renaissance Germany.* Charlottesville and London: University Press of Virginia.

Mary Milner. 1842. *Life of Isaac Milner.* London: Parker.

Philander Misaurus [pseud.]. 1699; 1720; 1735. *The Honour of the Gout.* London: printed for A. Baldwin; London, s.n.; London: R. Gosling.

B. Mitchell and H. Penrose, eds. 1983. *Letters from Bath 1766–1767 by the Rev. John Penrose.* London: Alan Sutton.

G. M. Mody and P. D. Naidoo. 1984. 'Gout in South African Blacks'. *Annals of Rheumatic Diseases.* xliii, 394–7.

Ellen Moers. 1960. *The Dandy: Brummel to Beerbohm.* London: Secker and Warburg.

H. J. Montoye, J. A. Faulkner, H. J. Dodge, W. M. Mikkelsen, P. W. Willis 3rd, W. D. Block. 1967. 'Serum Uric Acid Concentration among Business Executives'. *Annals of Internal Medicine.* lxvi, 838–49.

M. Mooney. 1757. *A Letter to a Physician Concerning the Gout and Rheumatism.* London: for the author.

Edward Duke Moore. 1864. *Memorandums and Recollections on Gout and Rheumatism, and their Treatment with a Few Practical Remarks on Sciatica and Lumbago.* London: J. Churchill.

Robert E. Moore. 1948. *Hogarth's Literary Relationships.* Minneapolis, Minn.: University of Minnesota Press.

Arthur D. Morris. 1989. *James Parkinson, His Life and Times*. Boston: Birkhauser.

David B. Morris. 1991. *The Culture of Pain*. Berkeley and Los Angeles, Calif.: University of California Press.

Richard Morton. 1694. *Phthisiologia: Or A Treatise of Consumptions. Wherein the Difference, Nature, Causes, Signs and Cure of All Sorts of Consumptions Are Explained*. London: S. Smith and B. Walford.

Walter Moyle. 1796. *Democracy Vindicated. An Essay on the Constitution and Government of the Roman State*. Ed. John Thelwall. Norwich: March.

Isadore G. Mudge and M. Earl Sears. 1910. *A Thackeray Dictionary*. London: George Routledge & Sons.

Richard Mullen. 1990. *Anthony Trollope: A Victorian in his World*. London: Duckworth.

Charles F. Mullett. 1946. 'Public Baths and Health in England, 16th–18th Century'. *Bulletin of the History of Medicine*. Supplement 5.

Ann Mullins. 1968. 'William Cadogan, a Physician in Advance of his Time'. *History of Medicine (London)*. October: 11–12.

Charles Murchison. 1862. *A Treatise on the Continued Fevers of Great Britain*. London: Parker & Bourn.

Charles Murchison. 1868. *Clinical Lectures on Diseases of the Liver, Jaundice and Abdominal Dropsy*. London: Longmans, Green.

P. Murray, ed. 1989. *Genius: The History of An Idea*. Oxford: Basil Blackwell.

Samuel Musgrave. 1779. *Gulstonian Lectures Read at the Royal College of Physicians*. London: T. Payne.

William Musgrave. 1703. *De Arthritide Symptomatica*. Exoniae: Farley for Yeo and Biship.

Daniel M. Musher. 1967. 'The Medical Views of Dr Tobias Smollett (1721–1771)'. *Bulletin of the History of Medicine*. xli, 455–62.

R. A. Mynors and D. F. Thomson, trans. 1974–94. *The Correspondence of Erasmus*, 11 vols. Toronto: University of Toronto Press.

Doreen Evenden Nagy. 1988. *Popular Medicine in Seventeenth-Century England*. Bowling Green, Oh: Bowling Green State University Popular Press.

Zdzistaw Najder. 1983. *Joseph Conrad: A Chronicle*. New Brunswick: Rutgers University Press.

Benjamin Nangle. 1934. *The Monthly Review*. Oxford: Oxford University Press.

Anna K. Nardo. 1991. *The Ludic Self in Seventeenth-Century English Literature*. Albany, NY: State University of New York Press.

Thomas Nash. 1600. *A Pleasant Comedie, Called Summers Last Will and Testament*. London: Simon Stafford.

Lucien Nass. 1914. *Curiosites Medico-Artistiques*. Paris: Librairie le Francois. 57–9.

R. S. Neale. 1981. *Bath 1680–1850: A Social History*. London: Routledge & Kegan Paul.

Gilbert Nelson. 1727. *The Nature, Cause and Symptoms of the Gout*. London: T. Warner.

G. Nelson. 1728. *A Short Account of Certain Remedies Used in the Cure of the Gout*. London, s.n.

Virgil Nemoianu. 1989. 'Illness and Style: The Case of Bramble's Hypochondria'. In *A Theory of the Secondary: Literature, Progress and Reaction*. Baltimore, Md: Johns Hopkins University Press.

M. Neuburger. 1932. *The Doctrine of the Healing Power of Nature Throughout the Course of Time*. Trans. J. Boyd. New York, s.n.

Melvyn and Joan New, eds. 1978. *The Florida Edition of the Works of Laurence Sterne: 'Tristram Shandy'*. vol. ii. Gainesville, Fla: University Press of Florida.

Malcolm Nicolson. 1988. 'The Metastatic Theory of Pathogenesis and the Professional Interests of the Eighteenth-Century Physician'. *Medical History*. xxxii, 277–300.

Marjorie Hope Nicolson. 1946. *Newton Demands the Muse: Newton's Opticks and Eighteenth Century Poets*. Princeton, NJ: Princeton University Press.

Marjorie Hope Nicolson. 1959. *Mountain Gloom and Mountain Glory: The Development of the Aesthetics of the Infinite*. Ithaca, NY: Cornell University Press.

Marjorie Hope Nicolson. 1960. *The Breaking of the Circle*. New York: Columbia University Press.

Marjorie Hope Nicolson and G. S. Rousseau. 1968. *'This Long Disease, My Life': Alexander Pope and the Sciences*. Princeton, NJ: Princeton University Press.

P. Niebyl. 1971. 'The Non-Naturals'. *Bulletin of the History of Medicine*. xlv, 486–92.

Andrew Nikiforuk. 1992. *The Fourth Horseman. A Short History of Epidemics, Plagues and Other Scourges*. London: Fourth Estate.

C. H. von Noorden. 1910. *Technique of Reduction Cures and Gout*. New York: Treat.

J. E. Norton, ed. 1956. *The Letters of Edward Gibbon*, 3 vols. New York: The Macmillan Company.

J. O. Nriagu. 1983. 'Saturnine Gout Among Roman Aristocrats. Did Lead Poisoning Contribute to the Fall of the Empire?' *New England Journal of Medicine*. cccvii, 660–3.

Claud Nugent. 1898. *Memoir of Robert, Earl Nugent*. Chicago: H. S. Stone & Co.

Ronald L. Numbers and Darrel W. Amundsen, eds. 1986. *Caring and Curing. Health and Medicine in the Western Medical Traditions*. New York: Macmillan.

Vivian Nutton. 1985. 'Murders and Miracles: Lay Attitudes towards Medicine in Classical Antiquity'. In Roy Porter, ed. *Patients and Practitioners: Lay Perceptions of Medicine in Pre-Industrial Society*. Cambridge: Cambridge University Press, 23–54.

Vivian Nutton. 1993. 'Humoralism'. In W. F. Bynum and Roy Porter, eds. *Companion Encyclopedia of the History of Medicine*. London: Routledge, 281–91.

William B. Ober. 1979. *Boswell's Clap and Other Essays: Medical Analyses of Literary Men's Afflictions*. Carbondale, Ill.: Southern Illinois University Press.

William B. Ober. 1987. *Bottoms Up! A Pathologist's Essays on Medicine and the Humanities*. Carbondale and Edwardsville, Ill.: Southern Illinois University Press.

Robert Olby. 1993. 'Constitutional and Hereditary Disorders'. In W. F. Bynum and Roy Porter, eds. *Companion Encyclopedia of the History of Medicine*. London: Routledge, 412–37.

William Oliver, MD. 1751. *A Practical Essay on the Use and Abuse of Warm-Bathing in Gouty Cases*. Bath: T. Boddely.

William Oliver, MD. n.d. *Reflections on the Gout*. London.

Walter J. Ong. 1982. *Orality and Literacy: The technologizing of the Word*. London: Methuen.

Janet Oppenheim. 1991. *'Shattered Nerves': Doctors, Patients and Depression in Victorian England*. Oxford: Oxford University Press.

William Osler. 1892, 1st edn; 1898, 3rd edn. *The Principles and Practice of Medicine. Designed for the Use of Practitioners and Students of Medicine*. New York: Appleton; Edinburgh and London: Young J. Pentland.

Oxford English Dictionary, 1989, 2nd edn. 20 vols. Ed. J. A. Simpson and E. S. C. Weiner. Oxford: Clarendon Press.

Walter Pagel. 1958a. *Paracelsus: An Introduction to Philosophical Medicine in the Era of the Renaissance*. Basel: Karger.

Walter Pagel. 1958b. *William Harvey's Biological Ideas*. Basel: Karger.

Walter Pagel. 1976. *New Light on William Harvey*. Basel: Karger.

Walter Pagel. 1982. *Joan Baptista Van Helmont: Reformer of Science and Medicine*. Cambridge: Cambridge University Press.

Walter Pagel. 1984. *The Smiling Spleen: Paracelsianism in Storm and Stress*. Basel and New York: Karger.

Sir James Paget. 1853. *Lectures on Surgical Pathology*, 2 vols. London, Longman, Brown, Green and Longmans.

Sir James Paget. 1866. 'Gouty and Some Other Forms of Phlebitis.' *St Bartholomew's Hospital Reports*. ii, 82–92.

Sir James Paget. 1875. *Clinical Lectures and Essays*. Ed. Howard Marsh. London: Longman Green and Co.

Sir James Paget. 1887. 'The Morton Lecture on Cancer and Cancerous Diseases.' *British Medical Journal*. ii, 1091–4.

Thomas Palmer. 1696; 1984. *The Admirable Secrets of Physick and Chyrurgery*. Ed. T. R. Forbes. New Haven, Conn.: Yale University Press.

Emiliano Panconesi. 1992. 'Lorenzo il Magnifico: His Life and His Diseases.' 12th International Congress of Thrombosis. Florence: Scientific Press.

Erwin Panofsky. 1974. *Meaning in the Visual Arts*. Woodstock, New York: Overlook Press.

Theophrastus von Hohenheim Paracelsus. 1574. *Das Sechste Buch in der Artznei. Von den Tartarischen oder Stein Krankheiten*. Basel: Samuel Apiaro.

Theophrastus von Hohenheim Paracelsus. 1589–90. *Die Bucher und Schriften . . . , an tag Geben Durch J. H. Brisgoium*. Basel: C. Waldkirch.

Theophrastus von Hohenheim Paracelsus. 1923–33. *Sämtliche Werke*, 14 vols. Ed. Karl Sudhoff. Munich: O. N. Barth, R. Oldebring.

Theophrastus von Hohenheim Paracelsus. 1941. *Four Treatises of Theophrastus von Hohenheim Called Paracelsus*. Ed. Henry E. Sigerist. Baltimore, Md: Johns Hopkins University Press.

Theophrastus von Hohenheim Paracelsus. 1951. *Paracelsus: Selected Writings*. Trans. N. Guterman. New York: Pantheon Books.

Theophrastus von Hohenheim Paracelsus. 1975–77. *Sämtliche Werke*, 4 vols. Ed. Bernard Aschner. Leipzig: Zentralantiquariat der Deutschen Demokratischen Republik.

Ambroise Paré. 1545. *La Méthode de Traiter les Playes Faictes par Hacquebutes, et autres bastons a feu*. Paris: Gaulterot.

Ambroise Paré. 1634. *The Workes of that Famous Chirurgeon Ambrose Parey*. Trans. Thomas Johnson. London: Thomas Cotes and R. Young.

Lawrence Charles Parish. 1963. 'An Historical Approach to the Nomenclature of Rheumatoid Arthritis'. *Arthritis and Rheumatism*. vi, 138–58.

Lawrence Charles Parish. 1964. *Augustin-Jacob Landré-Beauvais 1772–1840: A Neglected Forerunner in the History of Rheumatoid Arthritis*. Boston, Mass.: Department of the History of Medicine at Tufts University School of Medicine.

Katherine Park. 1985. *Doctors and Medicine in Early Renaissance Florence*. Princeton, NJ.: Princeton University Press.

Katharine Park. 1992. 'Medicine and Society in Medieval Europe, 500–1500.' In Andrew Wear, ed. *Medicine in Society: Historical Essays*. Cambridge: Cambridge University Press, 59–90.

Geoffrey Parker. 1978. *Philip II: Library of the World Biography*. London: Hutchinson.

Edmund Parkes. 1860. *The Composition of the Urine in Health and Disease*. London: J. Churchill.

Edmund Parkes. 1864. *Manual of Practical Hygiene*. London: J. Churchill.

James Parkinson. 1801, 4th edn. *Medical Admonitions to Families Respecting the Preservation of Health, and the Treatment of the Sick, Also a Table of Symptoms Serving to Point out the Degree of Danger, and to Distinguish One Disease from Another*. London: H. D. Symonds.

J. Parkinson. 1805. *Observations on the Nature and Cure of Gout*. London: H. D. Symonds.

J. Parkinson. 1817. *An Essay on the Shaking Palsy*. London: Sherwood, Neely & Jones.

The Parliament-Kite. 1648. No. 8. 13 July. Full run: May – August 1648.

Caleb Hillier Parry. 1799. *An Enquiry into the Symptoms and Causes of the Syncope Anginosa Called Angina Pectoris*. Bath: R. Cruttwell.

Caleb Hillier Parry. 1815. *Elements of Pathology and Therapeutics*. Bath: R. Cruttwell.

Talcott Parsons. 1958. 'Definitions of Health and Illness in the Light of American Values and Social Structure'. In E. G. Jaco, ed. *Patients, Physicians and Illness*. Glencoe, Ill.: The Free Press, 165–87.

Gail Kern Paster. 1993. *The Body Embarrassed: Drama and the Disciplines of Shame in Early Modern England*. Ithaca, NY: Cornell University Press.

Frank Allen Patterson and French Rowe Fogle, eds. 1940. *An Index to the Columbia Edition of the Works of John Milton.* New York: Columbia University Press.

Paul of Aegina. 1834. *The Medical Works of Paulus Aegineta, the Greek Physician.* Trans. Francis Adams. London: J. Welsh, Treuttel, Wurtz.

Paul of Aegina. 1844. *The Seven Books of Paulus Aegineta.* 3 vols. Trans. Francis Adams. London: Printed for the Sydenham Society.

Gustav Pauli. 1901. *Hans Sebald Beham: Ein Kritisches verzeichniss seiner Kupferstiche Radirungen und Holzschnitte.* Strassburg.

B. Z. Paulshook. 1983. 'William Heberden and Opium – Some Relief to All'. *New England Journal of Medicine.* cccviii, 53–6.

Ronald Paulson. 1965. *Hogarth's Works.* New Haven: Yale University Press.

Ronald Paulson. 1967. *Satire and the Novel in Eighteenth-Century England.* New Haven: Yale University Press.

Ronald Paulson. 1967. *The Fictions of Satire.* Baltimore: Johns Hopkins.

Ronald Paulson. 1972. *Rowlandson: A New Interpretation.* New York and Oxford: Oxford University Press.

Ronald Paulson. 1979. *Popular and Polite Art in the Age of Hogarth and Fielding.* Notre Dame: University of Notre Dame.

Ronald Paulson. 1992. *Hogarth: Volume II, High Art and Low 1732–1750* New Brunswick, N.J. Rutgers University Press.

Frederick W. Pavy. 1862. *Researches on the Nature and Treatment of Diabetes.* London: Churchill.

Frederick W. Pavy. 1874. *Treatise on Food and Dietetics.* London: J. & A. Churchill.

Lynn Payer. 1989. *Medicine and Culture: Notions of Health and Sickness in Britain, the U.S., France and West Germany.* London: V. Gollancz.

Steven J. Peitzman. 1992. 'From Bright's Disease to End-Stage Renal Disease'. In Charles E. Rosenberg and Janet Golden, eds. *Framing Disease: Studies in Cultural History.* New Brunswick, NJ: Rutgers University Press, 3–19.

M. Pelling. 1993. 'Contagion/Germ Theory/Specificity.' In W. F. Bynum and Roy Porter, eds. *Companion Encyclopedia of the History of Medicine.* London: Routledge, 309–34.

Max Pensky. 1993. *Melancholy Dialectics: Walter Benjamin and the Play of Mourning.* Amherst, Mass.: University of Massachusetts Press.

William Pepper. 1910; repr. 1970. *The Medical Side of Benjamin Franklin.* NY.: Argosy-Antiquarian Ltd.

Perfect Passages. 1645. No. 43. 20 August. Full run: October 1644–March 1646.

Martin S. Pernick. 1985. *A Culculus of Suffering. Pain, Professionalism and Suffering in Nineteenth Century America.* New York: Columbia University Press.

Catherine Peters. 1987. *Thackeray's Universe: Shifting Worlds of Imagination and Reality.* London: Faber.

Catherine Peters. 1991. *The King of Inventors: A Life of Wilkie Collins.* London: Secker & Warburg.

M. Jeanne Peterson. 1978. *The Medical Profession in Mid-Victorian London.* Berkeley, Calif.: University of California Press.

R. T. Petersson. 1956. *Sir Kenelm Digby: The Ornament of England 1603–1665.* London: Jonathan Cape.

Petrarch. 1975–85. *Letters on Familiar Matters.* 3 vols. Trans. Aldo S. Bernardo. Baltimore, Md: Johns Hopkins University Press.

Petrarch. 1991. *Petrarch's Remedies for Fortune Fair and Foul,* 3 vols. Trans. and commentary Conrad H. Rawski. Bloomington, Ind.: Indiana University Press.

Thomas J. Pettigrew. 1809. *Surgical Observations on the Constitutional Origin and Treatment of Local Diseases and on Aneurisms.* London: Longman, Hurst, Rees and Orme.

Thomas J. Pettigrew. 1838–40. *Medical Portrait Gallery.* London: Fisher, Whittaker.

Henry Pettit, ed. 1971. *The Correspondence of Edward Young 1683–1765.* Oxford: Clarendon Press.

Pharmacopoeia Londinensis. 1618, 1st edn. London: E. Griffin for J. Marriott.

Thomas Phelps. 1685. *A True Account of the Captivity of Thomas Phelps . . . Upon the Thirteenth Day of June 1685.* London: n.p.

'Philiatros'. 1655. *Natura Exeuterata: Or Nature Unbowelled by the Most Exquisite Anatomizers of Her. Wherein are Contained her Choisest Secrets Digested into Receipts Fitted For the Cure of All Sorts of Infirmities Whether Internal or External, Acute or Chronical That are Incident to the Body of Man.* London: H. Twiford.

E. D. Phillips. 1973. *Greek Medicine.* London: Thames & Hudson.

Philosophical Transactions of the Royal Society of London. 1660–1878.

Philosophical Transactions. 1685. 'An Abstract of a Letter of Mr Anthony Leewenhoek Fellow of the R. Society . . . the Chalk Stones of the Gout'. 15(3), 23 February: 891–2.

Philosophical Transactions. 1728. 'VI. An Extract of a Letter of Signior Michele Pinelli, concerning the causes of the Gout translated from the Stalean by John James Scheutzer, M.D.' 35 (403). July, August, September: 491–4.

Jean Piaget. 1972. *Play and Development: A Symposium with Contributions by Jean Piaget [and others].* Ed. Maria W. Piers. New York: Norton.

Daniel Pick. 1989. *Faces of Degeneration: Aspects of a European Disorder c. 1848–1918.* Cambridge and New York: Cambridge University Press.

George Pickering. 1976. *Creative Malady.* New York: Delta.

Gilbert A. Pierce. 1965. *The Dickens Dictionary.* London: Chapman & Hall, Ltd.

H. G. Piffard. 1876. *. . . Diseases of the Skin.* London: Macmillan.

Stuart Piggott. 1950. *William Stukeley: An Eighteenth-Century Antiquary.* Oxford: Clarendon Press.

S. Piggot, ed. 1974. *Antiquaries. . . . Stuart Piggott.* London: Mansell.

Philip Pinkus. 1980. *Grub Street Stripped Bare.* London: Constable.

Willibald Pirckheimer. 1617. *The Praise of the Gout, Or, The Gouts Apologie. A Paradox, Both Pleasant and Profitable, Written First in the Latine Tongue, by that Famous and Noble Gentleman Bilibaldus Pirckheimerus Councellor unto two Emperours, Maximillian the first and Charles the First. And now Englished by William Est, Master of Arts.* London: printed by G. P. for John Budge.

Robert Pitt, M.D. 1703, 3rd edn. *The Craft and Frauds of Physic Expos'd.* London: Childe.

Robert Pitt, M.D. 1704. *The Antidote: or the Preservative of Health and Life and the Restorative Physick to Its Sincerity and Perfection.* London.

Raffaela Piva. 1985. *Le 'Confortevolissime' Terme – Interventi pubblici e privati a Battaglia e nelle terme Padovane fra sette e ottocento. A cura di Fiorenzo toffanin.* Battaglia terme: Edizioni La Galiverna.

Pliny the Elder. 1949. *Historia Naturalis.* Trans. H. Rackham. London: William Heinemann.

Pliny the Younger. 1972, 1975. *Letters and Panegyncus,* 2 vols. Trans. Betty Radice. London: William Heinemann Ltd.

J. H. Plumb. 1967. *The Growth of Political Stability in England, 1675–1725.* London: Macmillan.

J. G. A. Pocock. 1972. *Politics, Language and Time: Essays in Political Thought and History.* London: Methuen.

J. G. A. Pocock. 1975. *The Machiavellian Moment. Florentine Political Thought and the Atlantic Republican Tradition.* Princeton, NJ: Princeton University Press.

J. G. A. Pocock, ed. 1981. *Three British Revolutions, 1641, 1688, 1776.* Princeton: Princeton University Press.

J. G. A. Pocock. 1985. *Virtue, Commerce and History: Essays on Political Thought and History.* Cambridge and New York: Cambridge University Press.

R. H. Popkin, ed. 1988. *Millenarianism and Messianism in English Literature and Thought 1650–1800*. Leiden: E. J. Brill.

Dorothy Porter and Roy Porter. 1988. 'What Was Social Medicine? A Historiographical Essay'. *Journal of Historical Sociology*. i, 90–106.

Dorothy Porter and Roy Porter. 1989. *Patient's Progress: Doctors and Doctoring in Eighteenth-Century England*. Cambridge: Polity Press.

Roy Porter, ed. 1985. *Patients and Practitioners: Lay Perceptions of Medicine in Pre-Industrial Society*. Cambridge: Cambridge University Press.

Roy Porter. 1986. 'The Scientific Revolution: A Spoke in the Wheel?' In Roy Porter and Mikulás Teich, eds. *Revolution in History*. Cambridge: Cambridge University Press, 290–316.

Roy Porter. 1987. 'Medicine and Religion in Eighteenth-Century England: A Case of Conflict?' *Ideas and Production: Issue Seven – History of Science*. Cambridge: Cambridgeshire College of Arts & Technology, 4–17.

Roy Porter, ed. 1987. *Man Masters Nature*. London: BBC Publications, 65–76.

Roy Porter. 1988; 1804, 1st edn. 'Introduction' to *Thomas Trotter: An Essay on Drunkenness*. London: Routledge.

Roy Porter. 1989a. *Health for Sale: Quackery in England 1650–1850*. Manchester: Manchester University Press.

Roy Porter. 1989b. '"The Whole Secret of Health": Mind, Body and Medicine in *Tristram Shandy*'. In John Christie and Sally Shuttleworth, eds. *Nature Transfigured*. Manchester: Manchester University Press, 61–84.

Roy Porter. 1989c. 'Death and the Doctors in Georgian England.' In R. Houlbrooke, ed. *Death, Ritual and Bereavement*. London: Routledge, 77–94.

Roy Porter, ed. 1990. *The Medical History of Waters and Spas* (London: *Medical History*, Supplement 10.

Roy Porter. 1991a. 'Civilization and Disease: Medical Ideology in the Enlightenment'. In J. Black and J. Gregory, eds. *Culture, Politics and Society in Britain 1660–1800*. Manchester: Manchester University Press, 154–83.

Roy Porter. 1991b. *Doctor of Society: Thomas Beddoes and the Sick Trade in Late Enlightenment England*. London: Routledge.

Roy Porter. 1992a. 'Addicted to Modernity: Nervousness in the Early Consumer Society'. In J. Melling and J. Barry, eds. *Culture in History*. Exeter: Exeter Studies in History, 180–94.

Roy Porter. 1992b. 'The Case of Consumption'. In Janine Bourriau, ed. *Understanding Catastrophe*. Cambridge: Cambridge University Press, 179–203.

Roy Porter, ed. 1992. *The Popularization of Medicine, 1650–1850*. London: Routledge.

Roy Porter. 1993a. 'Diseases of Civilization'. In W. F. Bynum and Roy Porter, eds. *Companion Encyclopedia of the History of Medicine*. London: Routledge, 585–602.

Roy Porter. 1993b. 'Pain and Suffering'. In W. F. Bynum and Roy Porter, eds. *Companion Encyclopedia of the History of Medicine*. London: Routledge, 1574–91.

Roy Porter. 1993c. 'Consumption: Disease of the Consumer Society?' In John Brewer and Roy Porter, eds. *Consumption and the World of Goods*. London: Routledge, 58–84.

Roy Porter. 1994. 'Gout: Framing and Fantasizing Disease.' *Bulletin of the History of Medicine*, lxviii, 1–28.

Roy Porter, ed. 1994. *Medicine and the Enlightenment*. Amsterdam: Rodopi.

Roy Porter. 1995. '"Perplex'd with Tough Names": The Uses of Medical Jargon'. In Peter Burke and Roy Porter, eds. *Languages and Jargons: Contributions to a Social History of Language*. Cambridge: Polity Press, 42–63.

Roy Porter. 1996. '"Laying Aside Any Private Advantage": John Marten and Veneral Disease'. In Linda E. Merians, ed. *The Secret Malady: Venereal Disease in Eighteenth Century Britain and France*. Lexington, Ky: University Press of Kentucky, 51–67.

Roy Porter. 1998. 'Gout and the Quacks'. In K. Bayertz and Roy Porter, eds. *Essays in Honour of Mikulàs Teich*. Amsterdam: Rodopi.

Roy Porter and Dorothy Porter. 1988. *In Sickness and in Health: The British Experience 1650–1850*. London: Fourth Estate.

Roy Porter & Mikulás Teich, eds. 1986. *Revolution in History*. Cambridge: Cambridge University Press, 290–316.

Roy Porter and Mikulás Teich, eds. 1992. *The Scientific Revolution in National Context*. Cambridge: Cambridge University Press.

Roy Porter and Mikulás Teich, eds. 1995. *Drugs and Narcotics in History*. Cambridge: Cambridge University Press.

Roy Porter and Andrew Wear, eds. 1988. *Problems and Methods in the History of Medicine*. London: Croom Helm.

Roy Porter and Lesley Hall. 1995. *The Facts of Life: The Creation of Sexual Knowledge in Britain from 1650 to 1950*. New Haven, Conn.: Yale University Press.

F. A. Pottle and C. H. Bennett, eds. 1936. *Boswell's Journal of a Tour in the Hebrides*. London: W. Heinemann.

Marie-Christine Pouchelle. 1990. *The Body and Surgery in the Middle Ages*. Trans. Rosemary Morris. New Brunswick: Rutgers University Press.

F. N. L. Poynter and W. J. Bishop, eds. 1956. *A Seventeenth Century Doctor and his Patients: John Symcotts, 1592–1662*. Luton: Bedfordshire Historical Society.

Mary Louise Pratt. 1991. *Imperial Eyes: Studies in Travel Writing and Transculturation*. London: Routledge.

William H. Prescott. 1906. *The Complete Works of William H. Prescott: History of the Reign of the Emperor Charles the Fifth*. New York: Thomas Y. Crowell.

Robert Proctor. 1989. *Racial Hygiene: Medicine Under the Nazis*. Cambridge, Mass., Harvard University Press.

William Prout. 1815. 'On the Relation Between the Specific Gravities of Bodies in their Gaseous State and the Weights of their Atoms,' *Annals of Philosophy*, vi, 321–30.

William Prout. 1818. 'Description of an Acid Principle Prepared from the Lithic or Uric Acid'. *Philosophical Transactions*. cix, 420–8.

William Prout. 1821. *An Inquiry into the Nature and Treatment of Gravel, Calculus, and Other Diseases Connected with a Deranged Operation of the Urinary Organs*. London: Baldwin, Cradock & Joy.

Samuel Pye. 1757. 'An Uncommon Crisis of the Gout'. *Medical Observations and Inquiries*, vol. i. London: W. Johnston.

Richard Quain. 1882. *A Dictionary of Medicine*, 3 vols. London: Longman's, Green and Co.

Peter Quennell, ed. 1948. *The Private Letters of Princess Lieven to Prince Metternich, 1820–1826*. London: J. Murray.

Claude Quétel. 1990. *The History of Syphilis*. Trans. Judith Braddock and Brian Pike. Oxford: Basil Blackwell.

M. M. Quinones. 1966. *Robert Adams and his Role in the History of Rheumatoid Arthritis*. Basel: Institute of the History of Medicine.

Bernardino Ramazzini. 1940. *De Morbis Artificum Bernardini Ramazzini Diatriba: Diseases of Workers*. Trans. Wilmer Cave Wright. Chicago: University of Chicago Press.

George Randolph, M.D. 1752. *An enquiry into the medicinal virtues of Bath-water. . . .* London: J. Nourse.

Mary Claire Randolph. 1941. 'The Medical Concept in English Renaissance Satiric Theory: Its Possible Relationships and Implications.' *Studies in Philology*. 38: 125–57.

D. Rannie, ed. 1898. *Remarks and Collections of Thomas Hearne*, vol.iv. Oxford: printed for the Oxford Historical Society at the Clarendon Press.

L. J. Rather. 1959. 'Towards a Philosophical Study of the Idea of Disease.' In *The Historical

Development of Physiological Thought, Ed. Chandler McC. Brooks and Paul F. Cranefield. New York: Hafner Pub. Co., 351–73.

L. J. Rather. 1968. 'The "Six Things Non-Natural": A Note on the Origins and Fate of a Doctrine and a Phrase'. *Clio Medica*. iii, 337–47.

L. J. Rather. 1978. *The Genesis of Cancer: A Study in the History of Ideas*. Baltimore: Johns Hopkins University Press.

Claude Rawson. 1994. *Satire and Sentiment 1660–1830* (Cambridge: Cambridge University Press.

Pierre-Francois Rayer. 1935, 2nd edn. *A Theoretical and Practical Treatise on Diseases of the Skin*. Trans. R. Willis. London: J. B. Ballière.

Pierre-Francois Rayer. 1840. *Treatise on Diseases of the Kidney*. Paris: J. B. Balliere.

Joad Raymond, ed. 1993. *Making the News: An Anthology of the Newsbooks of Revolutionary England 1641–1660*. Foreword by Christopher Hill. Moreton in Marsh, Gloucestershire: The Windrush Press.

Conyers Read. 1955. *Mr. Secretary Cecil and Queen Elizabeth*. London: Cape.

Conyers Read. 1960. *Lord Burghley and Queen Elizabeth*. London: Cape.

Bruce Redford, ed. 1992–4. *The Letters of Samuel Johnson*, 5 vols. Oxford: Clarendon Press.

Richard Reece. 1803. *Domestic Medical Guide*. London: Longman & Reed.

W. T. Reich, ed. 1978. *Encyclopedia of Bioethics*, 4 vols. New York: Free Press.

Emil Reicke. 1930. *Willibald Pirckheimer: Leben, Familie und Persönlichkeit*. Jena: E. Diederichs.

B. L. Reid. 1965. 'Smollet's Healing Journey.' *The Virginia Quarterly Review*. 41: 549–70.

John Rendle-Short. 1960a. 'Infant Management in the 18th Century with Special Reference to the Work of William Cadogan.' *Bulletin of the History of Medicine*. xxxiv, 97–122.

John Rendle-Short. 1960b. 'William Cadogan: Eighteenth Century Physician'. *Medical History*. iv, 288–309.

Henri Rendu. 1890. *Lecons de Clinique Médicale*, 2 vols. Paris: O. Doin.

W. Renwick. [1771]. *An Attempt to Restore the Primitive Natural Constitution of Mankind, and to Increase Conjugal Procreation. To which are added Cursory Observation on the Gout, together with the Correspondence between Mr. Hawes and the Author relative to the Interment of the Dead. The Author's principal Remarks on that Subject having been omitted in the Pamphlet lately published by the former Gentleman*. London: printed for the author.

Myra Reynolds. 1903. *The Poems of Anne Countess of Winchilsea*. Chicago, Ill.: University of Chicago Press.

Rhazes. 1848. *A Treatise on the Small-pox and the Measles*. Trans. from the Arabic. London: Sydenham Society.

Christopher Ricks, ed. 1987. *The Poems of Tennyson*. Berkeley, Calif.: University of California Press.

Paul Ricoeur. 1977. *The Rule of Metaphor: Multi-disciplinary Studies of the Creation of Meaning in Language*. Trans. Robert Czerny. Toronto: University of Toronto Press.

John M. Riddle. 1985. *Dioscorides on Pharmacy and Medicine*. Austin, TX.: University of Texas Press.

Walther Riese. 1953. *The Conception of Disease, its History, its Versions and its Nature*. New York: Philosophical Library.

James C. Riley. 1989. *Sickness, Recovery and Death: A History and Forecast of Ill Health*. Iowa City: University of Iowa Press.

John Ring. 1811. *A Treatise on the Gout*. London: Callow.

John Ring. 1816. *An Answer to Dr Kinglake: Showing the Danger of his Cooling Treatment of the Gout*. London: for the author.

Francis Riollay. 1778. *A Letter to Dr. Hardy . . . on the Origin of Gout*. Oxford.

G. Risse. 1978. 'Health and Disease: History of the Concepts'. In W. T. Reich, ed. *Encyclopedia of Bioethics*, 4 vols. New York: Free Press, ii, 579–85.

G. Risse. 1988. 'Brunonian Therapeutics: New Wine in Old Bottles'. In W. F. Bynum and Roy Porter, eds. *Brunonianism in Britain and Europe*. London: *Medical History*. Supplement 8, 46–62.

Lazare Rivière. 1678. *Of Pain in the Joynts, Called Arthritis, or the Gout*. London: G. Sawbridge.

Brenda D. Rix. 1987. *Our Old Friend Rolly: Watercolours, Prints and Book Illustrations by Thomas Rowlandson*. Toronto. Art Gallery of Ontario.

Caroline Robbins. 1959. *The Eighteenth-Century Commonwealthman*. Cambridge, Mass.: Harvard University Press.

K. B. Roberts. 1992. *The Fabric of the Body: European Traditions of Anatomical Illustration*. Oxford and New York: Clarendon Press.

Marie Mulvey Roberts and Roy Porter, eds. 1993. *Literature and Medicine During the Eighteenth Century*. London and New York: Routledge.

William Roberts. 1865. *A Practical Treatise on Urinary and Renal Diseases* (London: Walton and Maberly.

Sir William Roberts. 1892. *Chemistry and Therapeutics of Uric Acid and Gout*. London: Smith, Elder and Co.

William Robertson D.D., and William H. Prescott. 1586. *The History of the Reign of the Emperor Charles the Fifth, with an Account of the Emperor's Life After His Abdication*. Philadelphia: Lippincott.

Nicholas Robinson. 1753. *An Essay on the Gout, and All Gouty Affections Incident to Affect Mankind. Comprizing the Various Natures, Symptoms and Causes, Thro' Every Branch and Stage*. London: Edward Robinson.

J. Rodgers. 1978. 'Ideas of Life in "Tristram Shandy"'. PhD thesis, University of East Anglia.

Gerald P. Rodnan. 1961. 'A Gallery of Gout: Being a Miscellany of Prints and Caricatures from the 16th Century to the Present Day'. *Arthritis and Rheumatism*. iv, 27–46.

Gerald P. Rodnan. 1965. 'Early Theories Concerning Etiology and Pathogenesis of the Gout'. *Arthritis and Rheumatism*. viii, 599–610.

Gerald P. Rodnan. 1968. 'St. Wolfgang and Gout (Letter on Patron Saints of Gout and Request for Further Information on St. Wolfgang).' *British Medical Journal*. i, 581.

Gerald P. Rodnan and Thomas G. Benedek. 1963. 'Ancient Therapeutic Arts in the Gout'. *Arthritis and Rheumatism*. vi, 317–34.

Gerald P. Rodnan and Thomas G. Benedek. 1965. 'Cotton Mather on Rheumatism and the Gout: A Presentation of Chapters XII and XIII from The Angel of Bethesda'. *Journal of the History of Medicine*. xx, 115–39.

Gerald P. Rodnan and Thomas G. Benedek. 1970. 'Gout and the Spider'. *Journal of the American Medical Association*. ccxi, 2157.

S. Roe. 1981. *Matter, Life and Generation*. Cambridge: Cambridge University Press.

J. P. W. Rogers. 1986. 'Samuel Johnson's Gout'. *Medical History*. xxx, 133–44.

John Rogers. 1735. *Doctor Rogers's Oleum Arthriticum, or Specifick Oil for the Gout*. London: Alexander Cruden.

Pat Rogers. 1979. *Henry Fielding: A Biography*. New York: Charles Scribner's Sons.

Pat Rogers. 1981. 'The Rise and Fall of Gout'. *Times Literary Supplement*. 20 March: 315–16.

Richard Rolls. 1988. *The Hospital of the Nation: The Story of Spa Medicine and the Mineral Water Hospital at Bath*. Bath: Bird Productions.

E. C. R. Roose. 1885, 2nd edn. *Gout and its Relations to Diseases of the Liver and Kidneys*. London: H. K. Lewis.

Robert Root-Bernstein. 1993. *Rethinking AIDS: The Tragic Cost of Premature Consensus*. New York: Free Press.

Matthew Whiting Rosa. 1960. *The Silver-fork School: Novels of Fashion Preceding Vanity Fair*. New York: Columbia University Press.

George Rosen. 1970. 'Sir William Temple and the Therapeutic Use of Moxa for Gout in England'. *Bulletin of the History of Medicine*. xliv, 31–9.

Albert Rosenberg. 1953. *Sir Richard Blackmore: A Poet and Physician of the Augustan Age*. Lincoln, Nebr.: University of Nebraska Press.

Charles E. Rosenberg. 1962. *The Cholera Years: The United States in 1832, 1849 and 1866*. Chicago, Ill.: University of Chicago Press.

Charles E. Rosenberg. 1974. 'The Bitter Fruit: Heredity, Disease and Social Thought in Nineteenth Century America.' *Perspectives in American History*. viii, 189–235.

Charles Rosenberg. 1983. 'Medical Text and Medical Context; Explaining William Buchan's *Domestic Medicine*.' *Bulletin of the History of Medicine*. lvii, 22–4.

Charles E. Rosenberg. 1989. 'Disease in History: Frames and Framers.' *The Milbank Quarterly*. lxvii, 1–15.

Charles E. Rosenberg and Janet Golden, eds. 1992. *Framing Disease: Studies in Cultural History*. New Brunswick, N.J.; Rutgers University Press.

F. Rosner. 1969. 'Gout in the Bible and Talmud.' *Journal of the American Medical Association*. ccvii, 151–2.

Lisa Rosner. 1990. *Medical Education in the Age of Improvement: Edinburgh Students and Apprentices, 1760–1826*. Edinburgh: Edinburgh University Press.

Cecil Roth, ed. 1938. *Anglo-Jewish Letters*. London: Soncino Press.

Lawrence Rothfield. 1987. 'Gout as Metaphor'. In *History, Art, and Antiquity of Rheumatic Diseases*. Brussels: Elsevier and The Erasmus Foundation, 68–71.

Lawrence Rothfield. 1992. *Vital Signs: Medical Realism in Nineteenth-Century Fiction*. Princeton, NJ: Princeton University Press.

Berton Roueché. 1948. 'A Perverse, Ungrateful, Maleficent Malady.' *The New Yorker*. 13 March: 60–70.

G. S. Rousseau. 1966. 'Doctors and Medicine in the Novels of Tobias Smollett'. PhD thesis, Princeton University.

G. S. Rousseau. 1968. 'John Wesley's *Primitive Physick* (1747)'. *Harvard Library Bulletin*. xvi, 242–56.

G. S. Rousseau. 1976. 'Nerves, Spirits and Fibres: Towards Defining the Origins of Sensibility; with a Postscript'. *Blue Guitar*. ii, 125–53.

G. S. Rousseau. 1978a. 'John Hill: Universal Genius Manqué'. In J. A. Leo Lemay and G. S. Rousseau. *The Renaissance Man in the Eighteenth Century*. Los Angeles, Calif.: William Andrews Clark Library.

G. S. Rousseau. 1978b. 'Science'. In Pat Rogers, ed. *The Context of English Literature: The Eighteenth Century*. London: Methuen.

G. S. Rousseau. 1980. 'Psychology'. In G. S. Rousseau and Roy Porter, eds. *The Ferment of Knowledge*. Cambridge: Cambridge University Press, 143–210.

G. S. Rousseau. 1982. *Tobias Smollett. Essays of Two Decades*. Edinburgh: T. & T. Clark.

G. S. Rousseau. 1988. 'Mysticism and Millennialism: "Immortal Dr Cheyne."' In R. H. Popkin, ed. *Millenarianism and Messianism in English Literature and Thought 1650–1800*. Leiden: E. J. Brill, 81–126.

G. S. Rousseau. 1991a. *Enlightenment Borders: Pre- and Post-Modern Discourses: Medical, Scientific*. Manchester: Manchester University Press.

G. S. Rousseau. 1991b. 'The Discourses of Literature and Medicine: Theory and Practice (2)'. In *Enlightenment Borders: Pre- and Post-Modern Discourses: Medical, Scientific*. Manchester: Manchester University Press, 26–54.

G. S. Rousseau. 1991c. 'Towards a Semiotics of the Nerve'. In Peter Burke and Roy Porter, eds. *Language, Self and Society: The Social History of Language*. Cambridge: Polity Press, 213–75.

G. S. Rousseau. 1991d. 'Cultural History in a New Key: Towards a Semiotics of the Nerve'. In Joan H. Pittock and Andrew Wear, eds. *Interpretation and Cultural History*. London: Macmillan.

G. S. Rousseau. 1991e. *Perilous Enlightenment: Pre- and Post-Modern Discourses: Sexual*. Manchester: Manchester University Press.

G. S. Rousseau. 1993. 'Medicine and the Muses: An Approach to Literature and Medicine'. In Marie Mulvey Roberts and Roy Porter, eds. *Literature and Medicine during the Eighteenth Century*. London and New York: Routledge, 23–57.

G. S. Rousseau and Roy Porter, eds. 1987. *Sexual Underworlds of the Enlightenment*. Manchester: Manchester University Press.

G. S. Rousseau and Neil L. Rudenstine, eds. 1972. *English Poetic Satire: Wyatt to Byron*. New York and London: Holt, Rinehart & Winston.

G. S. Rousseau, ed. 1990. *The Languages of Psyche: Mind and Body in Enlightment Thought*. Berkeley, Calif.: University of California Press.

Margaret Rowbottom and Charles Susskind. 1984. *Electricity and Medicine: A History of their Interaction*. San Francisco, Calif.: San Francisco Press.

Thomas Rowlandson. 1971. *Medical Caricatures, with a forward by Morris H. Saffron*. New York: Editions Medicina Rara.

William Rowley. 1770. *An Essay on the Cure of Ulcerated Legs*. London: F. Newbery.

William Rowley. 1780. 'The Gout and Rheumatism Cured or Alleviated.' *Critical Review*. March: 239.

William Rowley. 1790, 2nd edn. *A Treatise on the Management of Female Breasts during childbed*. London.

William Rowley. 1792. *A Treatise on the Regular, Irregular, Atonic and Flying Gout*. London: J. Wingrave.

Martin J. S. Rudwick. 1976. *The Meaning of Fossils: Episodes in the History of Palaeontology*. New York: Scientific History Publications.

J. Ruhräh. 1925a. 'William Cadogan and his Essay on Gout'. *Annals of Medical History*. vii, 64–92.

J. Ruhräh. 1925b. *William Cadogan (His Essay on Gout)*. New York: P. B. Hoeber.

Benjamin Rush. 1947. *The Selected Writings of Benjamin Rush*. Ed. Dagobert D. Runes. New York: Philosophical Library.

J. A. Ryle. 1949. 'Social Pathology'. In Iago Galdston, ed. *Social Medicine: Its Derivations and Objectives*. New York: The Commonwealth Fund.

J. A. Ryle. 1994. *Changing Disciplines: Lectures on the History, Method, and Motives of Social Pathology*. New Brunswick, NJ: Transaction Publishers.

J. B. Ryley. 1887. *Electro-magnetism and Massage in the Treatment of Rheumatic Gout*. London: Renshaw.

Peter Sabor, ed. 1988. *Frances Burney, Cecilia, or Memoirs of an Heiress*. Oxford: Oxford University Press.

Hans Sachs. 1550; 1893. *Sämtliche Fabeln und Swänke*. Halle.

Oliver Sacks. 1981. *Migraine: Evolution of a Common Disorder*. London: Pan Books.

Dianne F. Sadoff. 1982. *Monsters of Affection: Dickens, Eliot, and Bronte on fatherhood*. Baltimore: Johns Hopkins University Press.

W. Salmon. 1671. *Synopsis Medicinae*. London: C. Jones.

W. Salmon. 1693a. *The Compleat English Physician: Or, the Druggist's Shop Opened*. London: for Matthew Gilliflower.

W. Salmon. 1693b. *Seplasium. The Compleat English Physician*. London: Gilliflower & Sawbridge.

W. Salmon. 1703. *The Country Physician, or A Choice Collection of Physick Fitted for Vulgar Use*. London: J. Taylor.

W. Salmon. 1710. *Botanologia. The English Herbal*. London: N. Rhodes & J. Taylor.

Agnivesa's Caraka Samhita. 1976. Trans. Ram Karan Sharma and Vaidya Bhagwan Dash. Varanasi, India: Chowkhamba Sanskrit Series Office.

Louis A. Sass. 1992. *Madness and Modernism: Insanity in the Light of Modern Art, Literature and Thought*. New York: Basic Books.

Hymen Saye. 1934. 'Translation of a Fourteenth Century French Manuscript Dealing with Treatment of Gout'. *Bulletin of the Institute of the History of Medicine*. ii, 112–22.

John Scarborough. 1969. *Roman Medicine*. Ithaca, NY: Cornell University Press.

Elaine Scarry. 1985. *The Body in Pain*. Oxford: Oxford University Press.

John Scat. 1779. An Enquiry into the Origin of the Gout.' *Critical Review*. November: 347–54.

R. Schafter. 1989. 'Narratives of the Self'. In A. M. Cooper, Otto F. Kernberg and Ethel Spector Person, eds. *Psychoanalysis: Toward the Second Century*. New Haven, Conn.: Yale University Press.

C. W. Scheele. 1776. '[Investigations of Bladder Stones: Swedish]', *Kongliga Vetenskaps Academiens Nya Handlingar*. xxxvii, 327–32.

C. W. Scheele. 1777. *Chemische Abhandlung von der Luft und dem Fever*. Uppsala: Magn. Swederus.

C. W. Scheele. 1786. *The Chemical Essays of C. W. Scheele Translated . . . with Additions*. Ed. and Trans. Thomas Beddoes. London: J. Murray.

Ferdinand Schevil. 1950. *The Medici*. London: V. Gollancz.

Londa Schiebinger. 1989. *The Mind Has No Sex? Women in the Origins of Modern Science*. Cambridge, Mass.: Harvard University Press.

Londa Schiebinger. 1993. *Nature's Body: Gender in the Making of Modern Science*. Boston, Mass.: Beacon Press.

Maurice A. Schnitker. 1936. 'A History of the Treatment of Gout'. *Bulletin of the Institute of the History of Medicine*. iv, 89–120.

Robert M. Schuler. 1979. *English Magical and Scientific Poems to 1700: an annotated bibliography*. New York: Garland

Eugene Schuyler. 1890. 'Smollett in Search of Health'. In *Italian Influences*. New York: Charles Scribner's Sons, 220–44.

J. Scot. 1780. *An Enquiry into the Origin of the Gout*. London: T. Becket.

Sir Walter Scott. 1821–4. *Lives of the Novelists,. Prefaces to Ballantyne's Library . . .* 4 vols.

Sir Walter Scott. 1824. *St. Ronan's Well*. 3 vols.

Sir Walter Scott. 1894. *Count Robert of Paris. Volume II: The Surgeon's Daughter*. Boston: Estes and Lauriat.

Sir Walter Scott. 1914. *The Antiquary*. Edinburgh: Nelson.

Sir Walter Scott. a. 1894. *Count Robert of Paris, vol. ii: The Surgeon's Daughter*. Boston, Mass.: Estes & Lauriat.

Sir Walter Scott. b. 1995. *The Antiquary*. Ed. David Hewitt. Edinburgh: Edinburgh University Press.

Sir Walter Scott. c. 1995. *St Ronan's Well*. Ed. Mark A. Weinstein. Edinburgh: Edinburgh University Press.

Charles Scudamore, MD. 1816; 1817, 2nd edn; 1819. *A Treatise on the Nature and Cure of Gout and Rheumatism, Including general considerations on Morbid States of the Digestive Organs and some remarks on Regimen and Practical Observations on Gravel*. London: Longman, Hurst, Rees, Orme & Brown; London: for the author.

Charles Scudamore, MD. 1823, 4th edn. *A Treatise on the Nature and Cure of Gout and Gravel*. London: printed for the author and sold by Longman, Hurst, Rees, Orme & Brown.

Charles Scudamore, MD. 1833a, 2nd edn. *A Treatise on the Composition and Medical Properties of the Mineral Waters of Buxton, Matlock, Tunbridge Wells . . . and the Beulah Spa, Norwood*. London: Longman, Rees, Orme, Brown, Green & Longman's.

Charles Scudamore. 1833b; 1835, 2nd edn. *A Further Examination of the Principles of the Treatment of Gout*. London: Longman, Rees.

Andrew Scull. 1987. 'Desperate Remedies: A Gothic Tale of Madness and Modern Medicine'. *Psychological Medicine*. xvii, 561–77.

Eve Kosofsky Sedgwick. 1985. *Between Men: English Literature and Male Homosexual Desire*. New York: Columbia University Press.

John Sekora. 1977. *Luxury: The Concept in Western Thought, Eden to Smollett*. Baltimore, Md: Johns Hopkins University Press.

John H. Sena. 1975. 'Smollett's Matthew Bramble and the Tradition of the Physician–Satirist'. *Papers on Language and Literature*. xi: 380–96.

Seneca. 1917–28. *Epistulae morales*, 3 vols. Trans. R. M. Gummere. London: W. Heinemann.

Daniel Sennert. 1611. *Institutonum Medicinae Libri V*. Wittenberg: W. Meisner for Z. Schürer.

Daniel Sennert. 1619. *De Febribus*. Wittenbergae: Apud Zachariam Schurerum.

Daniel Sennert. 1628–36. *Practicae Medicinae*. Wittenberg: A. Rothius.

Daniel Sennert. 1632, 1660. *De arthritide tractatus*. Paris: Societas. Trans. as *A Treatise of the Gout*. London: Peter Cole.

Steven Shapin. 1994. *A Social History of Truth: Civility and Science in Seventeenth-Century England*. Chicago, Ill.: University of Chicago Press.

Steven Shapin and Simon Schaffer. 1985. *Leviathan and the Air-Pump*. Princeton, NJ: Princeton University Press.

George Bernard Shaw. 1926. *The Doctor's Dilemma*. London: Constable.

John Shebbeare. 1772. *A Candid Enquiry into the Merits of Dr Cadogan's Dissertation on the Gout . . . With an Appendix in Which is Contained a Certain Cure for the Gout*. London: S. Hooper.

W. J. Sheils, ed. 1982. *The Church and Healing*. Oxford: Basil Blackwell for the Ecclesiastical History Society.

Charles L. Short. 1959. 'Rheumatoid Arthritis: Historical Aspects'. *Journal of Chronic Diseases*. x, 367–87.

Thomas Short, M.D. 1750. *Discourses on Tea, Sugar, Milk, Made-Wines, Spirits, Tobacco, &c. with Plain and Useful Rules for Gouty People*. London: Printed for T. Longman.

Edward Shorter. 1992. *From Paralysis to Fatigue. A History of Psychosomatic Illness in the Modern Era*. New York: Free Press.

Edward Shorter. 1994. *From the Mind into the Body: The Cultural Origins of Psychosomatic Symptoms*. New York: Free Press.

H. Shute. 1807–8. *Dissertation on Gout*, vol. lvii. Archives of the Royal Medical Society of Edinburgh.

David E. Shuttleton. 1992. '"My Own Crazy Carcase": The Life and Works of Dr George Cheyne, 1672–1743'. PhD thesis, University of Edinburgh.

Henry Sigerist. 1943. *Civilization and Disease*. Ithaca: Cornell University Press.

Kenneth Simons. 1985. *The Ludic Imagination: A Reading of Joseph Conrad*. Ann Arbor, Mich.: UMI Research.

Sir John Sinclair. 1807. *The Code of Health and Longevity. Or, A Concise View, of the Principles Calculated for the Preservation of Health, and the Attainment of Long Life . . .* Edinburgh: for A. Constable & Co.

N. G. Siraisi. 1990. *Medieval and Early Renaissance Medicine*. Chicago, Ill.: Chicago University Press.

Osbert Sitwell. 1945. *Left Hand, Right Hand! An Autobiography*, vol. i: *The Cruel Month*. London: Macmillan.

Paul Slack. 1979. 'Mirrors of Health and Treasures of Poor Men: Uses of the Vernacular Medical Literature of Tudor England'. In C. Webster, ed. *Health, Medicine and Mortality in the Sixteenth Century*. Cambridge: Cambridge University Press, 237–74.

Alan G. R. Smith, ed. 1990. *The Anonymous Life of William Cecil, Lord Burghley*. Lewiston, Me: E. Mellen Press.

Charlotte Smith. 1989. *The Old Manor House*. Oxford: Oxford University Press.

Daniel Smith. 1772, 1st edn. *Observations on Doctor Williams's Treatise upon the Gout*. Bristol: Farley.

Daniel Smith. 1772. 'A Letter to Dr. Cadogan. . . .' *Critical Review* July: 68–9.

E. A. Smith. 1990. *Lord Grey 1764–1845*. Oxford: Clarendon Press.

Henry Smith. 1598. *Four Sermons*. London: P. Short.

J. Smith. 1786. *Observations on the . . . Cheltenham Waters. . . .* Cheltenham: Harward.

Nowell C. Smith, ed. 1953. *The Letters of Sydney Smith*, 2 vols. Oxford: Clarendon Press.

Roger Smith. 1992. *Inhibition: History and Meaning in the Sciences of Mind and Body*. London: Free Association Books; Berkeley and Los Angeles, Calif.: University of California Press.

Virginia S. Smith. 1985. 'Cleanliness: The Development of an Idea and Practice in Britain 1770–1850'. PhD thesis, University of London.

Tobias Smollett. 1990. *The Expedition of Humphry Clinker*. Ed. Thomas R. Preston. Athens and London: The University of Georgia Press.

Albert Henry Smyth, ed. 1906. *The Writings of Benjamin Franklin, 1780–1782*, vol. viii. London: Macmillan.

H. Smythson. 1781. *The Compleat Family Physician*. London: Harrison.

Albert J. Solnit, Donald J. Cohen and Peter B. Neubauer, eds. 1993. *The Many Meanings of Play: A Psychoanalytic Perspective*. New Haven, Conn., and London: Yale University Press.

Susan Sontag. 1978. *Illness as Metaphor*. New York: Farrar, Straus & Giroux.

Susan Sontag. 1989. *AIDS as Metaphor*. Harmondsworth: Allen Lane.

Soranus of Ephesus. 1927. *Sorani Gynaeciorum Libri IV*. Ed. Johannes Ilberg. Leibzig: Berolini: B. G. Teubneri.

P. M. Spacks. 1976. *Imagining a Self*. Cambridge, Mass.: Harvard University Press.

R. D. Spector, ed. 1994. *Smollett's Women: A Study in Eighteenth-Century Masculine Sensibility*. New York: Greenwood Press, 1994.

Edmund Spenser. 1633. *A View of the Present State of Ireland*. Dublin.

Francis Spilsbury. 1775, 1780. *A Treatise on the Method of Curing the Gout, Scurvey, Leprosy . . .* London: s.n.

Francis Spilsbury. 1778. *Physical Dissertations on the Scurvy and Gout*. London: J. Wilkie.

T. L. S. Sprigge, ed. 1968–81. *The Correspondence of Jeremy Bentham*, 5 vols. London: Athlone.

R. Squirrell, M. D. 1820. *Essay on Indigestion and its Consequences; or, Advice to Persons Affected by Debility of the Degestive Organs, Gout, Nervous Disorders, Dropsy, etc.* n.p.: n.p.

Jean Starobinski. 1992. *The Remedy in the Disease: Critique and Legitimation of Artifice in the Age of Enlightenment*. Cambridge: Polity Press.

John Steel. 1985. *Robert Southey – Mr Rowlandson's England*. Woodbridge: Suffolk, England.

R. Ted Steinbock. 1993a. 'Gallstones (Cholelithiasis)'. In Kenneth F. Kiple, ed. *The Cambridge World History of Human Disease*. Cambridge: Cambridge University Press, 738–40.

R. Ted Steinbock. 1993b. 'Osteoporosis'. In Kenneth F. Kiple, ed. *The Cambridge World History of Human Disease*. Cambridge: Cambridge University Press, 909–10.

George Steiner. 1963. *The Death of Tragedy*. London: Faber.

Laurence Sterne. 1813–14. *The Works of Laurence Sterne*. vol. 2. New York.

Laurence Sterne. 1967. *The Sentimental Journey*. Ed. Graham Petrie. Harmondsworth: Penguin.

J. N. Stevens. 1758. *An Essay on the Disease of the Head and Neck . . . Dissertation on the Gout and Rheumatism*. Bath: for J. Leake.

J. N. Stevens reviewed by James Kirkpatrick, M. D. 1758. 'An Essay on the Diseases of the Head and Neck to which is added a Dissertation on the Gout and Rheumatism.' *Monthly Review*. August: 145–50.

L. Stevenson. 1965. '"New Diseases" in the Seventeenth Century'. *Bulletin of the History of Medicine*. xxxix, 1–21.

William Stevenson. 1779. *A Successful Method of Treating the Gout by Blistering. With An Introduction Consisting of Miscellaneous Matter*. Bath: Cruttwell.

William Stevenson. 1781, 2nd edn. *Cases in Medicine. . . .* Newark: Tomlinson.

Antonio Fabio Sticotti. 1769. *Garrick ou les acteurs anglois, ouvrage contenant des reflexions sur l'art dramatique, sur l'art de la representation, et le jeu des acteurs, traduit de l'anglois*. Paris: Lacombe.

Sir William Stirling-Maxwell. 1875, 4th edn. *The Cloister Life of Emperor Charles V.* London: John C. Nimmo.

F. G. Stokes, ed. 1931. *The Blecheley Diary*. London: Constable.

L. Strachey and R. Fulford. 1938. *The Greville Memoirs 1814–1860*, 8 vols. London: Macmillan.

Ralph Straus. 1910. *Robert Dodsley: Poet, Publisher and Playwright*. London: John Lane.

L. A. G. Strong. 1955. *Dr Quicksilver 1660–1742*. London: Melrose.

William Stukeley. 1723. *Of the Spleen . . . Particularly the Vapours*. London.

William Stukeley. 1734; 1736, 2nd edn. *Of the Gout, in Two Parts. First a Letter to Sir Hans Sloan . . . about the Cure . . . by Oyls Externally Apply'd; Secondly, A Treatise on the Cause and Cure of the Gout*. London: Roberts.

William Stukeley. 1740. *Stonehenge, A Temple Restor'd to the British Druids*. London: W. Innys and R. Manby.

Karl Sudhoff, ed. 1922–33. *Paracelsus: Sämtliche Werke*, 14 vols. Munich: R. Oldebourg.

A. Sutherland. 1763. *Attempts to Revive Antient Medical Doctrines. . . .* London: Millar.

Gerard van Swieten. 1744–73. *Commentaries Upon the Aphorisms of Dr H. Boerhaave*, 18 vols. London: for John and Paul Knapton.

Jonathan Swift. 1937. 'Bec's Birthday'. In *The Poems of Jonathan Swift*, 3 vols. Ed. Harold Williams. Oxford: Clarendon Press.

Thomas Sydenham. 1666. *Methodus Curandi Febres*. Amstelodami: Gerbrandum Schlagen.

Thomas Sydenham. 1676. *Observationes Medicae*. Londini: Kettilby.

Thomas Sydenham. 1683. *Tractatus de podagra et hydrope*. Londini: Gualt. Kettilby.

Thomas Sydenham. 1705, 4th edn. *The Whole Works of That Excellent Practical Physician*. London: R. Wellington.

Thomas Sydenham. 1850. *A Treatise on Gout, and Dropsy*, in *The Works of Thomas Sydenham*. Trans. R. G. Latham from the Latin edition of Dr Greenhill. London: Sydenham Society.

Franciscus dele Boë Sylvius. 1671. *Praxeos Medicae Idea Nova*. Leiden: Le Carpentier.

Charles Symmons. 1806. *The Life of John Milton*. London: T. Bensley.

Thomas S. Szasz. 1957. *Pain and Pleasure: A Study of Bodily Feelings*. London: Tavistock Publications.

Charles H. Talbot. 1967. *Medicine in Medieval England*. London: Oldbourne; New York: American Elsevier.

Reay Tannahill. 1975. *Flesh and Blood: A History of the Cannibal Complex*. New York: Stein and Day.

F. Kräupl Taylor. 1970–71. 'A Logical Analysis of the Medico-Psychological Concept of Disease.' *Psychological Medicine*. i, 356–64.

F. Kräupl Taylor. 1976. 'The Medical Model of the Disease Concept.' *British Journal of Psychiatry.* cxxviii, 588–94.

F. Kräupl Taylor. 1979. *The Concepts of Illness, Disease and Morbus.* Cambridge: Cambridge University Press.

James Spottiswoode Taylor. 1922. *Montaigne in Medicine: Being the Essayist's Comments on Contemporary Physic and Physicians; His Thoughts on Many Material Matters Relating to Life and Death; An Account of His Bodily Ailments and Peculiarities and of His Travels in Search of Health.* London: Humphrey Milford.

Owsei Temkin. 1961. 'The Scientific Approach to Disease: Specific Entity and Individual Sickness'. In A. C. Crombie, ed. *Scientific Change.* London: W. Heinemann, 629–47.

Sir William Temple. 1681, 2nd edn. 'An Essay on the Cure of the Gout'. *Miscellanea.* London: E. Gellibrand, 189–238.

William Makepeace Thackeray. 1886. *Miscellaneous Essays, Sketches and Reviews and Contributions to "Punch".* London: Smith, Elder & Co.

William Makepeace Thackeray. 1972. *The History of Pendennis.* Ed. Donald Hawes. Harmondsworth: Penguin.

Melchisédec Thévenot, ed. 1663–72. *Relations de divers voyages curiex, qui n'ont point esté publiées, etc.* Paris: De L'inprimene de Iaques Langleis.

Phillip Thicknesse. 1780. *The Valetudinarian's Bath Guide.* London: Dodsley.

Phillip Thicknesse. 1782. *An Epistle to Dr. William Falconer of Bath.* Bath: Pratt and Clinch.

Phillip Thicknesse. 1784; 1786, 2nd edn. *A Year's Journey through the Pais Bas, and Austrian Netherlands.* London: s.n. and London: John Debreh.

Phillip Thicknesse. 1787. *A Letter to Dr. James Makittrick Adair.* St. Catherine's Hermitage: for the author.

J. J. Thomas. 1975. 'Smollett and Ethical Sensibility.' Ph.D. dissertation, University of Iowa.

E. P. Thompson. 1963. *The Making of the English Working Class.* London: V. Gollancz.

E. P. Thompson. 1991. *Customs in Common.* London: Merlin Press.

Geraldine Thompson. 1973. *Under Pretext of Praise: Satiric Mode in Erasmus' Fiction.* Toronto: University of Toronto Press.

Thomas Thompson, MD. 1740. *An Historical, Critical and Practical Treatise of the Gout . . . Showing . . . Danger and Presumptions of all Philosophical Systems in Physick.* London: J. Hughs.

A. Thomson. 1807, 2nd edn. *The Family Physician.* London: R. Philips.

E. M. Tillyard. 1943. *The Elizabethan World Picture.* London: Chatto and Windus.

John Timbs. 1876. *Doctors and Patients.* London: Richard Bentley.

S.-A.-A.-D. Tissot. 1768. *An Essay on Diseases Incidental to Literary and Sedentary Persons.* London: E. & C. Dilly.

S.-A.-A.-D. Tissot. 1771. *An Essay on the Disorders of People of Fashion.* London: Richardson & Urquhart.

Paget Toynbee and Leonard Whibley, eds. 1935. *Correspondence of Thomas Gray*, 3 vols. Oxford: Clarendon Press.

R. R. Trail. 1970. 'Richard Morton (1637–98)'. *Medical History.* xiv, 166–74.

W. Treue. 1958. *Doctor at Court.* Trans. F. Fawcett. London: Weidenfeld & Nicolson.

E. J. Trimmer. 1967. *Rejuvenation: The History of an Idea.* London: Hale.

David Trotter. 1988. *Circulation: Defoe, Dickens, and the Economies of the Novel.* London: Macmillan.

Thomas Trotter. 1807. *A View of the Nervous Temperament.* London: Longman, Hurst, Rees & Orme.

Bryan S. Turner. 1984. *The Body and Society: Explorations in Social Theory.* Oxford: Basil Blackwell.

Bryan S. Turner. 1991. 'Recent Developments in the Theory of the Body.' In Mike Featherstone, Mike Hepworth and Bryan S. Turner, eds. *The Body. Social Process and Cultural Theory*. London: Sage, 1–35

William Turner. 1965. *The Names of Herbes* (1548). Facsimile with introduction by James Britten, B. Daydon Jackson and W. T. Stearn. London: Ray Society.

Theodore Turquet de Mayerne. 1676. *A Treatise of the Gout*. London: D. Newman.

Theodore Turquet de Mayerne. 1693. *La Pratique de Medecine . . . et un Traite de la Goutte.* Lyon: Anisson & Posuel.

James Tyson, M. D. 1895. 'Irregular or Atypical Gout: How shall we know it?' *Journal of the American Medical Association*. vol. 24: 870.

James Tyson, M. D. 1904. 'Alfred Baring Garrod.' *Journal of the American Medical Association*. 187(4): 299–300.

Graeme Tytler. 1982. *Physiognomy in the European Novel: faces and fortunes*. Princeton, N.J.: Princeton University Press.

E. A. Underwood. 1937. 'Medicine and Science in the Writings of Smollett'. *Proceedings of the Royal Society of Medicine*. xxx, 961–74.

University of California Medical Staff Conference. 1972. 'Hyperuricemia – Pathogenesis and Treatment.' *California Medicine*. 116(6). June: 38–44.

Sylvanus Urban. 1756. 'The Effect of Musk in curing the Gout in the Stomach . . .' *Gentleman's Magazine*. xxvi, May: 244.

Sylvanus Urban. 1756. 'The Gout: A Mock-Heroic Poem in Imitation of the Splendid Shilling'. *Gentleman's Magazine*. xxvi, December: 584.

G. Urdang. 1944. *Pharmacopoeia Londinensis of 1618*. Madison, Wis.: State Historical Society of Wisconsin.

Walter Vandereycken and Ron Van Deth. 1994. *From Fasting Saints to Anorexic Girls: The History of Self-Starvation*. London: Athlone Press.

C. A. Vandermonde. 1759. *Dictionnaire portatif de sante*. Paris: Vincent.

Otto van Veen [Vaenius]. 1607. *Imaginibus in aes incisis, notisque illustrata*. Antverpiae: Ex officina Hieronymi verdussen, auctoris aere & cura.

David Verey, ed. 1983. *The Diary of a Victorian Squire. Extracts from the Diaries and Letters of Dearman & Emily Birchall*. London: Alan Sutton.

M. M. Verney, ed. 1930. *The Verney Letters of the Eighteenth Century*. London: Benn.

Brian Vickers. 1968. *Francis Bacon and Renaissance Prose*. Cambridge: Cambridge University Press.

Brian Vickers. 1988. *In Defence of Rhetoric*. Oxford: Clarendon Press.

H. R. Viets. 1949. 'George Cheyne, 1673–1743.' Fielding H. Garrison Lecture. *Bulletin of the History of Medicine*. xxiii, 435–52.

Peter Virgin. 1994. *Sydney Smith*. London: HarperCollins.

Pide Vivignis. 1774. 'A Description of the Four Situations of a Gouty Person.' *Critical Review*. September: 239.

Ivan Waddington. 1984. *The Medical Profession in the Industrial Revolution*. Dublin: Gill & Macmillan.

Willoughby Francis Wade. 1863. *Notes on Clinical Medicine*. Birmingham: Josiah Allen.

Willoughby Francis Wade. 1893. *On Gout as a Peripheral Neurosis*. London: Simpkin, Marshall, Hamilton & Kent.

Peter Wagner. 1985. *Eros Revived: A Study of Eighteenth-Century Erotica*. London: Secker and Warburg.

Peter Wagner. 1986. *Lust and Love in the Rococo Period*. Nordlingen: Delphi

Peter Wagner, ed. 1989. *Christopher Anstey: The New Bath Guide*. Hildesheim: Georg Olms Verlag.

Peter Wagner. 1991. 'Hogarth's graphic palimpsests: intermedial adaptation of popular literature.' *Word & Image*. 7(4): 329–47.

Anthony Walker. 1686. *The Virtuous Woman Journal*. London: Nathaniel Ranew.

Stanley L. Wallace. 1962. 'A Wit and his Gout: The Reverend Sydney Smith'. *Arthritis and Rheumatism*. v, 610–15.

Stanley L. Wallace. 1968. 'Benjamin Franklin and the Introduction of Colchicum into the United States.' *Bulletin of the History of Medicine*. xlii, 312–20.

Stanley L. Wallace. 1973. 'Colchicum: The Panacea'. *Bulletin of the New York Academy of Medicine*. xlix, 130–5.

Margaret Waller. 1993. *The Male Malady: fictions of impotence in the French romantic novel*. New Brunswick, N.J.: Rutgers University Press.

Izaak Walton. 1927. *The Lives of John Donne . . .* London: World's Classics.

John Want. 1814a. 'Medical and Philosophical Intelligence'. *Medical and Physical Journal*. xxxii, 77–9.

John Want. 1814b. 'Mr Want in Answer to Dr Sutton'. *Medical and Physical Journal*. xxxii, 201–7.

John Want. 1814c. 'Case of the Paroxysm of Gout Removed by the Tincture of Colchicum'. *Medical and Physical Journal*. xxxii, 312–14.

John Want. 1814d. 'Cases Illustrative of the Modus Operandi of Colchicum'. *Medical and Physical Journal*. xxxii, 393–5, 491–3.

James Wardrop. 1851. *On the Nature and Treatment of the Diseases of the Heart, etc.* London: J. Churchill.

Ferdinando Warner. 1768. *A Full and Plain Account of the Gout; From Whence will be Clearly Seen the Folly, or the Baseness, of All Pretenders to the Cure of It*. London: T. Cadell.

John Harley Warner. 1986. *The Therapeutic Perspective. Medical Practice, Knowledge and Identity in America, 1820–1885*. Cambridge, Mass.: Harvard University Press.

J. W. Warter, ed. 1831. *Southey's Common-Place Book*. London: Longman, Brown, Green & Longmans.

Gilbert Watson. 1966. *Theriac and Mithidatium: A Study in Therapeutics*. London: The Wellcome Historical Medical Library.

Geoff Watts. 1992. *Pleasing the Patient*. London and Boston, Mass.: Faber & Faber.

Andrew Wear. 1985a. 'Historical and Cultural Aspects of Pain.' *Bulletin of the Society for the Social History of Medicine*. xxxvi, 7–21.

Andrew Wear. 1985b. 'Puritan Perceptions of Illness in Seventeenth-Century England'. In Roy Porter, ed. *Patients and Practitioners*. Cambridge: Cambridge University Press, 55–99.

Andrew Wear. 1987. 'Interfaces: Perceptions of Health and Illness in Early Modern England'. In Roy Porter and Andrew Wear, eds. *Problems and Methods in the History of Medicine*. London: Croom Helm, 230–55.

Andrew Wear. 1989. 'Medical Practice in Late Seventeenth- and Early Eighteenth-Century England: Continuity and Union'. In R. French and A. Wear, eds. *The Medical Revolution of the Seventeenth Century*. Cambridge: Cambridge University Press, 294–320.

Andrew Wear, ed. 1992. *Medicine in Society: Historical Essays*. Cambridge: Cambridge University Press, 59–90.

Andrew Wear. 1992. 'The Popularization of Medicine in Early Modern England'. In Roy Porter, ed. *The Popularization of Medicine, 1650–1850*. London: Routledge, 17–41.

Miles Weatherall. 1993. 'Drug Therapies.' In W. F. Bynum and Roy Porter, eds. *Companion Encyclopedia of the History of Medicine*. London: Routledge, 911–34.

Charles Webster. 1975. *The Great Instauration: Science, Medicine, and Reform 1626–1660*. London: Duckworth.

Judith Wechsler. 1982. *A Human Comedy: Physiognomy and Caricature in 19th Century Paris*. London: Thames and Hudson.

F. P. Wedeen. 1981. 'Punch Cures the Gout'. *Journal of the Medical Society of New Jersey*. lxxviii, 201–6.

F. P. Wedeen. 1984a. 'Irregular Gout: Humoral Fantasy or Saturnine Malady?' *Bulletin of the New York Academy of Medicine*. lx, 969–79.

F. P. Wedeen. 1984b. *Poison in the Pot: The Legacy of Lead*. Carbondale, Il.: Southern Illinois University Press.

A. Welles. 1803. *An Account of the Discovery and Operation of a New Medicine for Gout*. London: J. Johnson.

Benjamin Welles. 1669. *A Treatise of the Gout, or Joint Evil*. London: printed by J. M. for Henry Herringman.

Calvin Wells. 1964. *Bones, Bodies, and Disease: Evidence of Disease and Abnormality in Early Man*. New York: Frederick A. Praeger.

William Charles Wells. 1812. 'On Rheumatism of the Heart.' *Transactions of a Society for the Improvement of Medical and Chirurgical Knowledge*, iii, 373–425.

Richard Wendorf. 1990. *Elements of Life: Biography and Portrait-Painting in Stuart and Georgian England*. Oxford: Clarendon Press.

John Wesley. 1747. *Primitive Physick: Or, an Easy and Natural Method of Curing Most Diseases*. London: T. Trye.

William A. West. 1969. 'Matt Bramble's Journey to Health.' *Texas Studies in Literature and Language*. vol. 11: 1197–208.

A. N. Whitehead. 1926. *Science and the Modern World*. Cambridge: Cambridge University Press.

J. C. Whorton. 1982. *Crusaders for Fitness: The History of American Health Reformers*. Princeton, NJ: Princeton University Press.

Robert Whytt. 1751. *An Essay on the Vital and other Involuntary Motions of Animals*. Edinburgh: Hamilton, Balfour and Neill.

Robert Whytt. 1765. *Observations on Nervous, Hypochondriacal, or Hysteric Diseases*. Edinburgh: T. Becket and P. du Hondt.

J. Wiggins. 1718. *Quack Doctors: A Catalogue of Some Cures of the Gout. . . .* London.

P. R. Wilde. 1921. *Physiology of Gout, Rheumatism and Arthritis*. Bristol: J. Wright and Sons Ltd.

Basil Willey. 1962. *The Eighteenth Century Background: Studies on the Idea of Nature in the Thought of the Period*. London: Penguin in association with Chatto & Windus.

David Williams. 1778. *Unanimity in All Parts of the British Commonwealth, Necessary to its Preservation, Interest and Happiness*. London: Davis.

Greer Williams. 1959. *Virus Hunters*. New York: Knopf.

John Williams. 1774. *Advice to People Afflicted with the Gout*. London: T. Becket.

Ralph Williams. 1652, 2nd edn. *Physical Rarities, Containing the Most Choice Receipts of Physick, and Chyrurgerie, for the Cure of All Diseases*, London: W. L. and J. M.

A. F. M. Willich. 1799. *Lectures on Diet and Regimen*. London: Longman & Rees.

Thomas Willis. 1664. *De Cerebri Anatome*. London: J. Flesher.

A. Wilson. 1995. *The Making of Man Midwifery*. London: University College Press.

James Wilson. 1842. *A Practical Treatise on the Cure of Diseases by Water, Air, Exercise and Diet*. London: J. Churchill.

James Wilson. 1843. *Stomach Complaints and Drug Diseases: Their Causes, Consequences, and Cure by Water, Air, Exercise and Diet*. London: J. Churchill.

James Wilson and James Manby Gully. 1844, 4th edn. *The Practice of the Water Cure, With Authenticated Evidence of its Efficacy and Safety*. London: H. Baillière.

L. G. Wilson. 1993. 'Fevers.' In W. F. Bynum and Roy Porter, eds. *Companion Encyclopedia of the History of Medicine*. London: Routledge, 382–411.

John Wiltshire. 1991. *Samuel Johnson in the Medical World: The Doctor and the Patient*. Cambridge: Cambridge University Press.

John Wiltshire. 1992. *Jane Austen and the Body*. Cambridge: Cambridge University Press.

James Anderson Winn. 1992. *'When Beauty Fires the Blood': Love and the Arts in the Age of Dryden*. Ann Arbor, Mich.: University of Michigan Press.

D. A. Winstanley. 1935. *Unreformed Cambridge*. Cambridge: Cambridge University Press.

Clifton Wintringham. 1721. *An Essay on Contagious Diseases: more particularly on the small-pox, measles, putrid, malignant, and pestilential fevers.* York: Charles Bourne.

Robert Witty. 1677. *Gout Raptures. Astromaxia. Or an Historical Fiction of a War among the Stars* . . . Cambridge: John Hayes.

Robert Witty. 1685. *A survey of the heavens; being a plain description of the admirable fabrick and motions of the heavenly bodies* . . . *To which is added the Gout Raptures, augmented and improved in English, Latin and Greek verse.* London: printed for Richard Jones.

W. H. Wollaston. 1797. 'On Gouty and Urinary Concretions'. *Philosophical Transactions.* lxxxvii, 386–400.

Samuel Wood. 1775. *Structures on the Gout: With Practical Advice to the Gouty People of Great Britain.* London: for J. Bell and J. Sewel.

Carl Woodring, ed. 1990. *The Collected Works of Samuel Taylor Coleridge: Table Talk, Volume I.* London: Routledge.

J. Woodward. 1977. 'Towards a Social History of Medicine.' In J. Woodward and D. Richards, eds. *Health Care and Popular Medicine in Nineteenth-Century England: Essays in the Social History of Medicine.* London: Croom Helm, 15–55.

J. Woodward and D. Richards. 1977. *Health Care and Popular Medicine in Nineteenth-Century England: Essays in the Social History of Medicine.* London: Croom Helm.

Peter W. G. Wright and A. Treacher, eds. 1982. *The Problem of Medical Knowledge.* Edinburgh: Edinburgh University Press.

R. G. Wyndgaarden and W. N. Kelley. 1976. *Gout and Hyperuricaemia.* New York: Grune & Stratton.

John Wynter. 1725, 1st edn. *Cyclus Metasyncriticus; Or, an Essay on Chronical Diseases* . . . London: Innys.

Johann Heinrich Zedler. 1732–50. 'Arthritis'. In *Universal Lexicon.* Halle and Leipzig, cols 1707–17. London: for Johann Heinrich Zedler.

Theodore Zeldin. 1993. *A history of French Passions.* Oxford: Clarendon Press.

Theodore van Zelst. 1738. *Libellus Singularis, de Podagra.* . . . Amsterdam: Jansson-Waesberg.

H. von Ziemmsen, ed. 1870. *Cyclopaedia of the Practice of Medicine,* 17 vols. London: Sampson, Low, Marston, Searle & Irvington.

A. Zuckerman. 1965. 'Dr Richard Mead (1673–1754): A Biographical Study'. PhD thesis, University of Illinois.

Linda Zwinger. 1991. *Daughters, Fathers, and the Novel: The Sentimental Romance of Hetero-sexuality.* Madison: University of Wisconsin Press.

Index